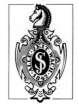

Search for the Causes of Schizophrenia

Edited by
H. Häfner, W. F. Gattaz, and W. Janzarik

With 35 Figures and 57 Tables

Springer-Verlag
Berlin Heidelberg New York
London Paris Tokyo

Prof. Dr. Dr. HEINZ HÄFNER
Prof. Dr. WAGNER FARID GATTAZ
Zentralinstitut für Seelische Gesundheit
J 5, 6800 Mannheim, Federal Republic of Germany

Prof. Dr. WERNER JANZARIK
Psychiatrische Klinik der Universität Heidelberg
Vossstraße, 6900 Heidelberg, Federal Republic of Germany

ISBN 3-540-17376-5 Springer-Verlag Berlin Heidelberg New York
ISBN 0-387-17376-5 Springer-Verlag New York Berlin Heidelberg

Library of Congress Cataloging-in-Publication Data. Search for the causes of schizophrenia. Bibliography: p.
Includes indexes. 1. Schizophrenia – Etiology. I. Häfner, H. (Heinz), 1926–   . II. Gattaz, W.F. (Wagner
Farid), 1951–   . III. Janzarik, W., 1920–. RC514.S366   1987. 616.89′82071   87-9504
ISBN 0-387-17376-5 (U.S.)

Typesetting, printing and bookbinding: Brühlsche Universitätsdruckerei, Giessen
2125/3130-543210

Contents

List of Contributors

You will find the address at the beginning of the respective contribution

Angermeyer, M.C. 331

Baron, M. 157

Beckmann, H. 241

Biehl, H. 98

Borst, U. 189

Burkovsky, G.V., 349

Carpenter, W.T., Jr. 214

Carlsson, A. 223

Cohen, R. 189

Crow, T.J. 260

Dohrenwend, B.P. 275

Ernberg, G. 107

Farmer, A.E. 143

Fleming, J.A. 88

Gasser, T. 250

Gattaz, W.F. 241, 250

Gottesman, I.I. 143

Gulbinat, W. 107

Häfner, H. 1, 47, 365

Hemsley, D.R. 179

Hirsch. S. 267

Jablensky, A. 107

Jakob, H. 241

Janzarik, W. 11

Jung, E. 98

Kabanov, M.M. 349

Katschnig, H. 353

Kohlmeyer, K. 250

Korabelnikov, K.V. 349

Kringlen, E. 123

Krumm, B. 98

Leff, J. 107, 317

Link, B.G. 275

Maurer, K. 98

McGuffin, P. 143

Nuechterlein, K.H. 297

Reynolds, G.P. 236

Sartorius, N. 107

Sass, H. 19

Schubart, C. 98

Shepherd, M. 29

Shrout, P.E. 275

Skodol, A.E. 275

Strauss, J.S. 75

Strömgren, E. 171

Tsuang, M.T. 88

Venables, P.H. 203

Wing, J.K. 39

Zubin, J. 114, 359

Introduction

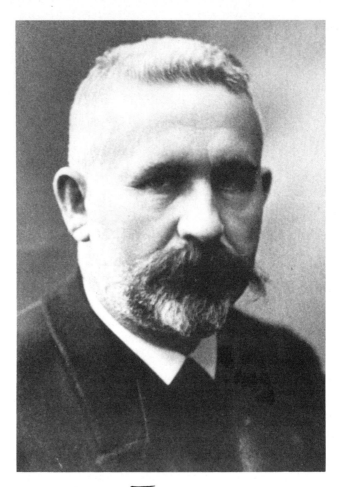

Schizophrenia is a frequently occurring and still often impairing mental disease. We are capable of successfully treating the psychotic episodes or the productive symptoms, but the course of the disease and the development of "unproductive" symptoms and impairment can be only modestly and sporadically influenced. Except for a reliable but unspecific indication that genetic factors strongly contribute to it, the aetiology of schizophrenia is still largely unknown. The scanty knowledge of the biological and psychological processes involved in the development of symptoms and dysfunctions – as well as in the individual attempts and failures to control them – is fragmentary and widely distributed over various disciplines. Efforts to integrate this knowledge in order to formulate and test promising hypotheses or pathogentic models at more than one level of approach are rare.

Probably one of the major challenges to psychiatric research is to advance the investigation of the aetiology of schizophrenia by creating and testing pathogenetic models that could explain why the symptoms, dysfunctions and impairments appear and disappear. We have tried to meet this challenge by inviting outstanding scientists from fields of active schizophrenia research to report on their findings, hypotheses and speculations to a small circle of expert participants and to have intensive discussions through working groups and disciplines. All contributions to this volume were presented at the symposium on the "Search for the Causes of Schizophrenia," which was jointly organised by the Central Institute of Mental Health, Mannheim and the Department of Psychiatry of the University of Heidelberg and was held at the Forum of Science of Heidelberg University from 24–26 September 1986.

This volume is not just one of the usual proceedings, but reflects the exceptional content and structure of the symposium. The contributions on the historical development of the disease construct, on classification research, on epidemiology and the course of schizophrenia, on population genetics, on studies of twins and adopted persons, on mathematical models for hereditary transmission, on experimental psychology and psychophysiology, on the pathology of the brain, on biochemistry and virology and on social psychology and family research represent the most essential approaches and methods of current research. Since the introduction of standardised, international, reliable methods of assessment, we have reached worldwide agreement on practicable research definitions of the diagnosis of schizophrenia. The schizophrenia studies conducted by the World Health Organization (WHO 1973, 1979) have made a decisive contribution to this development. For this reason, the prerequisites for schizophrenia research in gen-

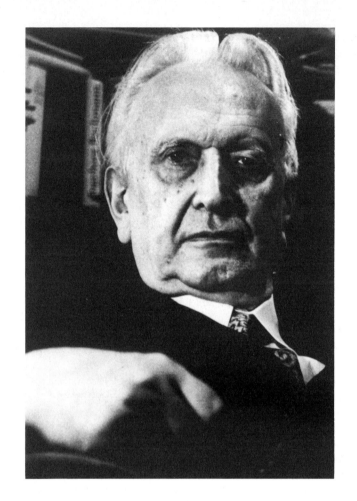

Karl Jaspers

eral and for an interdisciplinary symposium on this topic in particular were more favourable than ever before. The purpose of this enterprise was to give a state of our present knowledge, to initiate critical discussion on causal approaches and to bridge the gaps between the various disciplines and fields of work. The systematic elaboration of the programme, which has been taken as a basis for this volume, and the discussions of three to five precirculated papers on each of the topics by a renowned invited discussion participant – beyond the bounds of specialties and methods – have given this volume the character of a "state of the art" analysis of current schizophrenia research. We have included the papers of the discussion participants in this volume, since they are a most valuable contribution to the goals of our book.

There was not only sufficient reason for holding this symposium but also a special occasion to commemorate: the 600th anniversary of the University of Heidelberg. The oldest university in Germany, founded by Charles Rupert I of the Palatinate, was authorised by Pope Urban VI on 23 October 1385, with the issue of the papal bull "in supremae dignitatis." On 13 October 1386 it was opened with a solemn ceremony. The motto of the Anniversary was, "From tradition into the future." Nowhere else than at the University of Heidelberg is the tradition of schizophrenia research represented more strongly. Emil Kraepelin, Professor of Psychiatry at Heidelberg from 1891–1903, described the disease construct of "Dementia praecox" for the first time (Kraepelin 1896) and defined it by definite but partly variable characteristics of symptomatology and course. The concept of schizophrenia is still based on them. It is also to Kraepelin's merit to have stimulated the epidemiological, genetic and experimental research on the psychopathology and neuropathology of schizophrenia.

E. Bleuler's criticism that dementia praecox does neither lead stringently to dementia nor necessarily occur "praecox" (prematurely) has given more weight to the significance of psychotic symptomatology compared with more unspecific criteria like early age of first onset and unfavourable course. His proposal to rename "dementia praecox" into schizophrenia (Bleuler 1911) was readily accepted because of this.

Karl Jaspers, Resident at the Department of Psychiatry in Heidelberg from 1909–1915, Professor of Psychology at Heidelberg from 1916 onwards (Professor of Philosophy from 1921 until his forced retirement in 1937 and again from 1945–1948), published *General Psychopathology* (Jaspers 1913) when he was 30 years of age. He created a systematology of descriptive psychopathological phenomena for all mental disorders and especially for schizophrenic episodes and courses.

Kurt Schneider (1946), Professor of Psychiatry at Heidelberg from 1946–1955, who never did a quantitative study of diagnosis, gave precise definitions of those symptoms which define the nuclear syndrome of schizophrenia with high reliability on the basis of Karl Jasper's psychopathology. Standardised instruments still follow his suggestions, e.g. the PSE developed by Wing, Cooper and Sartorius (1974). This means that epidemiological, clinical and biological schizophrenia research of the present are also based on his contribution.

The history of the disease concept of schizophrenia and the importance of Kraepelin who performed his most essential work on this subject at the University of Heidelberg is dealt with by Werner Janzarik (see p. 11).

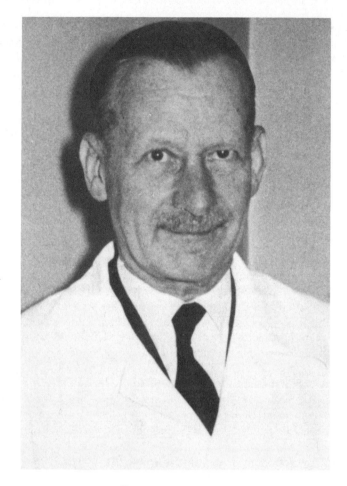

More than 90 years ago, Emil Kraepelin ventured to make assumptions on the aetiology of schizophrenia, but only a small part of them – the contribution of genetic factors to the disease risk – could be proven until now. Since Kraepelin's time we have accumulated a large amount of knowledge, and although we have not clarified the whole truth concerning the causes of schizophrenia, we may at least have come slightly closer to this goal by having successfully eliminated as many of the mistakes as possible through critical discussion of the papers presented, in search of false hypotheses – which Karl Popper (1979) considers to be the most important way to get nearer to the truth. We hope that the publication of these papers and discussions not only summarises the present state of our knowledge and ignorance of the causes of schizophrenia but may also contribute to the future development of research in this important field of psychiatry.

References

Bleuler E (1911) Dementia praecox oder die Gruppe der Schizophrenien. In: Aschaffenburg G (ed) Handbuch der Psychiatrie, Spezieller Teil, 4. Abt., 1. Hälfte. Deuticke, Leipzig
Jaspers K (1913) Allgemeine Psychopathologie. Springer, Berlin
Kraepelin E (1896) Psychiatrie: ein Lehrbuch für Studirende und Aerzte. 5 vollst. umgearb. Aufl. Barth, Leipzig
Popper K (1979) The growth of scientific knowledge. Klostermann, Frankfurt
Schneider K (1946) Klinische Psychopathologie, 1st ed. Thieme, Stuttgart
Wing JK, Cooper JE, Sartorius N (1974) Measurement and classification of psychiatric symptoms: an instruction manual for PSE and CATEGO programme. Cambridge University Press, London
World Health Organization (1973) The international pilot study of schizophrenia, vol 1. World Health Organization, Geneva
World Health Organization (1979) Schizophrenia. An international follow-up study. Wiley, Chichester

Part I
History, Classification, and Research Strategies

The Concept of Schizophrenia: History and Problems

W. Janzarik

The history of schizophrenia is the history of those psychopathological syndromes which were only gradually, and at a relatively late period, grouped under the new designation after numerous differentiations and reclassifications. The study of the psychoses termed endogenous, functional, or idiopathic, and in particular of the various types of schizophrenia, makes apparent fundamental problems in psychopathology. Only a limited number of aspects can be dealt with here. Proceeding from the history of the concept of schizophrenia, I shall concern myself primarily with questions of psychiatric systematology which are related to the development of the concept.

In the German-speaking area the new form of disease which was to lead to dementia praecox and the group of the schizophrenias appeared for the first time in 1865, in a lecture by Snell [27] on "Monomania as the Primary Form of Mental Disturbance." Griesinger [7], who also mentions Morel in this connection, was in agreement with Snell. In a lecture delivered in 1867 to commemorate the opening of the Berlin Clinic, he employed the synonymous term "primary insanity" (*primäre Verrücktheit*). Prior to that time, Griesinger [6], following the lead of his teacher Zeller, had recognized only affective and reversible disorders as primary. A disease process which Griesinger viewed as uniform may stop at these affective pathological states, i.e., at the affective and schizoaffective disorders of a later period. It is equally likely, however, that the process may continue, leading to irreversible conditions of debilitation and impairing cognition and volition. Griesinger had termed these secondary conditions of debilitation "insanity" (*Verrücktheit*) and "imbecility" (*Blödsinn*) and had described them in terms applicable to chronic schizophrenia. In 1867, with his assumption that insanity could become manifest even in the absence of the melancholia and mania previously thought to be necessary preliminary states, in other words, as a primary disorder, Griesinger abandoned the classification system of mental disorders hitherto traditional for him and his time.

In the years following Griesinger's death (in 1868) a new, comprehensive clinical entity established itself on the foundation of "primary insanity". Sander's [24] view, that the majority of institutionalized patients suffered from insanity and constituted the main focus of the publicly financed care of the mentally ill, was widely accepted. In 1878 Schüle [26] equated Kahlbaum's and Hecker's hebephrenia simply with the chronologically earliest appearance of insanity, and Westphal also included Kahlbaum's "catatonic" patients in this category. Thus as early as

Psychiatric Clinic, University of Heidelberg, Vossstraße 4, 6900 Heidelberg, Federal Republic of Germany

1878 the term "schizophrenia" might well have been employed as a synonym for "insanity" in Westphal's [28] sense.

There are a number of reasons for the fact that the bridge between insanity and dementia praecox was not erected until 20 years later. Although there existed a comprehensive new clinical picture whose description corresponded exactly to that of the later dementia praecox, there was as yet no binding medical term for it, but merely a vernacular expression. Once the boundaries of "primary insanity" had been defined, Griesinger's conception, so clear and consistent in its original formulation, lost its inner coherence and its power as a classificatory factor. Parts of the original conception continued to be applied, but to independent diseases. Side by side with these, the original conception remained in use, but now restricted to Kahlbaum's vesania typica.

The consequences for a uniform grouping of affective disorders, which – theoretically – could have been drawn even in the 1850 from Falret's *folie circulaire* and Baillarger's *folie á double forme*, were not recognized at that time. If they had been, the concepts of insanity, on the one hand, and *folie á double forme*, on the other, as two major groupings would have prevented the diagnostic confusion that followed Griesinger's death, and Kraepelin's dichotomy, in all its inspired simplicity, could have been formulated much earlier. But precisely this development was a long time in coming. The concepts of melancholia and mania, their roots traceable back to antiquity, had a different meaning, one that stood in the way of their being applied to purely affective disorders. "Melancholia" referred to a partial and "mania" to a generalized mental disturbance that also included "madness" (*Wahnsinn*), for example. It was only during the last third of the nineteenth century, when the two disorders became associated with periodic courses in which melancolic and manic states follow one another, that "melancholia" and "mania" were restricted to affective disorders. Prior to that time, there was "insanity" (*Verrücktheit*) on one side and a larger group of other mental disturbances on the other. Kahlbaum himself had barred the way to a simple solution with his attempt at nosological description. For a long time Kraepelin followed his lead along this deviant pathway, indicated by the concept of paranoia [4].

Thanks to the consistent observation of the courses of mental disorders, for which conditions were particularly favorable in the Heidelberg Clinic because of its institutional character at that time, Kraepelin finally succeeded in replacing a terminology that had become chaotic. His two groups of diseases gave precise form to the differentiation between "emotional" and "mental" disorders of the beginning of the nineteenth century. This appeared in the sixth edition of his textbook of 1899 [17], after the term "dementia praecox", adopted by Kraepelin in 1893, had acquired comprehensive significance. In 1908 Bleuler's synonymous term "schizophrenia," preferable both scientifically and linguistically replaced "dementia praecox" [4]. The semantic shift between the two terms arose only later.

Inasmuch as the recent history of the concept of schizophrenia is sufficiently familiar, I shall concern myself here only with the vicissitudes in the delineation of the two idiopathic categories, because they lead us to fundamental questions. On the one side are the schizophrenias, which have retained the character of dementia praecox or have been even more narrowly defined – for example, the "systematic schizophrenias" of Kleist and Leonhard, or wherever else there was a need to distinguish other atypical, reactive, schizophrenia-like, or other special forms from the basic group. On the other side we find Bleuler's very broadly defined concept of schizophrenia, which also included latent schizophrenia, and – for several decades – the extremely broad expansion of Bleuler's term in American psychiatry, which was dominated at that time by psychoanalysis. The Heidelberg School, oriented to Jaspers's psychopathology, and K. Schneider adopted a middle course, though closer to Bleuler and based not on Kraepelin's observation of courses, but rather on psychopathological phenomena of the type of first-rank symptoms. The scope of the one group defines the boundaries of the other. The oft-cited work by Pope and Lipinsky [23] illustrates the extent to which the neo-Kraepelin school of thought of the last decade has moved back to the narrow formulation of dementia praecox of the beginning of the century. Even Wilmanns [29] and Lange [20], both of them Kraepelin students, had included psychoses that were basically affective in character and accompanied by delusions, hallucinations, and catatonic phenomena, but without residual alteration, in the category of manic-depressive insanity. DSM-III [16] now speaks of manic and depressive episodes accompanied by mood-incongruent psychotic features, thus including first-rank symptoms, as typical affective disorders. In addition, beginning – after Wernicke – with Kleist, Leonhard, and Schröder, there have been the attempts, each with a new terminology, to narrow down the diagnosis of schizophrenia by recourse to an intermediate area that Kasanin termed schizoaffective, to paranoid disorders, other psychotic disorders, and paranoid and schizotypal personality disorders.

An entire book could be written about the transformations undergone by the concept of schizophrenia [13] during the course of the twentieth century. It would bear testimony to the clearly enhanced reliability recently achieved in diagnostic differentiation, but not to any convincing progress toward a nosology substantiated by objective findings. Diagnoses in the field of the idiopathic psychosyndromes are *conventions* that are obviously based on psychopathological phenomena and course criteria, conventions that can be neither right nor wrong, but at most reliable and useful. Diagnoses such as progressive paralysis or Huntington's chorea, which still properly refer to disease entities in the sense of the original nosological approach in psychiatry, are exceptions rather than the rule. The majority of psychiatric diagnoses reflect primarily the theoretical preliminary decisions and the methodological approaches on which the recognized conventions happen to be based at any given time. And to no small extent, such diagnoses also reflect the momentary power structures prevailing in the activity of psychiatric science.

The psychiatric systematology of the twentieth century is that of Kraepelin, even though the principle from which he derived his classification may have been oriented to a phantom. Kraepelin sought and found disease entities. These were clinical entities, derived from course observation in Kahlbaum's sense and, as recently pointed out by Pichot [22], also in the sense of French psychiatry. Certainly there was reason to expect neurophatological confirmation, but so far these expectations have not been fulfilled. What remains is the neurological disease model originally based on progressive paralysis and still exerting a certain amount of influence with its characteristic manner of thinking, which includes a one-sidedly biological view and at the same time the very antithesis of an exclusive psychogenesis. K. Schneider [25] stressed the conventional character of psychiatric diagnosis, but nevertheless postulated a somatic disease process for the psychopathological conventions he termed "cyclothymia" and "schizophrenia." Even the diagnoses cited in DSM-III will not be able to preserve their praiseworthy descriptive neutrality on the way to becoming disease entities, a way that is prescribed by the efforts toward validation.

But our respect for Kraepelin's monumental achievement should not be permitted to stand in the way of critical appraisal of a conception, long since taken for granted, concerning which Kraepelin [18] himself subsequently voiced certain doubts. If we abandon the disease model according to which specific disease processes that differ from known organic disorders lead to schizophrenic disturbances in one case and to affective disturbances in another, and restrict ourselves to the findings that are actually accessible in a given case, we will not progress beyond psychopathological syndromes which can be expanded into diagnoses for clinical use through the application of course criteria. Today, Kraepelin's guiding thought is reflected not only in the method of course observation, but also – and particularly – in exclusion criteria such as certain age limits, the mutual exclusiveness of the two idiopathic groups, and the required absence of any organic disorder, as well as in the endeavors toward validation in terms of a differential reaction to somatic therapy and a specific family pattern of distribution. Although the biological disease model is no longer explicitly adduced in substantiating the foundations of psychiatric systematology, nonetheless it determines the modes of thinking that still underlie a by now thoroughly pragmatic approach to the establishment of diagnostic classifications.

The outstanding importance of psychotropic drugs, which act upon certain neurotransmitters and receptors, in the therapy of schizophrenic as well as affective syndromes argues in favor of somatic deviations from the norm; *not*, however, in favor of specific disease processes. The disturbances in limbic and hypothalamic functions that can be assumed to be present here would correspond to the disturbances in drive and affectivity. Psychopathologically, these disturbances can be conceptualized as a restriction or expansion of the patient's "dynamic". Together with biorhythmic disturbances [2], they are characteristic of affective psychosyndromes and make themselves felt in the form of dynamic instability in productive schizophrenic episodes. In this connection we speak of "dynamic derailments" and see in them the psychotic core of idiopathic psychosyndromes, close to the point of attack of somatic therapy. The dynamic derailments would correspond to the primary mental disorders of *pre*-Kraepelin psychiatry, regarded as affective and reversible, but capable of progressing to secondary conditions of debilitation that are no longer reversible. From the standpoint of Kraepelin's disease model, this earlier conception, as Griesinger advocated it, was referred to in retrospect as the theory of unitary psychosis (*Einheitspsychose*).

For the purposes of a modified interpretation of unitary psychosis there are *no* clear boundaries, as far as dynamic derailments are concerned, between affective and schizophrenic syndromes. For example, affective disorders in particular, the majority of which are not characterized by florid phenomena such as delusions and hallucinations and whose psychopathological picture is determined by restriction or expansion of the patient's dynamic, show transitions in all directions. The diagnosis "schizophrenia" is based primarily on florid phenomena of the type of first-rank symptoms. When dynamic derailments are clearly apparent behind these phenomena, as is the case especially in acute psychotic episodes, and the instability approaches the phasic processes usual in affective disorders, above all the manic pole, then the symptoms may be subject to multiple interpretations. The schizoaffective intermediate area [15] in which psychopathological phenomena from both groups mingle is probably larger, after all, than we would like to believe in our present endeavors – in fashion once more – to establish an exact dividing line between affective and schizophrenic disorders.

There is still another problem that manifests itself in similar fashion in the case of affective syndromes, namely that a totality of psychopathological phenomena which is supplemented by course criteria and which, once organic causes have been excluded, is diagnosed as a schizophrenic disorder can just as well be the result of an organic disease process such as epilepsy or of the abuse of certain drugs. The convention based upon the assumption of an independent disease concept forbids us to speak of schizophrenia in the latter case. On the other hand, this convention is not necessarily binding. One can argue that the somatic dysfunction suspected behind the schizophrenic syndromes may be nonspecific and may have its origin in the patient's own predisposition, in somatic disease processes, or in the reaction to certain emotional strains. From this point of view, the somatic dysfunction triggered by any one of a number of factors would be less important than the patient's personality structure, which responds in the same way during the prodrome of what can be described as schizophrenic syndromes in the psychopathological sense. The pragmatics of therapy makes no distinction here in any case; schizophrenic amphetaminic psychoses and reactive psychoses are treated in exactly the same way, namely with neuroleptic drugs, as are schizophrenias regarded as "genuine."

From the point of view of the traditional disease model, the residual stages occurring during the course of schizophrenic disorders and originally regarded as typical only of dementia praecox are the direct result of a progressive disease process; however, this view is now subject to doubt. Residual stages are also observed during the course of affective disorders, but frequently they prove to be reversible; the residue that remains after the reversal of productive courses of the illness is often no more than a mild dynamic insufficiency already inherent in weaknesses in the patients personality prior to the onset of the disorders. A recent monograph by Mundt [21], on the apathy syndrome in schizophrenic patients of the Heidelberg Psychiatric Clinic, deals with these aspects. A great deal of what has been ascribed to a pathological process in the manifestation and development of schizophrenic syndromes seems to be rooted rather in the personality of the patient. In terms of my own model of structural dynamic coherency it would be necessary to inquire what is to be regarded as dynamic derailment in a schizophrenic syndrome, and what is contributed by the structural components carried over into the psychosis. It would have to be borne in mind that structure and dynamic are closely linked, so that pathogenetic courses, too, would have to be viewed as cyclical structural dynamic processes [12]. Particularly in the interpretation of chronic courses, emphasis would have to be placed not on the derailment of biological functions, but on the deformation of structure. If one adheres to recent diagnostic categories, the decision as to the chronicity of schizophrenic courses would also have to be based on axis II of DSM-III.

In closing, I shall deal briefly with the differentiation of the positive and negative symptoms of schizophrenia as a very recent development, based on the work of Wing as well as on that of Strauss, Carpenter, and Bartko, to which the *Schizophrenia Bulletin* devoted an entire number in 1985. This differentiation has been traced back to Jackson, and Berrios [3] traces it as far back as Reynolds, pointing out that the latter author's concept is more compatible with modern usage. The high degree of plausibility inherent in all simplifications has assured this differentiation widespread recognition in Germany as well. Crow [5], adducing the dopamine hypothesis, has classified positive symptoms as belonging to a (productive) type I and negative symptoms to a (deficient) type II of schizophrenic syndromes, and Andreasen [1] has developed an investigative tool for the determination of negative symptoms. British and American authors – albeit without being familiar with the earlier discussion – have taken up deliberations that were considered in psychiatric circles in Germany as long ago as 1922, when Gruhle [8] advanced his argument against the insufficiency hypothesis advocated by Berze, namely that in many cases of dementia praecox a plus in impulses in the sense of a hyperfunction could be observed. According to Gruhle, "some courses or phases of schizophrenia are marked by a plus, and others by a minus in psychic activity," similar to the hypo- and hyerphases of manic-depressive insanity.

The introduction of therapy with neuroleptic drugs has given new impetus to Gruhle's differentiation precisely because it is based not on individual symptoms, but rather on the overall mental state. Since 1959 my structural dynamic approach [11] has distinguished between a dynamic derailment of the instability type, whose productive phenomena respond well to neuroleptic drugs, and a dynamic insufficiency that is practically inaccessible to somatic therapy. Investigations by Huber [9] of changes resulting from cerebral atrophy, reported as early as 1957, and later studies by the same author on basic symptoms in schizophrenics have been disregarded by Anglo-American authors who have recently begun to concern themselves with related problems. Huber's most recently published monograph (Süllwold and Huber, 1986) [10], on the concept of basic disturbances, avoids one-sidedness in dealing critically with the differentiation of positive and negative schizophrenia.

There have been many detours and many false trails in the long history of the concept of schizophrenia, but at the same time there has been progress, particularly in the advances made in the therapeutic field and in the biological research, carried out along precise scientific lines, to which these advances have given rise. Among the especially noteworthy achievements of modern psychiatry has been the transformation of a body of experience accumulated over generations into empirically substantiated and objectively verifiable factual knowledge. At the same time, the plethora of data and detail has become so great that there may often be danger of losing sight of the larger context. For example, the authors who, under Zubin's lead, are now dealing with the currently very important questions connected with the vulnerability to schizophrenia are no longer aware of the fundamental concept which was evolved by Kretschmer [19] in 1918 on the basis of sensitive delusion of reference (*sensitiver Beziehungswahn*). Via an operational-ization of psychopathological phenomena, the empirical approach has led to reliable diagnostic differentiations, but not as yet to nosologically valid ones. Some initial steps have been taken in the direction of a convention concerning just what schizophrenia means, a convention that would transcend language barriers and traditional views. So far there is no conclusively defined disease known as "schizophrenia." The history of the concept is a history not of medical discoveries, but of the intellectual models on which the orientation of psychiatry is based.

Summary

Following a review of the historical development of the concept of schizophrenia since Griesinger's "primary insanity," consideration is given to the complex of problems that surround the diagnostic conventions based on psychopathological phenomena and course criteria, including the "positive" and "negative" symptoms of schizophrenia.

References

1. Andreasen NC (1982) Negative symptoms in schizophrenia. Arch Gen Psychiatry 39:784–788
2. Berner P (1982) Psychiatrische Systematik. Huber, Bern
3. Berrios GE (1985) Positive and negative symptoms and Jackson. Arch Gen Psychiatry 42:95–97
4. Bleuler E (1908) Die Prognose der Dementia praecox (Schizophreniegruppe). Allg Z Psychiatr 65:436–464
5. Crow TI (1980) Molecular pathology of schizophrenia: more than one disease process? Br Med J 280:66–68
6. Griesinger W (1861) Die Pathologie und Therapie der psychischen Krankheiten. Krabbe, Stuttgart
7. Griesinger W (1868/69) Vortrag zur Eröffnung der psychiatrischen Klinik zu Berlin am 2. Mai 1867. Arch Psychiatr Nervenkr 1:143–158
8. Gruhle HW (1922) Die Psychologie der Dementia praecox. Z Gesamte Neurol Psychiatr 78:454–471
9. Huber G (1957) Pneumencephalographische und psychopathologische Bilder bei endogenen Psychosen. Springer, Berlin Göttingen Heidelberg
10. Huber G (1986) In: Süllwold L, Huber G: Schizophrene Basisstörungen. Springer, Berlin Heidelberg New York Tokyo
11. Janzarik W (1968) Dynamische Grundkonstellationen in endogenen Psychosen. Springer, Berlin Göttingen Heidelberg
12. Janzarik W (1968) Schizophrene Verläufe. Springer, Berlin Heidelberg New York
13. Janzarik W (1978) Wandlungen des Schizophreniebegriffes. Nervenarzt 49:133–139
14. Janzarik W (1979) Die klinische Psychopathologie zwischen Griesinger und Kraepelin im Querschnitt des Jahres 1878. In: Janzarik W (Hrsg) Psychopathologie als Grundlagenwissenschaft. Enke, Stuttgart
15. Janzarik W (1980) Der schizoaffektive Zwischenbereich und die Lehre von den primären und sekundären Seelenstörungen. Nervenarzt 51:272–279
16. Koehler K, Saß H (1984) Diagnostisches und Statistisches Manual psychischer Störungen (DSM-III). Beltz, Wein heim

17. Kraepelin E (1899) Psychiatrie. Barth, Leipzig
18. Kraepelin E (1920) Die Erscheinungsformen des Irreseins. Z Gesamte Neurol Psychiatr 62:1–29
19. Kretschmer E (1966) Der sensitive Beziehungswahn. Springer, Berlin Heidelberg New York
20. Lange J (1922) Katatonische Erscheinungen im Rahmen manischer Erkrankungen. Springer, Berlin
21. Mundt C (1985) Das Apathiesyndrom der Schizophrenen. Springer, Berlin Heidelberg New York Tokyo
22. Pichot P (1983) Ein Jahrhundert Psychiatrie. Dacosta, Paris
23. Pope HG, Lipinski JF (1978) Diagnosis in schizophrenia and manic-depressive illness. Arch Gen Psychiatry 35:811–828
24. Sander W (1868/69) Über eine specielle Form der primären Verrücktheit. Arch Psychiatr Nervenkr 1:387–419
25. Schneider K (1967) Klinische Psychopathologie. Thieme, Stuttgart
26. Schüle H (1878) Handbuch der Geisteskrankheiten. Vogel, Leipzig
27. Snell L (1865) Ueber Monomanie als primäre Form der Seelenstörung. Allg Z Psychiatr 22:368–381
28. Westphal C (1878) Über die Verrücktheit. Allg Z Psychiatr 34:252–257 (Ref)
29. Wilmanns K (1907) Zur Differentialdiagnostik der „funktionellen" Psychosen. Zentralbl Nervenheilkd Psychiatr 30:569–588

The Classification of Schizophrenia in the Different Diagnostic Systems

H. SASS

Preliminary Remarks

The phenomenological-descriptive definition of schizophrenic syndromes has been decisively influenced by the clinical and psychopathological traditions in Heidelberg and by the Zürich school. This is the basis for most empirical searches for the causes of schizophrenia. Despite many reservations expressed by Kraepelin, Bleuler, Jaspers, and K. Schneider, the biological approach almost exclusively follows the theoretical model of the medical concept of disease. The natural history of schizophrenic syndromes, which were originally defined in terms of psychopathology and course, shall be elucidated by the discovery of pathogenetic mechanisms and a causal etiology. The task of psychopathology is seen largely in terms of optimizing the symptomatological definition of the schizophrenic syndromes in order to provide adequate samples for studies in biological research. The question of the fundamental relationships between a psychopathologically based classification of schizophrenia and the research strategies of exact sciences is seldom raised. This problem is to be a keynote of the following review.

Classical Conceptions of Schizophrenia

First of all, some positions of German-language psychiatry in our century with regard to the classification of schizophrenia will be sketched in continuation of the historical lines drawn out in the previous paper. Most comparisons of systems for diagnosis of schizophrenia are based on American and British concepts and definitions; however, the majority of these concepts are German in origin, at least as stated by Kendell (1985).

Four psychopathological conceptions are especially important for the time before systematic development of the operational criteria which constitute a crucial turning point in research and diagnosis: those of Kraepelin, E. Bleuler, the Heidelberg school of psychopathologists after Jaspers, and K. Schneider. The special positions of the Wernicke-Kleist-Leonhard line (Leonhard 1972) and C. Schneider's conception of schizophrenia (1939, 1942), which are of similar theoretical importance but have little influence today, cannot be considered here.

Kraepelin (1899) specified the classification of functional, idiopathic, or endogenous psychoses which is still valid today in the sixth edition of his textbook.

Psychiatric Clinic, University of Heidelberg, Vossstraße 4, 6900 Heidelberg, Federal Republic of Germany

In this grouping, he subsumed the catatonia of Kahlbaum (1874), the hebephrenia of Hecker (1871), the monomania of Snell (1865), and the primary madness of Griesinger (1868/69) under the designation "dementia praecox", which derives from Morel (1860), and contrasted this with the affective disorders of manic-depressive madness. The essence of his method of research was the study of the complete life history of the psychiatric patients above and beyond the notation of current psychopathological signs and symptoms. Koehler (1979 a) described Kraepelin's classification as a four-level dichotomy in the areas of terminology, nosology, clinical descriptive boundaries, and prognosis. Exceptions from the eminently important prognostic dichotomy were already discussed at an early stage and recognized by Kraepelin (Wilmanns 1907; Kirby 1913; Lange 1922), and were often illustrated by catatonic conditions (cf Saß 1981). An approach to the operationalization of the originally relatively narrow field of dementia praecox with symptomatological criteria is to be found in Landmark (1982) and in Berner et al. (1983). In conceptual terms, Kraepelin as well as Kahlbaum assumed that the disease entities had a biological foundation based on the idea of uniformity in terms of causes, symptoms, course, and outcome. In principle, modern validation strategies are clearly preformed in the "clinical method" of these authors.

The equally influential conception of E. Bleuler (1911) was developed in parallel with Kraepelin and shows much agreement with him. Bleuler's extension of the field of schizophrenia by the idea of latent schizophrenia has become important for all further classifications. This was also accepted by Kraepelin, who regarded some psychopathic personalities as undeveloped cases of dementia simplex. The concept of latent schizophrenia was frequently criticized because of its vagueness, but it has become the point of departure for fruitful research in the field of schizotypal and borderline personality disorder (Gunderson and Siever 1985; Saß and Koehler 1983) via the intermediates of pseudoneurotic schizophrenia (Hoch and Polatin 1949) and the schizophrenic spectrum concept (Kety et al. 1968; Kety 1985).

The differences between Kraepelin and E. Bleuler consist less in the clinical approach and diagnostic delimitation than in the development of a psychological theory by Bleuler which introduced the ideas of Freud into the psychopathology of schizophrenie (Bleuler and Jung 1908). They regarded its prominent symptoms, e.g., delusions, thought blocking, hallucinations, and negativism, as secondary and as a reaction of the psychosis to affect-laden complexes. The primary symptoms, especially the disturbances of association, were regarded as a more direct consequence of the somatic disease process. In the further development, M. Bleuler (1971) formulated from this the concept of a primary disorder centering on autism and splitting. Like Kraepelin, E. Bleuler assumed an unknown organic disease process of schizophrenia which has no direct relationship with the psychopathological symptoms: "We differentiate sharply between the physical illness and its symptoms, the latter in dementia praecox being almost exclusively psychic ... The disease itself, even when far advanced, need not produce any of the symptoms commonly considered as typical" (Bleuler and Jung 1908).

Concerning the consequences for further research in schizophrenia, Kraepelin's conception appears to be important above all for the classification, for example owing to its emphasis on descriptive symptomatology, the course of the illness, and genetics, three areas which are still crucial in modern diagnostic re-

search. On the other hand, owing to its psychological and theoretical speculations, Bleuler's conception is fruitful for psychodynamically oriented attempts at
understanding and treatment, and also for the development of neurophysiological and neuropsychological hypotheses in accordance with the explanatory model
of exact sciences.

After Kraepelin left for Munich, an active school of psychopathologists developed in Heidelberg under the brain pathologist Nissl. Besides the later philo-
sopher Jaspers, in particular Wilmans, Beringer, Gruhle, and Mayer-Groß belonged to this school. This group, which was broken up by the National Social-
ists, clinically applied the phenomenological method of Jaspers (1963). Their
studies culminated in the famous schizophrenia volume of Bumke's handbook,
in which the ideas of Kraepelin, Bleuler, Kretschmer, C. Schneider, and
K. Schneider were critically examined. The central sections on clinical picture and
differential diagnosis derived from Mayer-Groß (1932), who later introduced this
view of schizophrenia to Great Britain. Once more, the psychological extension
of Kraepelin's symptomatological description was involved, but not with the
strongly rejected psychoanalysis concentrating on contents, rather with the
phenomenological methods of introspection and a comprehending reconstruction of the experiences of the patient in order to subject his motives, reflections,
and feelings to a formal analysis.

The Heidelberg school's very broad concept of schizophrenia was based on
the assumption of an endogenous mental disorder of organic or toxic etiology but
with an unknown cause. With regard to the connection between the somatic level
and the psychopathological phenomena, the symptoms were considered to be in
principle nonspecific; there was also no theoretical-speculative distinction into
fundamental and accessory disturbances. For Mayer-Groß, the differential classification of symptoms which initially appear to be ubiquitous was, in the tradition of Jaspers, attained by phenomenological analysis of the way in which the
psychological conditions were experienced; in particular, the precise circumstances of the beginning of the disease were of interest. This differential criterion
of a specific experiential quality of the symptoms has lost significance in present
systems of classification, probably due above all to the question of reliability. Today, a formalized pattern of signs and symptoms of which the description is increasingly oriented to objective behavior appears to be more important than the
atmospheric background of subjective experiences which guided the diagnosis of
the Heidelberg phenomenologists.

K. Schneider (1925, 1959) also adhered to the postulate of schizophrenia as a
somatosis. However, since the biological causes were completely unknown, he advocated a purely psychopathological typology of the endogenous psychoses.
Once more, the experiential phenomena had special significance. For their differentiation with regard to schizophrenia, the disturbances of the sense of activity
were accorded a central place. The first-rank symptoms (FRS) have become
highly influential as a clinically and didactically very helpful operationalization
of symptomatological criteria for the diagnosis of schizophrenia. Together with
further experiential phenomena, termed second-rank symptoms, and other abnormalities of behavior and expression they rendered Schneider's schizophrenia
similar in extent to that of Bleuler and the earlier Heidelberg school.

Recently, empirical data and changed diagnostic conventions have led to a relativization of K. Schneider's criteria. The FRS are found only in a proportion of the cases diagnosed as schizophrenic, even in centers of psychiatry oriented toward K. Schneider (Koehler et al. 1977; Mellor 1970, 1982). Mellor (1982) argued that FRS are strongly associated with schizophrenia, but that they occur in a remarkable percentage of other conditions too; K. Schneider's belief that FRS invariably distinguish schizophrenia from cyclothymia appeared to be discredited. Kety (1980) stated even more rigorously: "K. Schneider established a new syndrome that may be more prevalent, have a more favorable outcome, and be more responsive to a wide variety of treatments, but it is not schizophrenia." However, it is to be pointed out that K. Schneider's recording of FRS is linked to a subtle phenomenological analysis of psychic experiences in accordance with Jaspers, such as is not always ensured in modern investigations.

Berner and Küfferle (1982) have associated the question of the specificity of FRS with the structural-dynamic psychopathological conception of Janzarik (1959, 1968). Both in the basic or primary symptoms of Bleuler and in the first-rank symptoms of K. Schneider, a dynamic derailment in the sense of Janzarik is assumed, mostly as a dynamic instability, so that the delimitation of schizophrenia is similar in both conceptions despite the theoretical differences. However, dynamic instability can occur in very different psychological disorders, and Berner and Küfferle (1982) conclude that FRS are an inadequate diagnostic tool only suitable for classifying dynamic instability states of a very heterogeneous origin.

Modern Systems of Classification

Two trends contributed to the crisis of psychiatric diagnosis at the end of the 1960s: on the one hand the antipsychiatric movement motivated by social change (Szasz 1962; Laing 1965), and on the other hand the scientific criticism of the weaknesses of the diagnostic process revealed, for example, in studies by Beck et al. 1962, the US/UK diagnostic project (Cooper et al. 1972), and the dubious experiment of Rosenhan (1973). Since schizophrenia was at the center of controversies in both lines of argumentation, various large-scale comparative investigations were suggested (e.g., WHO 1973), and in the meantime efforts to classify schizophrenia and its borderline syndromes have attained a pacemaker function for the greatly advanced diagnostic research.

The most important result was the development of operationalized systems of diagnosis which constitute a formalization of textbook knowledge and the present state of research expressed in symptomatological criteria. Koehler (1979 b) concluded: "*In summa*, the exact relationships of symptoms or other clinical characteristics such as race, sex, age at onset, precipitating factors, and personality features to various diagnostic categories are operationalized in terms of clear-cut rules of application by an unambiguous statement of inclusion and exclusion criteria."

Milestones in this development are, in the USA, the St. Louis criteria (Feighner et al. 1972), the RDC (Spitzer et al. 1975), and the DSM-III (Apa 1980);

in Great Britain, the PSE and CATEGO system (Wing et al. 1967, 1977); in France, the LICET S system (Pull et al. 1981); and in the German-speaking countries, the Vienna research criteria (Berner et al. 1983).

The in principle rather similar definitions of schizophrenia in the various classification systems differ in some details which are connected with the varying recourse to the elements of the classical conceptions. The differences concern the choice of symptom criteria, the structure of diagnostic algorithms, the temporal criteria, and the evaluation of affective syndromes. In the meantime, there are more than 10 comparative studies on the over a dozen definitions of schizophrenia in the different diagnostic systems (Bland and Orn 1979; Brockington et al. 1978; Endicott et al. 1982; Fenton et al. 1981; Hawk et al. 1975; Kendell et al. 1979; McGuffin et al. 1984; Stephens et al. 1982; Strauss and Carpenter 1974; Strauss and Gift 1977; Taylor 1972).

The investigation of joint frequencies and reliability of various criteria sets is concentrated on diagnostic problems in the narrow sense. Endicott et al. (1982) found as a whole a higher reliability than in earlier studies, with values between 0.65 and 1.0. The greatly differing rates of cases diagnosed as schizophrenia in a given sample are unsatisfactory. They ranged between 4% and 26% of a psychiatric population in the study by Endicott et al. (1982), in which RDC, DSM-III, and the criteria of Carpenter were close together, with rates between 11% and 14%. In a study by Brockington et al. (1978), the rate of diagnosis of schizophrenia in a series of 119 psychotic first admissions varied between 3.4% and 38%. RDC, CATEGO, Langfeldt's criteria, and the Carpenter system obtained good results with regard to concordance between different systems.

In the search for validating parameters for the different schizophrenia classifications, the prognostic criterion of Kraepelin plays a prominent role (Häfner 1982). Various studies show that there is a consistent tendency for the FRS to be weak in the prediction of outcome, whereas the RDC, Langfeldt's definition, Carpenter's system, the Feighner criteria, and DSM-III pick out prognostically unfavorable cases relatively well (Bland and Orn 1979; Brockington et al. 1978; Hawk et al. 1975; Stephens et al. 1982; Strauss and Carpenter 1974). Formerly, it was criticized that in systems with a 6 months criterion for the diagnosis of schizophrenia, pure prognosis constitutes not a validating criterion but rather a tautology, "since chronic patients are chronic" (Koehler 1979 b; Strauss and Carpenter 1974). It was interesting that according to Kendell's (1985) precise data analysis on this objection, the ability of the DSM-III criteria to predict poor long-term prognosis is due not only to the 6 months criterion, but largely to other elements of the definition.

As a further validating parameter, heritability was investigated, since so far there is strong evidence for a genetic transmission of schizophrenia. The question was examined as to which of the competing definitions of schizophrenia are suitable to identify the patients who possess genetically determined biological abnormality (Kendell 1985). McGuffin et al. (1984) have checked six definitions on heritability: RDC and the criteria of Feighner attained the highest values, whereas the FRS of K. Schneider displayed a heritability of 0 and thus had a similar result to that in prediction of prognosis.

If – beyond the comparison of detailed differences – major tendencies in classification of schizophrenia in recent years are looked for, the four following developments can be discerned:

1. The state of theoretical knowledge and comparative investigations shows that in the absence of firm criteria a definitive evaluation of the systems is not possible. According to Kendell (1985), the question may not be "What is right?" or "Which is best?" but only "Which shall I use?" The choice of diagnostic system depends on the problems raised: clinical therapeutic, prognostic, genetic, and other interests may lead to the use of different instruments in different situations. In view of this, it appears plausible to suggest that different classification systems be used in parallel in a transition stage (Kendell 1982; Strauss and Gift 1977; Young et al. 1982). Berner et al. (1983) advocate this polydiagnostic approach most consistently.

2. Above all in the USA, the field of schizophrenic disorders has become greatly reduced in size with a corresponding extension of the affective field. With different stringency, the classification systems mostly prescribe the diagnosis of an affective disease in combined occurrence of affective and schizophrenic disorders, which is a reversal of the hierarchical rule of Jaspers. On the other hand, RDC permits differentiation of an independent field of schizoaffective syndromes. A final classification of the syndromes with admixture of affective and schizophreniform symptomatology is apparently not possible at present either from a psychopathological or from a biological point of view. Nevertheless, the opening of the affective disorders at the expense of schizophrenia appears to be clinically reasonable, with regard especially to questions of pharmacotherapy and long-term prophylaxis with lithium, but also to the prognostic variability in conventional schizophrenia which has become the center of interest once more owing to the three large European follow-up studies (M. Bleuler 1972; Ciompi and Müller 1976; Ciompi 1984; Huber et al. 1979).

3. The development and improvement of operationalized classification systems in the 1970s has shown that high reliability is no guarantee of validity, so that attention is concentrated today more on the latter problem. For validation of mental diseases, the clinical description, laboratory study, family or genetic study, follow-up, and treatment response are regarded as important parameters (Robins and Guze 1970). For delimitation of the schizophrenic syndromes, two areas in particular stand out in addition to clinical symptomatology so long as the etiology is unclarified: the criterion of homogeneous outcome and the occurrence of similar disorders in the family. Kendell (1982, 1986), however, points out that the outcome validity is not identical with the etiological validity, for there are well-validated disease entities with quite different outcomes. Similar objections can be raised with regard to heritability, since certain factors which have not yet been adequately explored may have a modifying effect on the manifestation of the schizophrenic disorder, e.g., premorbid personality, biographical experiences, life events, or minor brain disease. The clinically important criterion of treatment response is also suitable for validation only to a limited extent, since many therapeutic measures are nonspecific. All in all, it must remain an open question as to whether the different results of the diagnostic systems in the detection of schizophrenic patients with regard to different validation parameters may not be based on the diagnostic diversity of the subjects selected.

4. A further trend in the classification of schizophrenia results from the advances in biological investigation and the validation paradigm connected therewith. In this line of research, the view that the schizophrenias are a group of etiologically heterogeneous disorders which break down into different nosological subgroups is increasingly prevailing. According to Haier (1980), the concept of schizophrenia as a unitary disease has diminished and heterogeneity is no longer regarded as a source of error variance to be eliminated, but is becoming the focus of study in subtyping investigations. The biological studies reveal an increasing number of subtle abnormalities in the neurophysiological, biochemical, and morphological field, and recently also the studies of in vivo neurotransmitter metabolism. The hierarchical rule of Jaspers is thus placed in question for a second time. It is becoming more and more uncertain where the boundary should be drawn between disorders of organic origin and idiopathic psychoses. Depending on this research approach, alternative subtyping suggestions instead of the four traditionally defined schizophrenic syndromes are gaining significance: e.g., the good- vs poor-prognosis schizophrenia (Robins and Guze 1970), the type I vs type II schizophrenia (Crow 1980), the contrasting of core schizophrenia vs schizophrenic spectrum (Kety et al. 1968), the differentiation of familial vs sporadic cases of schizophrenia (Murray et al. 1985), or the separation of an ADD psychosis (Bellak 1985).

Concluding Remarks

The emergence of these new subtypings once more raises the problems sketched at the beginning as to the relationship between psychopathological and biological approaches to research in the classification of schizophrenia. In the polydiagnostic approach, the traditional predominance of psychopathological criteria is preserved, but it already affords the possibility of a more flexible handling of the different classification systems. It is a similar step forward that in some of the newer conceptions of schizophrenia the biological parameters gradually become classification criteria of equal rank, e.g., the genetic characteristics in the model of Murray et al. (1985) or dopamine metabolism and structural alterations in the brain in the theory of Crow (1980). In continuation of this strategy, further efforts will be made to integrate the levels of psychopathological description and biological explanation in order to arrive at disease entities in accordance with the current validation paradigm.

Besides this, an alternative strategy is emerging in a review of research in this century. Various heuristically valuable models have been developed when the formulation of psychopathological theories was not too dependent on the frequently changing findings at the somatic level. The corollary of this also applies. Thus, for example, Heimann (1985) advocates the nosologically neutral study of protective pathophysiological mechanisms with which the body reacts to pathological cerebral processes. The highly advanced diagnostic rules in modern classification systems still do not guarantee adequate delimitation of investigation groups in biological research, especially since many of the psychopathological criteria are rather nonspecific. Thus, besides the strategies of integrating the psychopathological and biological research issues, a provisional emancipation from these strategies will also be necessary from time to time for the development of new concepts and classifications.

Summary

Considering the problematical relationship between psychopathological and biological research disciplines, some classic conceptions of schizophrenia and then the modern classification systems are discussed. The validation paradigm of schizophrenia research oriented on the exact sciences requires flexible classifications based on criteria from different levels of investigation.

References

American Psychiatric Association, Committee on Nomenclature and Statistics (1980) Diagnostic and statistical manual of mental disorders, 3rd edn. American Psychiatric Association, Washington DC

Beck AT, Ward C, Mendelson M, Mock J, Erbaugh J (1962) Reliability of psychiatric diagnoses: 2. A study of consistency of clinical judgements and ratings. Am J Psychiatry 119:210–216

Bellak L (1985) ADD psychosis as a separate entity. Schizophr Bull 11(4):523–527

Berner P, Küfferle B (1982) British phenomenology and psychopathological concepts. A comparative view. Br J Psychiatry 140:558–565

Berner P, Gabriel E, Katschnig H, Kiefer W, Koehler K, Lenz G, Sinhandl CH (1983) Diagnostic criteria for schizophrenia and affective psychoses. World Psychiatric Association, American Psychiatric Press, Washington D.C.

Bland RC, Orn H (1979) Schizophrenia: diagnosis criteria and outcome. Br J Psychiatry 134:34–38

Bleuler E (1911) Dementia praecox oder Gruppe der Schizophrenien. In: Aschaffenburg G (ed) Handbuch der Psychiatrie. Deuticke, Leipzig

Bleuler E, Jung CG (1908) Komplexe und Krankheitsursachen bei Dementia praecox. Zentralbl Psychiatr Nervenheilk 3:220–227

Bleuler M (1971) Klinik der schizophrenen Geistesstörungen. In: Meyer JE, Müller M, Strömgren E (eds) Psychiatrie der Gegenwart, vol II/1, 2nd edn. Springer, Berlin Heidelberg New York, pp 7–82

Bleuler M (1972) Die schizophrenen Geistesstörungen im Lichte langjähriger Katamnesen und Familiengeschichten. Thieme, Stuttgart

Brockington IF, Kendell RE, Leff JP (1978) Definitions of schizophrenia: concordance and prediction of outcome. Psychol Med 8:387–398

Ciompi L (1984) Is there really a schizophrenia? The long-term course of psychotic phenomena. Br J Psychiatry 145:636–640, 146:558–559

Ciompi L, Müller M (1976) Lebensweg und Alter Schizophrener. Eine katamnestische Langzeitstudie bis ins Senium. Springer, Berlin Heidelberg New York

Cooper JE, Kendell RE, Sharpe L, Copeland JRM, Simon R (1972) Psychiatric diagnosis in New York and London. Oxford University Press, London (Maudsley monograph no 20)

Crow TJ (1980) Molecular pathology of schizophrenia: more than one dimension of pathology? Br Med J 280:66–68

Endicott JN, Fleiss J, Cohen J, Janel W, Simon R (1982) Diagnostic criteria for schizophrenia. Arch Gen Psychiatry 39:884–889

Feighner JP, Robins E, Guze SB, Woodruff RA, Winokur G, Munoz R (1972) Diagnostic criteria for use in psychiatric research. Arch Gen Psychiatry 26:57–63

Fenton WS, Mosher LR, Matthews SM (1981) Diagnosis of schizophrenia. A critical review of current diagnostic systems. Schizophr Bull 7(3):452–476

Griesinger W (1868/69) Vortrag zur Eröffnung der Psychiatrischen Klinik zu Berlin am 2. Mai 1867. Arch Psychiatr Nervenkr 1:143–158

Gunderson W, Siever LJ (1985) Relatedness of schizotypal to schizophrenic disorders: editor's introduction. Schizophr Bull 11(4):532–537

Häfner H (1982) Beziehungen zwischen Diagnose und Verlauf bei der Schizophrenie. In: Beckmann H (ed) Biologische Psychiatrie. Thieme, Stuttgart, pp 14–18

Haier RJ (1980) The diagnosis of schizophrenia. A review of recent developments. Schizophr Bull 6(3):417–428

Hawk AB, Carpenter WT, Strauss JS (1975) Diagnostic criteria and five-year outcome in schizophrenia. Arch Gen Psychiatry 32:343–347

Hecker E (1871) Die Hebephrenie. Ein Beitrag zur klinischen Psychiatrie. Arch Pathol Anat Berlin 52:394–429

Heimann H (1985) Specifity and nonspecifity – a major problem in biologically oriented psychopathology. Psychopathology 18:82–87

Hoch P, Polatin R (1949) Pseudoneurotic forms of schizophrenia. Psychiatr Q 23:248–276

Huber G, Gross G, Schüttler R (1979) Schizophrenie. Verlaufs- und sozialpsychiatrische Langzeituntersuchungen an den 1945–1959 in Bonn hospitalisierten schizophrenen Kranken. Springer, Berlin Heidelberg New York

Janzarik W (1959) Dynamische Grundkonstellationen in endogenen Psychosen. Springer, Berlin Göttingen Heidelberg

Janzarik W (1968) Schizophrene Verläufe. Eine strukturdynamische Interpretation. Springer, Berlin Heidelberg New York

Jaspers K (1963) General psychopathology. University Press, Manchester

Kahlbaum KL (1874) Die Katatonie oder das Spannungsirresein. Eine klinische Form psychischer Krankheit. Hirschwald, Berlin

Kendell RE (1982) The choice of diagnostic criteria for biological research. Arch Gen Psychiatry 39:1334–1339

Kendell RE (1985) Which schizophrenia? In: Huber G (ed) Basisstadien endogener Psychosen und das Borderline-Problem. Schattauer, Stuttgart, pp 145–156

Kendell RE (1986) The classification and phenomenology of schizophrenia. In: Kerr A, Snaith P (eds). Contemporary issues in schizophrenia. Geskell, London, pp 119–123

Kendell RE, Brockington IF, Leff JP (1979) Prognostic implications of six definitions of schizophrenia. Arch Gen Psychiatry 35:25–31

Kety SS (1980) The syndrome of schizophrenia: unresolved questions and opportunities for research. Br J Psychiatry 136:421–436

Kety SS (1985) Schizotypal personality disorder. An operational definitional of Bleuler's latent schizophrenia? Schizophr Bull 11(4):590–594

Kety SS, Rosenthal D, Wender PH, Schulsinger F (1968) The types and prevalence of mental illness in the biological and adoptive families of adopted schizophrenics. In: Rosenthal D, Kety SS (eds) The transmission of schizophrenia. Pergamon, Oxford, pp 345–362

Kirby GH (1913) The catatonic syndrome and its relation to manic depressive insanity. J Nerv Ment Dis 40:694–707

Koehler K (1979a) The diagnosis of schizophrenia, part I. Historical background of modern research criteria. Weekly Psychiatry Update Series 11(3):1–7

Koehler K (1979b) The diagnosis of schizophrenia, part II. Reliability and validity of modern research criteria. Weekly Psychiatry Update Series 12(3):1–7

Koehler K, Guth W, Grimm G (1977) First-rank symptoms of schizophrenia in Schneider-oriented German centers. Arch Gen Psychiatry 34:810–813

Kraepelin E (1899) Psychiatrie. Ein Lehrbuch für Studirende und Ärzte. Barth, Leipzig

Kraepelin E (1920) Die Erscheinungsformen des Irreseins. Z Gesamte Neurol Psychiatr 62:1–29

Laing RD (1965) The divided self. Penguin, London

Landmark I (1982) A manual for the assessment of schizophrenia. Acta Psychiatr Scand [Suppl 298] 65

Lange J (1922) Katatonische Erscheinungen im Rahmen manischer Erkrankungen. Springer, Berlin

Leonhard K (1972) Aufteilung der endogenen Psychosen in der Forschungsrichtung von Wernicke und Kleist. In: Kisker KP, Meyer JE, Müller M, Strömgren E (eds) Klinische Psychiatrie 1, 2nd edn. Springer, Berlin Heidelberg New York, pp 183–212 (Psychiatrie der Gegenwart vol I/1)

Mayer-Groß W (1932) IV. Die Klinik. V. Erkennung und Differentialdiagnose. In: Wilmanns K (ed) Die Schizophrenie. (Bumke Handbuch der Geisteskrankheiten, Band 9: Spez. Teil 5) Julius Springer Berlin, pp 293–594

McGuffin P, Farmer AE, Gottesman IJ, Murray AM, Revely AM (1984) Twin concordance for operationally defined schizophrenia: confirmation of familiality and heritability. Arch Gen Psychiatry 41:541–545

Mellor CS (1970) First-rank symptoms of schizophrenia. Br J Psychiatry 117:15–23

Mellor CS (1982) The present status of first-rank symptoms. Br J Psychiatry 140:423–424

Morel BA (1860) Traité des maladies mentales. Masson, Paris

Murray RM, Lewis SW, Revely AM (1985) Towards an aetiological classification of schizophrenia. Lancet 1:1023–1026

Pull CB, Pull MC, Pichot P (1981) Licet-S: Une liste intégrée de critères d'evaluation taxinomique pour les psychoses non-affectives. Psychiatr Biol Ther 1(1):33–37

Robins E, Guze SB (1970) Establishment of diagnostic validity in psychiatric illness: its application to schizophrenia: Am J Psychiatry 126:983–987

Rosenhan D (1973) On being sane in insane places. Science 179:250–258

Saß H (1981) Probleme der Katatonieforschung. Nervenarzt 52:373–382

Saß H, Koehler K (1983) Borderline-Syndrome: Grenzgebiet oder Niemandsland. Nervenarzt 54:221–230

Schneider C (1930) Die Psychologie der Schizophrenie. Thieme, Leipzig

Schneider C (1942) Die schizophrenen Symptomverbände. Springer, Berlin

Schneider K (1925) Wesen und Erfassung der Schizophrenien. Z Neurol 99:542–547

Schneider K (1959) Clinical psychopathology. Grune and Stratton, New York

Snell L (1865) Über Monomanie als primäre Form der Seelenstörung. Allg Z Psychiatr 22:368–381

Spitzer RL, Endicott J, Robins E (1975) Research diagnostic criteria for a selected group of functional psychoses, 2nd edn. Biometrics Research Division, New York

Stephens JH, Astrup C, Carpenter WT, Shaffer JW, Goldsberg J (1982) A comparison of nine systems to diagnose schizophrenia. Psychiatry Res 6:127–143

Strauss JS, Carpenter WT (1974) Characteristic symptoms and outcome in schizophrenia. Arch Gen Psychiatry 30:429–434

Strauss JS, Gift TE (1977) Choosing and approach for diagnosing schizophrenia. Arch Gen Psychiatry 34:1248–1253

Szasz TS (1962) The myth of mental illness. Secker & Warburg, London

Taylor MA (1972) Schneiderian first rank symptoms and clinical prognostic features in schizophrenia. Arch Gen Psychiatry 26:64–67

Wilmanns K (1907) Zur Differentialdiagnostik der „funktionellen" Psychosen. Zentralbl Nervenheilk 30:569–588

Wing JK, Birley JLT, Cooper JE, Graham P, Isaacs AD (1967) Rehability of a procedure for measuring and classifiying "present psychiatric state". Br J Psychiatry 113:499–515

Wing JK, Nixon J, von Cranach M, Strauss A (1977) Further developments of PSE and CATEGO system. Arch Psychiatr Nervenkr 224:151–160

World Health Organization (1973) Report of the International Pilot Study on Schizophrenia, vol 1. WHO, Geneva

Young MA, Tanner MA, Meltzer HY (1982) Operational definitions for schizophrenia. What do they identify? J Nerv Ment Dis 170:443–447

Formulation of New Research Strategies on Schizophrenia

M. Shepherd

I should begin by defining my terms of reference. When Professor Häfner first invited me to look into a crystal ball and formulate new research strategies in schizophrenia, I asked him whether my contribution was to be delivered in a session devoted to astrological psychiatry. He replied, with characteristic discretion, that he preferred to think in terms of astronomical psychiatry, exemplified by a star-studded symposium. Eventually, however, he returned to earth to explain that my contribution might serve to bridge the gap between the two general introductory reviews and the more specific papers to follow. A transitional paper of this type should allow for both a backward glance to where we have come from and an anticipation of where we are going without trespassing on the areas to be cultivated over the next 2 days. To try and achieve this objective I propose to subdivide my paper into three sections: definition, outcome and causation.

In presenting this conspectus, however, I am conscious of the fact that any visitor who speaks about schizophrenia in Germany, particularly in Heidelberg, must choose his words with care. In his *Die Pathologie und Therapie der psychischen Krankheiten* [8], the book that Ludwig Binswanger justly called the Magna Carta of psychiatry, Wilhelm Griesinger comments that "mental illness is only a symptom... our classification depends on the symptomatological method by which alone can any classification be effected". Some of the fruits of the symptomatological method in respect to the schizophrenias were demonstrated to me at an early stage of my career by the late Wilhelm Mayer-Groß, to whom I turned for guidance concerning information about the disorder. He advised me to read the ninth volume of Bumke's handbook and learn about what he called "Heidelberg schizophrenia". In this volume, I came to realise, resides the evidence of how much of the groundwork of our knowledge of the schizophrenic syndrome was laid in Heidelberg, associated with such names as Karl Jaspers, Hans Gruhle, Kurt Schneider and, of course, Emil Kraepelin.

Since the publication of that volume in 1932, however, the preoccupations of psychiatrists in Germany appear to have changed. Ten years ago Professor Janzarik's paper "The Crisis in Psychopathology" [10] mentioned the "disinterest and insecurity in tune with the spirit of modern times" and last year, in his retrospective survey of the past 40 years of German psychiatry [17], Professor J. E. Meyer identified seven themes as dominant during this period: (1) the era of "shock" treatment, (2) the introduction of psychotropic drugs, (3) *Daseinsanaly-*

The Bethlem Royal Hospital, Institute of Psychiatry, University of London, De Crespigny Park, London SE 5 8AF, United Kingdom

se, (4) the separation of psychiatry from neurology, (5) the Enquête Commission report, (6) psychiatry and psychotherapy and (7) psychiatry and National Socialism. It is noteworthy that several of these topics are primarily of German national interest and that Professor Meyer mentions schizophrenia only twice, once in relation to insulin coma therapy and once in relation to neuroleptic drugs. If this may be taken as an overview of the situation during a difficult period of destruction and reconstruction, the situation in other countries was very different, much of it being concerned with the first of my three categories, namely definition.

Definition

From the late 1930s the torch of the German tradition was carried elsewhere, and helped light the fires of investigation throughout Europe and North America. By the early 1950s Manfred Bleuler was able to publish a massive review article of some 1100 articles, most of them published in the UK, the USA, France or Italy, which he entitled "Research and Changes in the Study of Schizophrenia, 1941–1950" [5]. The great majority of these studies, however, paid little regard to the need for agreement on terminology, concepts or communication, and, significantly, the principal factor prompting Bleuler to undertake this daunting task was the First International Congress of Psychiatry held in Paris in 1950, when, as he pointed out, there emerged "the realisation of the dangerous fact that we can no longer understand one another".

The justice of this verdict was endorsed in 1957 at the Second International Congress, which was devoted entirely to schizophrenia. Some of you may recall that the foyer of the conference building was dominated by a large pyramid of books with one enormous volume entitled *Schizophrenia: New Knowledge* at the apex. Laying hands on it was no easy task, but one day I managed to ascend the biblio-mountain and bring the book down to ground level. It proved to be a pre-publication copy whose cover enclosed several hundred pages of blank paper! This mighty volume – impressive in appearance but empty of content – symbolized much of the meeting. A glance at the procedings shows why this was so, for many disputations among the eminent clinicians on the subject of diagnosis was conducted in a manner reminiscent more of a mediaeval school of theology than of a scientific meeting. Indeed, one of the symposia was devoted appropriately to the concepts of St. Thomas Aquinas and Aristotle. The divine rights of the *Ordinarius* were stoutly defended and an outspoken participant reflected the spirit of the occasion as follows: "You say this is a case of schizophrenia. Do you mean schizophrenia as Dr. X., my chief, uses it or are you referring to schizophrenia as construed by your chief, Dr. Y?" [23].

This state of affairs was evidently no longer good enough, even for Heidelberg schizophrenia. One year later, in 1958, the WHO invited Erwin Stengel to examine the Tower of Babel which housed the schemata of classification in use at the time. Looking to the future, Stengel pointed out that while a scientifically based nosology depends ultimately on causal knowledge, communication can be greatly improved by widespread use of operational concepts and definitions which, in turn, demand a common language and an acceptable nomenclature. With regard to the schizophrenias Stengel was explicit:

Schizophrenia, then, as an operational concept, would not be an illness, or a specific reaction type, but an argued operational definition for certain types of abnormal behaviour ... The question, therefore, which a person or group of persons trying to reach agreement on a national or international classification ought to answer is not what schizophrenia ... is, but what interpretation should be placed on these concepts for the purpose of communication [22].

If this seems a modest objective it does no more than echo Kraepelin's own retrospective assessment of his own system: "I should like to emphasise that some of the clinical pictures outlined are no more than attempts to present part of the material observed in a communicable form" [13].

It was against this background that in the early 1960s the WHO initiated a large-scale programme to standardise psychiatric diagnosis, classification and statistics, aiming to obtain international agreement on the use of one public system rather than on a multiplicity of private systems. This became known as Programme A, for which I must bear some responsibility as the organiser of the initial study on schizophrenia in 1965 which served as the prototype for the series. In the light of subsequent developments, incidentally, it is worth recalling that there were no American psychiatrists at that meeting, an invitation having failed to attract a single senior psychiatrist with sufficient interest in nosology to attend. It would have been difficult then to predict the appearance of DSM-III only 15 years later.

The original WHO study, based on video tapes and written case histories, was focused on observer variation in the assessment of schizophrenia [21]. The findings demonstrated that the factors leading to disagreement and difficulty in communication derive from three principal sources, namely (1) variations in clinical observation and perception, (2) variations in the inferences drawn from these data, and (3) variations in the individual classificatory schemata employed. By the same token, it became apparent that variation in the first two of these categories could be reduced substantially by the introduction of a multidimensional system of classification which was recommended for public statistical purposes so as to do justice to the multifactorial nature of the condition. These objectives became more urgent as a result of the surge of biological investigations that followed the introduction of psychotropic drugs. The report of a WHO Scientific Group on "Biological Research in Schizophrenia" at about the same time made the point explicitly:

If it is possible to obtain an accurate detailed description of the patient's behaviour and present state and of changes in these factors over a period of time, it would apear to be unnecessary to insist on obtaining rigid agreement among different investigators on a precise diagnostic classification. The main requirement is that collaborating investigators in different centres should establish empirically that, despite theoretical differences, they can use the same clinical measuring instruments and arrive at similar quantitative conclusions concerning aspects of a patient's present state ... Given a sufficient number of reliable indices of this kind, correlations can be sought between individual clinical symptoms and syndromes and biological data. Agreement on a system of clinical diagnosis can then become a goal rather than pre-condition for collaborative ... studies of schizophrenia [20].

The past 15 years have witnessed the flowering of this approach, resulting in a plethora of studies which make use of clinical data, computer-derived syndromes, numerical taxonomy and ingenious statistical analysis. No doubt this acknowledgement of the need for numeracy represents a form of progress; there are very few tables and figures in the 783 pages of the ninth volume of Bumke's handbook. Far more of this concern, however, has to do with *reliability*, i.e. the consistency with which a measure assesses a given trait, than with *validity*, i.e. the extent to which the measure actually measures the trait. Bartko and Carpenter identified the importance of this distinction 10 years ago:

Establishing validity of a concept such as schizophrenia might be achieved by finding that patients so diagnosed can be distinguished from other patient groups by certain genetic, biochemical, psychological, course or treatment variables. However, to the extent that schizophrenic patients cannot be reliably diagnosed, one cannot expect to find a consistent set of validating data. Hence, even if a concept is valid, reliability in its use is required to assure communicative value and to provide the foundation for scientific evaluation [3].

Underlying this approach, then, is the assumption that the schizophrenic syndrome can be defined provided that a satisfactory method of dealing with its phenomenological heterogeneity can be devised. Dr. Carpenter and his colleagues have neatly summed up the sources of the confusion in astronomical terms (though in a manner quite different from that of Professor Häfner) by identifying four categories [6]. First comes the antimatter approach, whereby heterogeneity is reduced through the annihilation of all cases failing to meet predetermined criteria. Secondly, the black hole approach, which consigns all annihilated cases to the black hole of affective illness. Thirdly, the satellite approach, assuming the existence of the two Kraepelinian planets and defining atypical disorders as satellites of uncertain provenance. Finally, the nova approach, assuming the possibility of more than two major stars and of heterogeneity as a mode of discovery in its own right.

A host of investigators are now employing their telescopes and space probes in the universe of phenomenology to try and decide between these alternatives, a choice which must influence research strategy. Relatively few of these workers, however, focus their attention on outcome, to which I now turn as my second category.

Outcome

The importance of outcome as the natural history of disease was emphasised by Griesinger as part of his argument against the notion of an ontological theory of illness. "The nature, the concept of disease", he worte, "emerges only from the entire history of the disease … i.e. the gradual progression of qualitative dysfunction… In this way a *natural history* of the process of a disease will be observed, but in an entirely different sense from that given by the natural history school" [9].

Not the least of the advantages attaching to this standpoint is that it lends itself to empirical clinical research. Richard Warner's interactionist model, adapted from that of Strauss and Carpenter, incorporates the prodromal phase of illness in its natural history [24] (Fig. 1).

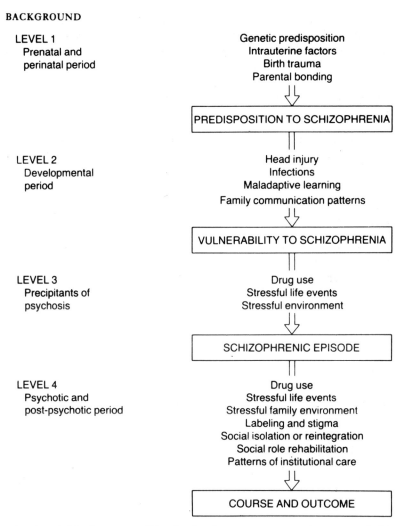

BACKGROUND

LEVEL 1
Prenatal and
perinatal period

Genetic predisposition
Intrauterine factors
Birth trauma
Parental bonding

PREDISPOSITION TO SCHIZOPHRENIA

LEVEL 2
Developmental
period

Head injury
Infections
Maladaptive learning
Family communication patterns

VULNERABILITY TO SCHIZOPHRENIA

LEVEL 3
Precipitants of
psychosis

Drug use
Stressful life events
Stressful environment

SCHIZOPHRENIC EPISODE

LEVEL 4
Psychotic and
post-psychotic period

Drug use
Stressful life events
Stressful family environment
Labeling and stigma
Social isolation or reintegration
Social role rehabilitation
Patterns of institutional care

COURSE AND OUTCOME

Fig. 1. Interactional model for factors possibly affecting the onset, course, and outcome of schizophrenia

Most of the individual items specified in this model are either clinical, psychological or social. As individual beads on an interactionist thread they are discussed in some detail at this symposium. Their potential significance has become more evident with the growing awareness that the diagnosis of schizophrenia is not synonymous with a poor prognosis. Eugen Bleuler wrote in 1908: "As yet I have never released a schizophrenic in whom I could detect signs of the disease; indeed, there are very few in whom one would have to search for such signs" [4]. Nonetheless, less than 30 years later Ødegaard pointed out that subsequent follow-up studies have indicated that the picture had changed [18]. To date, however, these studies have been bedevilled by defects which have rendered the findings ambiguous.

It is now clear that the design of a study aiming to elucidate the natural history of schizophrenia must take account of at least four factors: (1) the identification of all cases in a defined population during a fixed period of time; (2) the application of standardised diagnostic procedures with criteria of known reliability; (3) prospective follow-up procedures, preferably from the onset of first attachment for at least 5 years, with interim as well as end-point assessments and, preferably, uniform treatment regimes throughout the follow-up period; (4) standardised and independent clinical and social measures of outcome.

Of these criteria, the first remains the most difficult to satisfy. The identification of schizophrenia is traditionally made by hospital contact, on the assumption that in conditions of adequate medical care the patients suffering from the disorder will make contact with the mental health services. It may be recalled, however, that Kraepelin, in the fifth edition of his textbook, pointed out that there were probably many people who had suffered an attack of dementia praecox which had not been sufficiently severe to bring them to specialist attention [12]. In this context, particular interest attaches to Watts' virtually unique report on the long-term fate of a cohort of schizophrenics in his general practice population of 15 000 over the period 1946–1983 [26]. The diagnosis of all patients was confirmed by referral to a psychiatric institution, and there was a sharp fall in such referrals over the 5 years. Overall, furthermore, the outcome was much better than is generally assumed.

No hospital-based investigation has so far met all four specified criteria, but we have gone some way to doing so in a 5-year prospective clinical and social follow-up study carried out on a representative cohort of 121 patients living within a stable, delimited population of an English county. An outline of this study has already been published [25] and here I would make only a few points relevant to this symposium.

The first of these relates to clinical outcome, which, again, belies the uniformly gloomy prognosis recorded by the early workers (Fig. 2). So marked a variation between good and poor prognostic groups raises questions in its own right, and a multivariate analysis was carried out to try and account for the differences. In the event, most of the variance could not be satisfactorily explained in terms of the variables included. Here is clearly a challenging area for new research strategies, whether they be focused on more complex psychosocial factors like "expressed emotion" or biological factors like the immunoglobulin concentrations studied by Pulkinnen in relation to outcome [19].

Mention may also be made of two striking sex differences. The first of these was the more favourable outcome enjoyed by females, a finding which has been confirmed by several other workers [14]. Most obviously, twice as many women experienced complete 5-year remission, while more than twice as many men underwent a deteriorating course. Further, the average period of hospital care was 3 times longer among men than women over the quinquennium, though the same proportion of both sexes (35%) displayed a relapsing course. Social functioning was consistently better among women on all variables.

The other sex difference relates to the age of onset of schizophrenic symptoms. By the age of 30 approximately 70% of the men had exhibited clinical symptomatology, compared with only 42% of the women. The incidence rates are nonethe-

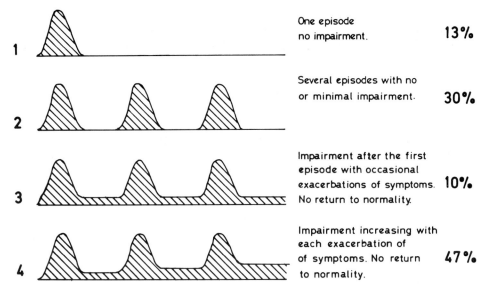

1   One episode no impairment.   **13%**

2   Several episodes with no or minimal impairment.   **30%**

3   Impairment after the first episode with occasional exacerbations of symptoms. No return to normality.   **10%**

4   Impairment increasing with each exacerbation of of symptoms. No return to normality.   **47%**

Fig. 2. Five-year follow-up of schizophrenics: course of illness. $n = 102$

less equal in the two sexes. There is, therefore, the unusual profile of a condition with an identical cumulative sex incidence and a similar symptom picture, but dissimilar age of onset and outcome. Among the tentative explanations which have been advanced to account for these sex differences are stress, drug compliance and the protective effects of natural oestrogens. None of these associations has been established, however, and all of them call for further investigation in the formulation of new research strategies.

Causation

Finally, a few words about causation. Here we can do worse than return once more to Griesinger, who recognised that the definition and classification of all mental illness must ultimately be based on causal factors but drew a fundamental distinction between aetiology and pathogeny. Of the former he wrote:

The conclusion, post hoc ergo propter hoc, depends ... on a simple empirical (statistical) knowledge of the fact that these particular circumstances (for example, hereditary disposition) very frequently coincide with, or precede, the commencement of the insanity ... the province of *aetiology* in the narrow sense is only to enumerate empirically the known circumstances of causation [8].

This is the province of what has been called clinical cartography or, more often, clinical epidemiology. By contrast, Griesinger states that it is the task of *pathogeny* to explain "the physiological connection between cause and effect, to show the particular mechanical act by means of which insanity is induced through a given circumstance...", a task towards which we have hitherto done little more

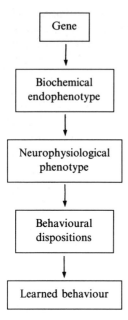

Fig. 3. Meehl's causal chain

than prepare the way". This is the province of biological science, and is conducted in or using the resources of the laboratory.

Traditionally, the quest for pathogenic causes has been in terms of a single, prepotent factor – a toxin, an infectious agent, a metabolic defect, a dietary deficiency. The evidence bearing on the genetic determinants of the schizophrenic syndrome, however, makes it necessary to consider a more complex multifactorial model, acknowledging that we may be confronted with either clinical diversity in genetic unity or genetic diversity in clinical unity. One of the most persuasive models of this type was advanced by Paul Meehl some years ago [16]. Meehl proposed what he termed a "causal chain from gene through biochemical endophenotype (e.g. synaptic slippage) to behavioural dispositions to the ultimate learned behaviour" (Fig. 3).

Central to this notion is the postulate that "clinical schizophrenia as such cannot be inherited because it has behavioural and phenomenal contents which are learned". What is inherited is what he calls "schizotaxia", a "subtle neurointegrative defect" associated with a "schizotypic" personality organisation. It is this schizotaxia, according to Meehl, which represents the endophenotype which will eventually be identified in biochemical and neurophysiological terms. If environmental and interpersonal factors are favourable and there are also robust personality traits, the individual remains a well-compensated schizotype with no evidence of mental disease but with faint signs of what Meehl calls "cognitive slippage and other minimal neurological aberrations". This theoretical model has since received some support from empirical findings, including those of Kety and his coworkers on the Danish twin-study data [11].

The causal chain is extended in Warner's model, to which I have already alluded [24]. Here "predisposition" and "vulnerability" make their appearance up to the outbreak of the schizophrenic episode and other factors bearing on outcome are identified. Much of the remainder of this symposium will be devoted to the pathogenic and the aetiological links in this long, sequential chain. Future research will, I suggest, be concerned with the interaction between pathogeny and aetiology and, doubtless, among them and other, as yet unidentified factors. Meanwhile, I would emphasise that in the absence of an established biological marker for the clinical investigator, the significance of all such factors – whether they be life events or viruses, family communication or season of birth – depends on the strength of an association and is therefore essentially epidemiological. Ideally, therefore, a representative population is needed within which it could be possible to study both these associations and the clinical features of the covert as well as the overt disorder.

In this task there is a key role for the clinican alongside the biological and epidemiological investigator, especially in the assessment of psychological dysfunction, still the elusive core of the schizophrenic syndrome. There, if anywhere, is where an operational definition of "thought disorder", Meehl's "cognitive slippage", has to be established. Psychological inquiry has already demonstrated that thought disorder is in part a form of perceptual aberration; that it is less specific than was formerly believed; that it is readily modifiable by operant techniques; and that most controlled experiments provide results that are unreliable and non-replicable. Recent work [15] suggests that neurological findings are less promising than studies of psychological constructs like the Thought Disorder Index [2] but it is, I think, instructive to learn from Allen's recent report that while both sophisticated clinical and experimental tests failed to discriminate between the speech of non-speech-disordered schizophrenics and the speech of normal subjects, an experienced clinician was able to do so without being able to identify the factors contributing to his own success [1]. This would seem to indicate a need to examine clinical acumen still more carefully, in the light of the newer neuropsychological techniques.

Finally, I would also mention another source of information for clinical inquiry, namely the patient, for whom the exclusion of the diagnosis of schizophrenia is as important as its confirmation. Let me conclude by citing a former patient of my own, one of the foremost living creative writers who was originally admitted to a psychiatric institution in her teens with a diagnosis of schizophrenia. There she remained for 3–4 years, was treated with 200 ECT's and narrowly escaped prefrontal leucotomy. By chance we were able to see her some years later and eliminate the diagnosis on clinical grounds. Since then she has remained well and in her recently published autobiography she describes the impact of the clinical verdict:

I myself had suddenly been stripped of a garment I had worn for 12 or 13 years – my schizophrenia ... I remembered how ... I had accepted it, how in the midst of the agony and terror of the acceptance I found the unexpected warmth, comfort, protection: how I had longed to be rid of the opinion but was unwilling to part with it, and even when I did not wear it openly, I always had it by for an emergency, to put on quickly, for shelter from the cruel world. And now it was gone ... banished officially by experts. I could never turn to it again for help [7].

Her comment has, I would maintain, some relevance to the definition, outcome and causation of schizophrenia and for any research strategy that may be adopted.

References

1. Allen HA (1985) Can all schizophrenic speech be discriminated from normal speech? Br J Clin Psychol 24:209–210
2. Arboleda C, Holzman PS (1986) Thought disorder in children at risk for psychosis. Arch Gen Psychiatry 42:1004–1012
3. Bartko JJ, Carpenter WT (1976) On the methods and theory of reliability. Nerv Ment Dis 163:307–317
4. Bleuler E (1908) Die Prognose der Dementia praecox – Schizophreniegruppe. Allg Z Psychiatr 65:436–464
5. Bleuler M (1955) Research and changes in concepts in the study of schizophrenia. Bull Isaac Ray Med Library 3 (1,2):1–132
6. Carpenter WT, Heinrichs DW, Wagman AMI (1985) On the heterogeneity of schizophrenia. In: Alpert M (ed) Controversies in schizophrenia. Guilford Press, New York, pp 25–37
7. Frame J (1985) The envoy from Mirror City. Women's Press
8. Griesinger W (1845) Die Pathologie und Therapie der psychischen Krankheiten. Krabbe, Stuttgart
9. Griesinger W (1872) Herr Ringseis und die naturhistorische Schule. Arch Physiol Heilk 1:43–66
10. Janzarik W (1976) The crisis in psychopathology. Nervenarzt 47:73–80
11. Kety SS (1972) Prospects for research in schizophrenia – an overview. Neurosci Res Prog Bull 10(4):456–467
12. Kraepelin E (1896) Psychiatrie, 5th edn. Barth, Leipzig
13. Kraepelin E (1920) Die Erscheinungsformen des Irreseins. Z Gesamte Neurol Psychiatr 62:1–29
14. Loranger AW (1984) Sex difference in age of onset of schizophrenia. Arch Gen Psychiatr 41:157–161
15. Marcus J, Hans SL, Mednick SA, Schulsinger F, Michelson F (1985) Neurological dysfunctioning in offspring of schizophrenics in Israel and Denmark. Arch Gen Psychiatr 42:753–761
16. Meehl PE (1962) Schizotaxia, schizotypy, schizophrenia. Am Psychol 17:827–838
17. Meyer JE (1985) Psychiatrie im XX. Jahrhundert: ein Rückblick. Gotze, Göttingen
18. Ødegaard Ø (1967) Changes in the prognosis of functional psychoses since the days of Kraepelin. Br J Psychiatry 113:813–822
19. Pulkinnen E (1977) Immunoglobins, psychopathology and prognosis in schizophrenia. Acta Psychiatr Scand 56:173–182
20. Report of a WHO Scientific Group (1980) Biological research in schizophrenia. WHO Tech Rep Ser 450
21. Shepherd M, Brooke EM, Cooper JE, Lin TY (1968) An experimental approach to psychiatric diagnosis. Acta Psychiatr Scand [Suppl 210]
22. Stengel E (1959) Classification of mental disorders. Bull WHO 21:601
23. Surya NC (1959) Some remarks concerning an anthology of psychiatric definitions. In: Second International Congress for Psychiatry, Congress Report IV. Orell Fussli, Zurich, pp 275–278
24. Warner R (1985) Recovery from schizophrenia. Routledge & Kegan Paul, London
25. Watt DC, Katz K, Shepherd M (1983) The natural history of schizophrenia: a 5-year prospective follow-up of a representative sample of schizophrenics by means of a standardised clinical and social assessment. Psychol Med 13:663–670
26. Watts CAH (1985) A long-term follow-up of schizophrenic patients: 1946–1983. J Clin Psychiatry 46(6):210–216

History, Classification, and Research Strategies: Discussion

J. K. WING

Both Professor Janzarik and Professor Saß have referred to the fact that the phenomenological concepts that most psychiatrists use when they consider the differential diagnosis of schizophrenia are German in origin. Both feel that the early history of the development of these concepts is highly relevant to current controversies. They are right on both counts. Their papers are welcome as a contribution to a literature with which many psychiatrists worldwide are unfamiliar.

My comments are concerned with the phenomena – the symptoms and signs – of psychiatric disorder, not simply with the rules for making a diagnosis. There is a tremendous preoccupation with such rules at the moment, and, as Robert Kendell (1985) has pointed out, there is an uncomfortably wide variety of sets of operational criteria to choose from. Professor Shepherd quoted Manfred Bleuler's comment on the International Congress of Psychiatry in 1950, at which he realised "that we can no longer understand each other". I am by no means certain that there was less confusion before the war or that there is more now. Sir Aubrey Lewis, in his foreword to the glossary and guide to classification of mental disorders in the International Classification of Diseases (1978) pointed out that "accurate observation is still the gate that needs the closest guard ... Since the disorders listed in this glossary are identified by criteria that are predominantly descriptive, its use should encourage an emphasis on careful observation". Michael Shepherd reminded us of WHO's Programme A. That study showed, and the US-UK Diagnostic Project (1972) later confirmed, that getting agreement on the phenomena reduced diagnostic disagreement, even without the application of operational rules.

In my view, the great achievement of "Heidelberg psychiatry" was the limpid exposition of phenomenology by Karl Jaspers and Kurt Schneider. Professor Janzarik (1984) has described the regular exchange of letters between them during the years 1921–1955, as their concepts of clinical psychopathology developed. His account of this relationship is particularly important in view of the fact that Kurt Schneider's name is rarely mentioned nowadays, except to belittle, often on the basis of rather uncertain understanding, one of his many important concepts – that of first-rank symptoms.

The differential definitions of symptoms in the glossary of the Present State Examination (PSE), which forms the basis and origin for the whole system, owe

Institute of Psychiatry and London School of Hygiene, MRC Social Psychiatry Unit, London SE5 8AF, United Kingdom

a great deal (particularly in the case of the psychotic symptoms) to the Heidelberg school. Those who use the system seem often to be interested only in the very final stage of the CATEGO classification and to want to use this as though it were a prescriptive diagnosis. I have never seen it like that (Wing 1983). The reliable description of phenomena is the central issue. In the successor system (known as SCAN) that we are now developing, the simulated "diagnoses" (ICD10 and DSMIIIR) will be labelled as such, with appropriate warnings as to their limitations and advantages, while the reference or research classification will be seen for what it is.

One reason for giving priority to the phenomena is that thereby we are doing justice to what patients and their relatives are most concerned about. This is immensely important. One of the nicest things said to me about the PSE, by a psychiatrist who was using it in a different language and a different culture, was that patients had the feeling that their problems were being taken seriously, that many of the questions suggested in the PSE schedule were worded just as patients themselves described them. But an equally central reason for being interested in the phenomena is that by understanding how patients experience them, we may be able to help them live with their symptoms and impairments when we are unable to prevent them occurring.

Thus far, then, I am in full agreement with Professors Janzarik and Sass. The phenomena of mental disorders should be our starting point, and also the material to which we return when our efforts to classify them, to find causes, pathology and effective methods of treatment and prevention seem to be getting nowhere. But both lecturers are less enthusiastic when they turn their attention to methods of empirical investigation that have been developed in other parts of the world. Perhaps the problem is that they are still thinking in terms of disease entities – a diagnosis of schizophrenia has to be ruled out, for example, if there is coexisting temporal lobe epilepsy.

But this search for a kind of inviolable Platonic entity is most unlikely to succeed. It rarely has in medicine. Disease theories should be put forward only to be tested, to be made to compete against each other and, very often, to be discarded (Wing 1978). This is the discipline of science. In order to test theories, the hypotheses must be formulated with precision. If they are untestable, it does not necessarily mean that they are false, but they cannot claim to have passed a rigorous test and must wait their turn.

I have already indirectly addressed the problem of reliability vs validity, raised by all three lecturers. Improving the reliability of rating symptoms may well be more likely to improve the validity of classification than laying down operational rules. In the International Pilot Study of Schizophrenia (IPSS), many of the examples of first-rank symptoms rated in patients with clear-cut mania were actually examples of incorrect rating. For example, an elated patient said that his thoughts were so powerful they must be God's thoughts. This "as if" phenomenon is not uncommon in affective psychoses. The same sort of problem is raised by the negative impairments. However various combinations of symptoms and signs are classified, if the underlying phenomena can be trusted their profiles will indicate whether and to what extent the classifying rules differ. Validity is, of course, a matter of testing hypotheses.

Edward Hare (1982), in a thoughtful discussion of the epidemiology of schizophrenia, suggested that diagnostic precision was not essential to the discovery of causes. He gave the examples of dementia paralytica and pellagra. Professor Janzarik mentions Huntington's chorea in a similar context. But much depends on accidents of history such as whether the appropriate investigative techniques are available, in which case a blunderbuss approach, or even one based on a completely false theory, might well prove successful if there is a single substantial cause. But the argument has less force if there are multiple causes, as in hypertension or coronary heart disease, or if the supposed disease "entity" turns out to be composed of several conditions with some manifestations in common. Either or both of these possibilities may apply in schizophrenia. Certainly no single causative factor has emerged, and the differences between diagnostic schools demonstrated by the US-UK studies and the IPSS were such as to render incomparable most research based on the varied criteria used. Fortunately, both studies showed that by using a standardised assessment of the clinical phenomena leading to a reference classification, in addition to psychiatric diagnosis, substantial clarification could be achieved (Wing et al. 1974).

Edward Hare's gleanings from the literature on the epidemiology of schizophrenia hardly constitute a harvest. There is a small but definite genetic predisposition (or perhaps the word should be "predisposition"). The age and sex distribution is unlike that of any other major psychiatric disorder. Schizophrenia begins earlier and runs a more sinister course in men than in women. (The study by David Watt and colleagues mentioned by Michael Shepherd is the latest in a long line of investigations to demonstrate this.) People who later become schizophrenic tend to be born during the winter months. These are three "small nuggets of knowledge dredged from a sea of ignorance" as Manfred Bleuler once observed of the literature on primary prevention.

One encouraging suggestion made by Michael Shepherd is that the course of "schizophrenia" is less severe than once was thought. Kraepelin's data suggested to him that only about 17% of inpatients treated at the Heidelberg Clinic were reasonably well socially adjusted many years later. Mayer-Groß, following up, in 1926, patients admitted to the same clinic in 1912 and 1913, found that some 35% had made social recoveries, while 5% were socially disabled but out of hospital. There was, however, a high death rate of 43% (Mayer-Groß 1932). Another study in which Michael Shepherd was involved (Harris et al. 1956) showed that 45% of patients admitted for deep insulin treatment between 1945 and 1950 were living independently, another 12% were dependent and 9% were severely affected but outside hospital. Our own 5-year follow-up of patients first admitted from three catchment areas in 1956 found 56% independent, with no or only moderately severe symptoms (Brown et al. 1966).

As Shepherd says, it is very difficult to compare the results of follow-up studies because of the lack of comparability of diagnostic criteria or methods of assessing course and outcome. But one thing is clear – the course is not one of inevitable deterioration and it does seem to have improved somewhat during the century. Manfred Bleuler's summary of his own personal series, which is not dissimilar to the results of Huber and of Ciompi, is that about 25% of all patients recover completely, with no need of further phenothiazine treatment. There is an intermediate group of at least 50% whose symptoms continue to fluctuate over decades. Of the remaining 25%, only 10% suffer irremediable lifelong invalidism. Bleuler suggests that the proportions with the best and the worst prognoses have not much changed during his long professional career.

If the prognosis has improved somewhat, I am inclined to agree with Manfred Bleuler that this is due primarily to the better social conditions in which schizophrenic patients live. This improvement began long before the introduction of the phenothiazines, and affected chiefly the level of negative impairment. The phenothiazines suppress symptoms sufficiently to allow most patients to live outside hospital, but this involves a risk of repeated breakdown. In other words, there is an interaction between the social environment and whatever disorder of cerebral structure and function underlies "schizophrenia". This interaction involves both the positive symptoms and the negative impairment.

It is interesting that Professor Janzarik and Professor Saß consider only biological theories in their lectures. The new non-invasive techniques of brain imaging will certainly be powerful tools for theory testing and theory construction, but the relationship between the positive and negative aspects of schizophrenia demands other types of theory as well. My own guess has long been that cognitive disorder could be the link (Wing and Brown 1970). Part, at least, of the negative impairment is due to the patient's reaction to his or her own difficulties in communication. Socially understimulating conditions provide a tempting means of reducing this distress and the process can easily go too far. On the other hand, an intrusive social environment can force someone with schizophrenia into public exposure of the underlying thought disorder. Patients have themselves spoken of their strategies for coping with these problems and we can learn from them (Wing 1975).

I do not, however, think that negative impairments can be entirely explained in this way, nor that positive symptoms are entirely reactive. There is a basic level of each type of manifestation that is impervious to environmental conditions and that can fluctuate "spontaneously". These are the two principal groups of manifestation of schizophrenia described by Emil Kraepelin and Eugen Bleuler. Each group has been described as "primary", although the grounds for making a decision either way have always been complex and contradictory. There have been many attempts to dismember the concept. Seymour Kety, as Professor Saß reminds us, argued that the first-rank syndrome described by Kurt Schneider "is not schizophrenia". On the other hand, Dr. Zubin considers that the negative syndrome, thought by Eugen Bleuler to be basic, is "in large part an artifact" (1986).

This brings me to Professor Janzarik's final statement that "there is no conclusively defined disease known as 'schizophrenia'". I think he means that schizophrenia as a disease entity is dead and gone. If so, it began in Heidelberg and it has ended here. We need not mourn. However, I give "schizophrenia", as the starting point for a long series of disease theories (most of which will be wrong, as nearly all have been up to now), a good prognosis. The rewards of discovering that there are, indeed, a few interlinked pathologies underlying the phenomena described as schizophrenic by Emil Kraepelin, Eugen Bleuler, Karl Jaspers, and Kurt Schneider, would be so great that I cannot see the concept being abandoned for a long time to come.

In their different ways, all three lecturers and their discussant are providing evidence for the robust nature of the concept. This conference will no doubt follow our lead. This may be an unsatisfactory measure of validity, but, for the moment, it is not entirely negligible.

References

Brown, GW, Bone M, Dalison B, Wing JK (1966) Schizophrenia and social care. London, Oxford University Press

Hare EH (1982) Epidemiology of schizophrenia. In: Wing JK, Wing L (eds) Psychoses of uncertain aetiology, Chap 8. Cambridge: The University Press, pp 42–48

Harris A, Norris V, Linker I, Shepherd M (1956) Schizophrenia: a prognostic and social study. Br J Prev Soc Med 10:107

Janzarik W (1984) Jaspers, Kurt Schneider und die Heidelberger Psychopathologie. Nervenarzt 55:18–24

Kendell RE (1985) Which schizophrenia? In: Huber G (Hrsg) Basisstadien endogener Psychosen und das Borderline-Problem. Schattauer, Stuttgart

Lewis AJ (1978) Foreword in: Mental disorders: glossary and guide to their classification in accordance with the ninth revision of the ICD. WHO, Geneva

Mayer-Groß W (1932) Die Schizophrenie. In: Bumke O (Hrsg) Handbuch der Geisteskrankheiten, Bd IX. Springer, Berlin

Wing JK (1975) Schizophrenia from within. National Schizophrenia Fellowship, 78/79, Surrey, Surbiton, Victoria Road

Wing JK (1977) The management of schizophrenia in the community. In Usdin G (ed) Psychiatric medicine, Chap 10. Brunner/Mazel, New York

Wing JK (1978) Reasoning about madness. Oxford University Press, London

Wing JK (1983) Use and misuse of the PSE. Br J Psychiatry 143:111–117

Wing JK, Brown GW (1970) Institutionalism and schizophrenia. University Press, Cambridge

Wing JK, Cooper JE, Sartorius N (1974) The measurement and classification of psychiatric symptoms. University Press, Cambridge

Zubin J (1986) Mögliche Implikationen der Vulnerabilitätshypothese für das psychosoziale Management der Schizophrenie. In: Böker W, Brenner HD (Hrsg) Bewältigung der Psychiatrie. Verlag Hans Huber, Bern, S 29–41

Part II
Epidemiology and Course of Schizophrenia

Epidemiology of Schizophrenia

H. HÄFNER

The hope of finding some indication of causal relations by investigating the distribution of cases over populations and time has brought forth an almost indeterminable number of epidemiological studies of schizophrenia. Their modest results were reported in several reviews (Mishler and Scotch 1963; Dunham 1965; Sanua 1970; Cooper 1978; Torrey 1980; Eaton 1985). I shall confine myself here to some findings which may point to or speak against causal models.

Distribution of Morbidity in Populations over Time and Space

Prevalence

Prevalence rates are relevant for estimating needs of care. Besides the risks of onset and relapse, several other components – such as life expectancy after onset – contribute to the value of "prevalence". This is why in general prevalence rates are not suited for testing aetiological hypotheses. For the same reason, the uneven distribution of prevalence rates over countries (Table 1) does not permit the deduction that the risk of onset varies correspondingly in these populations. If one compares these figures with those reported in methodologically sound studies that were conducted before 1960 (Yolles and Kramer 1969), the ranges of the rates do not show much variation.

Table 1. Range of results from prevalence studies of schizophrenia (rate per 1000 population). Data taken from Eaton (1985)

	Maximum	Minimum
Point prevalence	8.3 (Ireland)	0.6 (Ghana)
Period prevalence (1 year)	7.0 (Baltimore)	1.7 (Czechoslovakia)
Lifetime prevalence	3.7 (India)	0.9 (Taiwan)

Central Institute of Mental Health, J5, 6800 Mannheim 1, Federal Republic of Germany

Incidence

Do incidence rates as an indicator of the morbid risk vary, or are they stable over countries and cultures? It is difficult to estimate incidence figures of schizophrenia by population studies. In the Lundby field study, Hagnell (1966) found five onsets of schizophrenia in a total of 24 400 man-years, yielding an incidence rate around 0.2 per 1000 people per year. Accordingly, one would have to examine 100 000 people in order to find about 20 cases. For this reason one has to use date from first contact with psychatric facilities exclusively serving a defined population – in spite of some sources of error implied in such a proceeding – in particular if trends over time are investigated.

Table 2 presents crude incidence rates from 19 studies. With few exceptions the data are taken from case registers. At a minimum of 0.08 per 1000 people in South Verona, Italy, and a maximum of 0.69 per 1000 in Rochester, United States of America, the annual incidence rates show a marked tendency to form two clusters: in the Scandinavian countries, United Kingdom, Italy and Australia they cluster around 0.1–0.2; in United States of America, Federal Republic of Germany and Ireland, around 0.5–0.7.

Table 2. Incidence studies of schizophrenia

Place	Reference	Year	Rate per 1000 people
Norway	Astrup (1982)	1926–1930	0.23[a]
Norway	Astrup (1982)	1977/1978	0.24[a]
Iceland	Helgason (1977)	1966/1967	0.27
Aberdeen, UK	Robertson (personal communication)	1980	0.19
Camberwell, UK	Wing and Fryers (1976)	1969–1973	0.13
Salford, UK	Wing and Fryers (1976)	1969–1973	0.13
Southampton, UK	Gibbons et al. (1983)	1980	0.25
Denmark	Munk-Jørgensen (1987)	1972	0.12
Victoria, Australia	Krupinski (personal communication)	1978	0.16
Netherlands	Giel et al. (1980)	1978/1979	0.11[b]
South Verona, Italy	Tansella et al. (1985)	1983	0.08[c,d]
Detroit, USA	Dunham (1965)	1958	0.52[g,h]
Maryland, USA	Warthen et al. (1967)	1963	0.50
New Haven, USA	Hollingshead and Redlich (1958)	1950	0.30[g,h]
Texas, USA	Jaco (1960)	1950	0.35[g,h]
Rochester, USA	Babigian (1975)	1975	0.69
Mannheim, FRG	Häfner and Reimann (1970)	1965[e]	0.54
Mannheim, FRG	Häfner (own data)	1974–1980[f]	0.59
Oberbayern, FRG	Dilling et al. (1975)	1974/1975[e]	0.48

Sources: Häfner and an der Heiden (1986); Eaton (1985); Munk-Jørgensen (1987)
[a] "Lifetime expectancy rate", hospitalised cases only, schizophrenia and "reactive psychoses"
[b] Including ICD 297, 0–297.9; 298.3–298.9
[c] Rate for first-ever contacts
[d] Rate for schizophrenia and other functional psychoses
[e] Survey based on comparable sources of data collection
[f] Data from the cumulative psychiatric case register of the Central Institute of Mental Health, Mannheim, Federal Republic of Germany
[g] Rate calculated with population over 15 years of age as denominator
[h] Incomplete collection of outpatient data

Is the true incidence of schizophrenia in one group really three or four times higher than in the other, or does it reflect some kind of multinational alliances of diagnosing? We may summarise the result of all incidence studies of schizophrenia by quoting Sartorius et al. (1986):

In spite of nearly a century of research ... the question about the rates of occurrence of schizophrenic disorders in geographically and culturally different age groups and the two sexes within such populations, has not been answered satisfactorily.

In order to obtain satisfying answers some prerequisites must be fulfilled:

1. In sufficiently large, stable and demographically well-prepared populations, cases of first onset should be collected as completely as possible over a defined period of time (case finding)

2. Diagnoses should be assessed by using transculturally standardised instruments (case identification)

3. In addition to the age at first contact, the age at first onset of the psychosis should be ascertained

4. The rates should be calculated, standardising for age, per age group, and additionally, methods for estimating the lifetime risk should be applied, such as Strömgren's (1935) or survival methods, and be based on life tables of the most recent date (Thompson and Weissman 1981)

The first study in which these requirements were met successfully was the "WHO Collaborative Study on Determinants of Outcome of Severe Mental Disorders" (Sartorius et al. 1986). Its findings represent the most essential progress

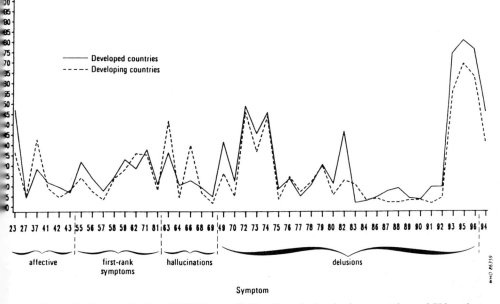

Fig. 1. Profiles on 44 selected PSE items of 586 patients in developing countries and 783 patients in developed countries, all meeting "broad" diagnostic criteria for schizophrenia and related disorders (Sartorius et al. 1986)

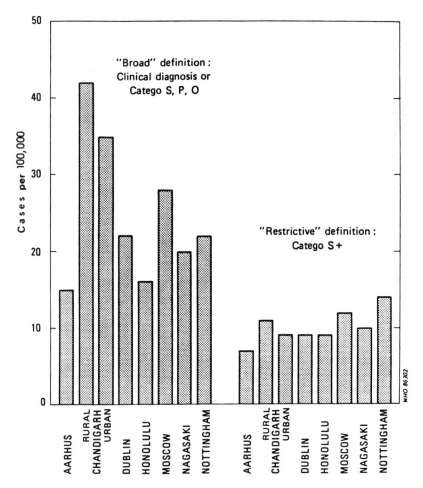

Fig. 2. Incidence rates per 100000 population aged 15–54 (both sexes), for the "broad" and for the "restrictive" definition of schizophrenia (Sartorius et al. 1986)

that has been made in the epidemiology of schizophrenia during the past 50 years.

In 12 research centres situated in ten countries (Aarhus/Denmark, Agra and Chandigarh/India, Cali/Columbia, Dublin/Ireland, Honolulu and Rochester/ United States of America, Ibadan/Nigeria, Moscow/USSR, Nagasaki/Japan, Nottingham/United Kingdom, Prague/Czechoslovakia; coordination: WHO Headquarters, Geneva), a total of 1379 persons aged 15–54 years who had been given the clinical diagnosis of schizophrenia (ICD 9 no. 295, 297, 298.3, 298.4, 298.8 or 298.9) were examined (for design and results of the study see also Sartorius et al., this volume). Patients at first onset meeting the ICD and CATEGO criteria for schizophrenia had remarkably similar symptom profiles in both developed and developing countries (Fig. 1).

Up to the present, the incidence rates have been calculated on the basis of data from eight centres in seven countries. For the clinical diagnosis of schizophrenia and for the CATEGO criteria S, P and O, i.e. a "broad" diagnostic definition, the crude annual incidence rates per 1000 population (aged 15–54 years) range from about 0.15 in Aarhus to about 0.42 in the rural area of Chandigarh (Fig. 2).

The number of CATEGO S$^+$ cases in a population with schizophrenic nuclear syndrome, which is generally defined by productive symptoms of first rank (Schneider 1950), naturally do not include all cases of schizophrenia occurring in this population. In the "WHO Collaborative Study on Determinants of Outcome of Severe Mental Disorders" this restrictive definition is applied to approximately half the cases given the clinical diagnosis of schizophrenia. However, we can begin with the fact that this restrictive definition, independent of whether it includes only the characteristic or the severest cases, is a reliable indicator of the disease frequency. The broader the definition of the diagnosis, the higher will be the proportion of uncertain cases among the incidence figures. Under this cover, the number of phenocopies, i.e. similar syndromes of different cause, will be unquantifiably large. Thus we can extrapolate from geographically stable rates of CATEGO S$^+$ syndromes to geographically stable rates of schizophrenia, whatever that might be.

Changes in the Morbid Risk over Longer Periods

Nine studies dealt with changes in the morbid risk of schizophrenia over periods longer than 30 years (Goldhamer and Marshall 1949; Astrup 1956, 1982; Kramer et al. 1967; Ødegard 1971; Dunham 1976; Eaton 1980; Torrey 1980; Krupinsky and Alexander 1983). The interpretation of the data, which range over periods between 38 (Kramer et al. 1967) and 130 years (Krupinski and Alexander 1983), is not consistent: six of the nine studies mentioned came to the conclusion that there has been a stable trend in the rates of schizophrenia (Goldhamer and Marshall 1949; Dunham 1976; Kramer et al. 1967; Ødegard 1971; Astrup 1982; Krupinsky and Alexander 1983), while three stated a slight rise (Astrup 1956; Torrey 1980; Eaton 1980). One of the authors, Astrup (1982), corrected the interpretation of his own data in a later study by taking the age variable precisely into account.

Six of the studies referrred to show considerable shortcomings. Only three of them sufficiently meet methodological requirements for their results to be considered valid: Ødegard (1971); Astrup (1982); Krupinsky and Alexander (1983).

By means of the National Norwegian Case Register Ødegard investigated all first admissions for schizophrenia over a period of 40 years. Later Astrup extended this period to 63 years, 1916–1978. Diagnoses were based on the Kraepelinean definition of dementia praecox, before ICD 6 was introduced. The rates were calculated in consecutive 5-year birth cohorts in relation to the same five birth years of the Norwegian population and thus were controlled for age and cohort effects. Over a period of 63 years, the rates varied a little, ranging between an initial value of about 0.18–0.19 and a final value of about 0.20–0.25 per 1000 for males and females; from 1946 on these included the so-called reactive psychoses also.

Krupinsky and Alexander used data on all admissions for schizophrenia to the psychiatric hospitals of the State of Victoria, Australia, over 130 years, 1848–1978. They controlled the factor of "definition of diagnosis" by applying DSM III criteria for retrospective diagnosing of samples, each consisting of 100 admissions in successive periods of time. They, too, found a fairly stable trend of age-corrected admission rates for schizophrenia.

Ødegard (1971) summarised the results of long-term trend studies of the morbid risk of schizophrenia by saying:

> The astonishing stability of first admission rates over half a century indicates that in the countries investigated the true incidence of schizophrenia remained essentially unchanged.

Although these results were obtained by investigating only two populations so far (Norway and Victoria), it has significance because it was supported even by less reliable data and has never been falsified by reliable data.

Discussion

The small variability of the clearly defined morbid risk of schizophrenia over decades, countries and cultures reduces the hope of transcultural psychiatry for contributing to our knowledge of its aetiology. Also, the plausibility of other aetiological hypotheses is affected: it is rather unlikely that sociocultural factors and stressfull environmental events – should they be of a specific nature and should they influence the morbid risk to a relevant extent – are evenly distributed over countries, cultures and relatively long periods of time. The present state of epidemiological knowledge does not support sociocultural models of aetiology. However, they are still of great heuristic value for explaining the variability of the course of the disease – and thereby for explaining the prevalence rates – which obviously depends on environmental factors much more than the risk of falling ill with schizophrenia. It is also difficult to interpret these findings as supporting the assumption of a uniform infectious aetiology (Murray and Reveley 1983; Crow 1983, 1984). If one compares the distribution of schizophrenia with that of bacterial or viral infections like cholera or poliomyelitis (Fig. 3), there are clear differences. Infectious diseases are unevenly distributed over time and space, revealing paths of spread and waves of frequency, partially due to the immunisation of the population during every outbreak.

Processes of spreading, which lead to a geographically uneven distribution and to changes over time, are not only found in rapidly communicable diseases, but also in deseases with an extremely slow course and spread. Even multiple sclerosis, a disease of as yet unknown aetiology, which – similar to schizophrenia – develops in episodes with intervals of improvement or takes a chronic course, displays a characteristic pattern of distribution (Fig. 4).

It mainly occurs in regions with a dense population and a moderate climate (McAlpine et al. 1972). Its pattern of distribution makes the assumption of a viral

cases per 100,000

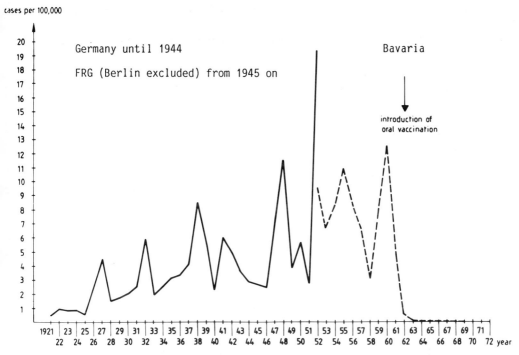

Fig. 3. Wavelike course of poliomyelitis from 1919 until the introduction of oral vaccination

aetiology more plausible than the even distribution of the morbid risk of schizophrenia.

As Jablensky recently pointed out, there is one rather uniform syndrome with a heterogeneous aetiology: severe and moderately severe mental retardation (IQ $\leq$ 60). Its pattern of distribution over geographical areas and time is almost analogous to that of schizophrenia (Table 3). How can we explain the even distribution of the morbid risk when the restrictive definition of CATEGO S$^+$ is applied for "caseness"? If we start from Kraepelin's concept, which distinguishes schizophrenia clearly from other comparable diseases not only by characteristic syndromes and types of course but also by a supposedly homogeneous aetiology, the arrangement of first onsets of schizophrenic syndromes would be a sufficiently reliable indicator of an almost evenly distributed disease of "schizophrenia". This first assumption is, however, improbable for two reasons. (1) The precise distinction between S$^+$ schizophrenia and similar syndromes is probably not natural but a reasonable artefact resulting from precisely basing the definition mainly on dichotomous symptoms (e.g. first rank symptoms) and a stable algorithm of diagnostic attribution. (2) The even distribution of a monocausal morbid risk is somewhat contradictory to experience.

If, however, we apply a broader definition of the schizophrenic syndrome such as the clinical diagnosis of "schizophrenic syndrome" including brain dysfunctions or the unprecise category of "schizophrenia spectrum disorder", then the distinction between these and the neighbouring mental disorders becomes in-

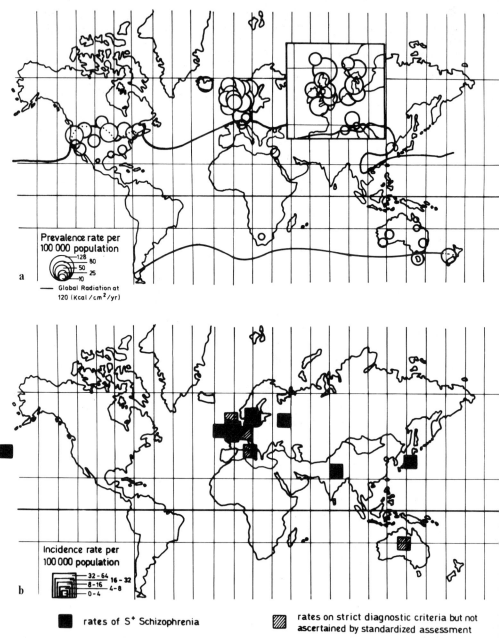

Fig. 4. a World distribution of multiple sclerosis (prevalence). The *size* of the circles is proportional to the prevalence, with the *largest circles* representing 128 cases/100 000 population. The *wavy line* divides the world by levels of solar irradiation as well as a mean temperature of 15.6 °C (60 °F). Adapted from McAlpine et al. (1972). **b** World distribution of schizophrenia (annual incidence rates)

Table 3. Prevalence rates of mental retardation (severe and moderately severe grades combined) among children and young persons in urban and rural areas (rates per 1000 population). (Based on Dupont 1981 and additional material)

Reference	Country	Age range 10–14 years
Lewis (1929)	England	0.37[d]
Lemkau et al. (1942)	USA	0.33[d]
Goodman et al. (1956)	USA	0.36[d]
Kushlick (1961)	England	0.27[d]
Goodman and Tizard (1962)	England	0.36[d]
Scally and McKay (1964)	N. Ireland	0.36
Imre (1967)	USA	0.47
Innes et al. (1968)	Scotland	0.23
Birch et al. (1970)	Scotland	0.37[a,d]
Flynn (1970)	Ireland	0.49
Wing (1971)	England	0.37[d]
Brask (1972)	Denmark	0.37[d]
Sorel (1974)	Netherlands	0.73[b,d]
Bernsen (1976)	Denmark	0.45
Martindale (1977)	England	0.4[d]
Thomas (1978)	England	0.41[d]
Liepmann (1979)	FRG	0.42[c,d]
Cooper and Lackus (1984)	FRG	0.37[c,d]

The author is grateful to Professor Brian Cooper for making this table available
[a] Age group   8–10 years
[b] Age group 10 years
[c] Age group   7–16 years
[d] Urban

creasingly vague. This supports a second, namely a dimensional model with different threshold values, similar to the model on which the defintion of severe or moderately severe mental retardation as low marginal values of the total distribution of the intelligence quotient (IQ) is based (Fig. 5 a). If an indicator like IQ is normally and rather evenly distributed in various populations and over long periods of time, the conventional way of determining a threshold value leads to case rates that show a stable distribution over time and space.

If we assume that the distribution of a positive trait in the population (as IQ measures) is – in direct analogy – applicable to a schizothymia or schizophrenia dimension, we would have to construct something like "mental stability". At the extreme end of the distribution we would then have thresholds for different definitions of schizophrenia – analogous to the thresholds of mental retardation on the IQ curve. this assumption, which is similar to Antonovsky's speculative construct of a "mental ease/mental disease dimension" (Antonovsky 1979), has not yet been sufficiently supported by empirical findings.

The assumption of a negative dimension seems more plausible: a liability to or vulnerability for schizophrenia that is normally distributed over the population. The morbid risk of schizophrenia would then be high where it attains high

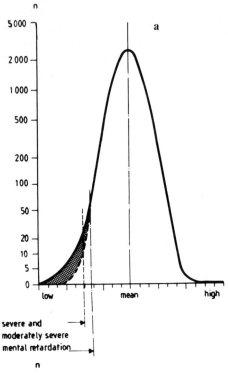

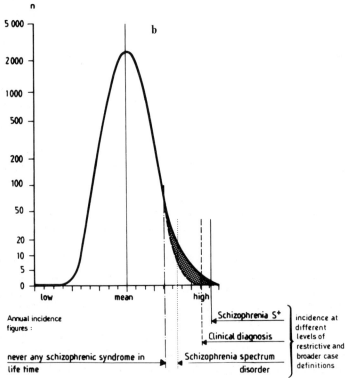

Fig. 5. a Distribution of IQ with threshold values for mental retardation. **b** Speculative model: distribution of vulnerability for schizophrenia with threshold values for different definitions of schizophrenia

values and be accordingly low where it tends towards zero. If this assumption were true, one would have to ask first, what kind of characteristics should be distributed this way? Should it be manifest behaviour dimensions, the extremes of which would be a psychosis or should it be latent liabilities like the vulnerability for schizophrenia? It could also be possible that a transphenomenal liability is associated with manifest personality traits or psychophysical characteristics either in a direct, linear way or by way of threshold values.

If we first inquire into manifest behaviour dimensions or into traits that are characteristic of the schizophrenic syndrome and might be found in the population in an intensity which decreases when their frequency increases, we are confronted with a lack of knowledge. However, we cannot rule out that – formulated at different levels of case definition – characteristics including fear of social proximity, lack of social competence, insufficient information processing, loss of customary hierarchies and delayed modality shift or autonomous hyperarousal on adverse stimuli may be distributed in the population either as a single phenomenon or as a multiple dimension which attains maximum values in schizophrenics or individuals liable to schizophrenia. The personality dimension of "psychoticism" (Eysenck), which is characterised by aggressiveness, egocentricity, coldness, tough-mindedness and empathy, has failed to be a valid construct of a dimensionally distributed schizophrenia factor, as had Ernst Kretschmer's schizothymia dimension before.

In fact, schizophrenia or high vulnerability values seem to be associated with specific and stable personality traits. Contrary to mental retardation, however, the schizophrenic psychosis takes an episodic course. Owing to this, the analogy of the distribution of manifest symptoms of a schizophrenic psychosis to the distribution of IQ deficits remains unsatisfactory. For this reason, the second assumption mentioned – the distribution of a liability to or vulnerability for schizophrenia with or without direct relation to manifest traits – seems more plausible than the first assumption. Under this second assumption the extent of the vulnerability dimension or the level of the vulnerability threshold must be distributed normally and presumably evenly over populations.

Some of the manifest traits mentioned before, like the autonomous hyperarousal upon adverse stimuli or the delayed modality shift, might be indicators of a vulnerability dimension. Since at present the morbid risk is our only external measure of vulnerability for proving this hypothesis, direct testing of these assumptions has to cope with enormous difficulties. An indirect way of examining the hypothesis would be to prove that higher values for the vulnerability factors mentioned before are found more often in the families of schizophrenic patients.

The deviation of the IQ distribution from the ideal gaussian curve at extremely low values (see Fig. 5, hatched zone) illustrates a further analogy between the dimensional distribution patterns of mental retardation and those of schizophrenia. The deviation is accounted for by an accumulation of severe and moderately severe mental retardation which is due to a large number of different brain damages. There is some indication that the relatively uniform syndrome of schizophrenia or the underlying reaction pattern of the brain can be attributed to various causes or to a combination of several causes. Even though rare, the occurrence of schizophrenic symptoms in various brain disturbances or following amphetamine abuse speaks for this assumption.

Finally, a dimensional distribution of the vulnerability for schizophrenia or of manifest traits which – when attaining extremely high values – accompany the schizophrenic symptoms would show a further analogy to the IQ distribution in the population. IQ ist determined both genetically and by learning factors. The proportion of genetic factors is particularly high at the lower end of the scale as a consequence of the accumulation of hereditary diseases in this area. The same may apply to extremely high values of vulnerability for schizophrenia. If this analogy were applied literally, it would mean polygenia. Other models for genetic transmission are also consistent with the pattern of dimensional distribution .

The comparison between the distribution of the vulnerability for schizophrenia or of a manifest "schizothymia" factor and IQ distribution does not mean that the aetiology of schizophrenia or of schizophrenic impairment would have to be materially similar to that of mental retardation.

It has not yet been possible to validate a dimensional concept of schizophrenia. On the other hand, it must be said that so far these dimensional concepts have not been evaluated by means of promising markers and adequate methods. We must admit that this concept is speculative, but to test it is not at all a hopeless venture.

Sociodemographic Factors

Among first admissions for schizophrenia in the period 1931–1945 Ødegard (1946) found that the figures for unmarried males were 4.3 times higher and for unmarried females 3.7 times higher than those of the general population of the same birth years. After this period the frequency of marriage decreased in the Norwegian population, as it has in other developed countries. In the comparative period 1956–1965 the rate of unmarried females first admitted for schizophrenia was moderately increased by 4.5%, whereas that of males was distinctly higher by 7.7% compared to the rates found in the general population of the same birth years (Ødegard 1971). Surprisingly, the reproduction rate of schizophrenics displayed a similar trend: in a comparison of the periods 1965–1967 and 1949–1950, Propping et al. (1982) – avoiding methodological shortcomings of earlier studies – showed that the number of children borne by schizophrenic women decreased more than the number of births in the population of the same age. The overproportional reduction in reproductivity occurred even though the average length of hospital stays had been considerably shortened.

Ødegard's interpretation of the decline in marriages among schizophrenics prior to first admission corresponds to the selection hypothesis by which the reduced chances of social advancement are explained: the prepsychotic poverty of social contacts reduces the chance of getting married. In cultures demanding of males a more active mating behaviour, this impairment affects them more than females. The raised threshold of successful mating consequently leads to an enlarged increase in unmarried schizophrenic men. The marked deficit in births to schizophrenic women may be explained correspondingly.

The alternative explanation of the extremely low rate of married schizophrenic males starts from the assumption that marriage has a protective effect on the morbid risk. This assumption is contradicted by Eaton (1985). Like Ødegard (1953), he points to the fact that the disease rate of widowed people is similar to that of married people and that it is essentially lower than that of never-married or divorced/separated persons.

Socioeconomic Factors

If we review more than 50 years of socioepidemiological research on the question of possible causal relations between the morbid risk of schizophrenia and social class, we may state:

1. There are no valid findings which prove the so-called breeder hypothesis, the assumption of a causal relation between belonging to the lowest social class and the morbid risk of schizophrenia

2. Besides the increased risk of social drift after the onset of the disease, schizophrenics prior to onset on average seem not to have attained fully the social level corresponding to their social origin. The lag of social ascent in contrast to the comparable population seems already developed to a smaller extent in the parents of schizophrenics – selection hypothesis of social intra- und inter-generation mobility (Goldberg and Morrison 1963; Turner and Wagenfeld 1967; review, Häfner 1971; Eaton 1985). The processes which led to an uneven ecological and social distribution of schizophrenics may thus be interpreted as part of the general trend of downward mobility among the socially impaired and disabled in the history of cities (like Chicago or Mannheim) and populations (Häfner and an der Heiden 1986).

We may ask ourselves why such an enormous expenditure of research on the social epidemiology of schizophrenia done over decades has not before led to the insight that the fruitfulness of the breeder hypothesis is very limited. Let me give two answers. First, case finding was largely biased in many studies, and case identification was inaccurate with the exception of very few studies. Both deficiencies imply the risk of overestimating the case rates for the lower social classes. Secondly, as Ødegard (1975) stated, the construct of socioeconomic class or stratum is too imprecise to test hypotheses on the contribution of social factors to the risk of schizophrenia and to study possible explanations of selection processes among individuals with an increased risk of schizophrenia in social contexts. In his longitudinal studies of occupational and social mobility of schizophrenics prior to onset of the disease conducted from 1926–1965 on the basis of the National Norwegian Register of Psychoses, Ødegard demonstrated very clearly that the "selection hypotheses" are superior to the "breeder hypotheses" in explaining the sociocultural patterns of the distribution of schizophrenia. The fact that the majority of the social epidemiologists did not foresee his findings may be explained by the immunising power of a research paradigm against "rebellious" results that was favoured by the zeitgeist.

Epidemiology of the Course

Until recently the results of medium- and long-term follow-up studies of schizophrenia have shown a large variability. In their examination of 11 published studies Shapiro and Shader (1979) reported 7%–40% favourable courses. Reviewing 38 cases, Stephens (1978) found between 10% and over 60% patients recovered. In these studies outcome criteria varied greatly. In Switzerland and in the Federal Republic of Germany, Bleuler (1972), Ciompi and Müller (1976) and Huber et al. (1980) published clinical follow-up studies of schizophrenics covering very long periods of time. By means of standardised assessment instruments Berner et al. (1986) and Möller and v. Zerssen (1986) conducted prospective studies among nonrepresentative cohorts of first or readmitted schizophrenics over a 5-year period.

Most recently, quite a few prospective longitudinal studies were based on sufficiently representative samples of first onset patients to contribute to the epidemiology of the "natural course" of schizophrenia. Besides requiring a sample of clearly identifiable cases collected from a population with low mobility, generalised statements about the course of the disease should be based on standardised methods of assessment, on a prospective design with a sufficient number of reassessments (at least three) over a sufficiently long period (at least 5 years) and on clearly defined outcome criteria (see also Stephens 1978, Watt et al. 1983). As schizophrenic patients cannot be left without treatment over long periods on ethical grounds, treatment variables should be controlled in addition to the variables that are relevant for the course.

The number of studies of patients with first onset of schizophrenia which fulfill all these requirements is still small (Strauss and Carpenter 1977; Watt et al. 1983; Biehl et al. 1986). Owing to diverging criteria of the course and of different methods for assessing symptoms, impairment, disability and social outcome, the comparability of their results is very unsatisfying.

In Table 4 Maurer and Biehl (1986; Biehl et al. 1987) from our institute compared two of these studies by classifying their results into three simple categories of course and outcome. The consistency of the total results at high thresholds could only be obtained by means of an arbitrary definition of the threshold values for the classes "one/more than one episode" and "no/minimum impairment" vs "severe impairment". Nevertheless, the values for males and females considerably vary in the three categories. At low thresholds a consistency of the rates 5 years after first admission for schizophrenia could not be achieved in any of them. Since so far there is no agreement on precisely defined and assessable criteria of course and outcome – with the exception of the assessment dimensions used in the multinational WHO schizophrenia studies – the supposedly high consistency of outcome rates in schizophrenia reported in the European longitudinal studies can be attributed to a well-meant concordant interpretation of very soft data.

The marked differences in the course of schizophrenia between developing and developed countries (World Health Organization 1973, 1979; Sartorius et al. 1977; Jablensky 1984) call for an explanation of nation- or culture-specific data on its prognosis. All prospective studies underline the predictive power of the productive symptoms regarding the complete course of schizophrenia. In about 60%

Table 4. Comparison of 5-year course and outcome categories in two representative first admission studies

Reference	Outcome criteria	Males		Females		Total	
		n	%	n	%	n	%
Watt et al. (1983)	(a) One schizophrenic episode/ no impairment	4	15.4	7	31.8	11	23
	(b) More than one episode or productive symptoms at follow-up without or with minimum impairment	9	34.6	8	36.4	17	35.4
	(c) Impairment/disability with several episodes or chronic productive symptoms	13	50	7	32	20	43
	Total	26		22		48	
Maurer and Biehl (1986)	*High threshold*						
	(1) Good	8	19.5	5	18.5	13	19.1
	(2) Intermediate	11	26.8	14	51.9	25	36.8
	(3+4) Poor	22	53.7	8	29.6	30	44.1
	Total	41		27		68	
	Low threshold						
	(1) Good	7	17.9	5	18.5	12	18.2
	(2) Intermediate	7	17.9	7	25.9	14	21.2
	(3+4) Poor	25	64.1	15	55.6	40	60.6
	Total	39		27		66	

–80% of the cases, the occurrence of productive symptoms of S^+ type correctly predicts their persistence or recurrence. In about 30%–60% of cases impairment or disability or so-called minus symptoms can be predicted to develop within 5 years after the first onset of a "S^+ schizophrenia" syndrome.

As was shown by Strauss and Carpenter (1972, 1974, 1977, 1978), Tsuang et al. (1979; Tsuang and Dempsey 1979), Strauss and Carpenter (1981), Huber et al. (1979), Möller and v. Zerssen (1986) and Schubart et al. (1986), productive schizophrenic symptoms contribute very little towards explaining the outcome variance of unproductive or "minus symptoms", of disability and of the social course in schizophrenic patients. Prepsychotic behaviour and personality traits – summarised by Strauss and Carpenter (1981) under the terms of "level of social relations function" and "level of work function" – seem to have more predictive power. In nearly all predictive studies covering a 5-year period, the social class of the parents, sex, educational level, occupational career and social behaviour of a patient prior to onset have a large share in the explication of outcome variance (Strauss and Carpenter 1972, 1974, 1977, 1978; Huber et al. 1976, 1980; Möller and v. Zerssen 1986; Schubart et al. 1986). An analogous relationship seems to prove true for the prognosis of treatment success in schizophrenics (Hogarty et al. 1974).

The consequence to be drawn from these relationships is that the non-psychotic precursors of the psychosis should be considered in heuristic models for explicating the aetiology of schizophrenia. The frequency of deficits of social and cognitive competence prior to first onset of the psychosis (Schubart et al. 1986) led Ødegard to the assumption that the psychotic episodes and the precursory personality deficits were part of a homogeneous disease process. Huber (1966, 1983) considers them to be the real psychosis from which productive episodes emerge from time to time. This assumption makes it difficult to explain two facts: schizophrenic episodes are not necessarily preceded by social deficits, and in other chronic psychiatric and organic diseases a low level of work performance and social relations function is also a predictor of an unfavourable course, including social disability and occupational downward drift.

In contrast to this, the vulnerability models by Wing (1975), Zubin and Spring (1977) and others start with a genetic transmission of a specific vulnerability for schizophrenia which, due to unspecific stress factors, may result in a psychotic episode. The risk of "minus symptoms" or disability following the outbreak of the psychosis may then be increased or reduced by a series of unspecific factors like social deficits or insufficient coping resources. According to these models, prepsychotic deficits may be interpreted partly as characteristic features of a specific vulnerability and partly as unspecific aggravating factors.

The fact that the social and cognitive deficits often decrease when the psychosis fades away in old age rather than increase as is the case in senile dementia (Janzarik 1968; Ciompi and Müller 1976; Harding and Strauss 1985) would be compatible with such reaction models, which begin with a multifactorial aetiology and see psychotic episodes as a specific pathology. Psychotic disability is understood partly as an unspecific and heterogeneous pattern of adaptation to the experience of being vulnerable and sometimes psychotic and to a changed social environment.

If we assume, to simplify matters, that the disease of schizophrenia finds its specific expression in the psychotic episode – as an effect of an insufficiently clarified vulnerability – and that the development of an unspecific pattern of impairment and disability is largely dependent on personality and environmental factors, then the two main epidemiological findings mentioned would be in good agreement with (a) the essential influence of sociocultural factors on its course and outcome, and (b) the invariability of the risk of first onset across cultures and time periods.

We are still far away from confirming or rejecting these aetiological models. In particular the question, whether environmental factors and imprecise premorbid personality traits like deficits in social, educational and occupational behaviour are able to increase the risk of first onset, particularly when genetic factors are controlled, has not yet been fully answered. On the basis of a retrospective assessment of the premorbid personality in M. Bleuler's clinical schizophrenia study (1972) and Essen-Möller's (1955) epidemiological Lundby study, Zubin (1986) recently calculated the morbid risk of individuals whose premorbid adaptation was extremely bad to be 9.36, whereas that of better-adapted people only was 0.69 and that of premorbidly inconspicuous individuals was 0.67. Considering the lack of a control population and the insufficient reliability of the data on which these calculations were based, these values can be taken as an indication only. Controlled prospective studies of cohorts consisting of adolescents with poor social and educational performance and other unfavourable personality traits are now required, under control of indicators of genetic traits.

Let me now deal with two more specific epidemiological findings, the first of which – deviant birth seasonality – is presumably overestimated at present for its aetiological relevance, and the second of which – sex differences in the age of on-set – is rather underestimated.

Deviant Birth Seasonality

Compared to the seasonal distribution of births in the control population, schizo-phrenics exhibit a plus of about 10% in the winter or spring season and a minus of an equal size in the summer. In a recently published review Bradbury and Miller (1985) described 11 of 43 studies to be free from major shortcomings; 10 studies showed a significant seasonal birth excess, 9 of them in the winter or spring months. In an article published in the *Schizophrenia Bulletin*, Boyd et al. (1986) analysed 30 of the studies already reviewed by Bradbury and Miller and noted that – regardless of methodological shortcomings – 19 studies reported an excess of births in the winter and spring months that was significant at a level of at least 0.05, and 6 of these at a level of 0.01. Thus the results of studies with methodolog-ical shortcomings are rather consistent and support the validity of the findings. Table 5 gives a survey of studies conducted among sufficiently large numbers of cases. The months or quarters with significant schizophrenic birth excesses are marked, as are the levels of significance.

Before dealing with the question of the aetiological importance of this finding which may account for no more than about 10% of cases or for a contribution of this extent to a multifactorial risk, it should be examined whether the plus of winter births or the minus of summer births are really specific to schizophrenia. Watson et al. (1984) reviewed studies of birth seasonality effects and noted that 6 of the 11 studies among manic-depressive patients, 4 of 6 studies of neurotic dis-orders and 2 of 6 studies of personality disorders showed birth excesses (not nec-essarily significant) in the first part of the year. However, they could not confirm this trend on the basis of their own data. In addition to the methodological short-comings these investigations have in common with most of the schizophrenia studies on this subject, the lower reliability of the diagnosis and the smaller pro-portion of hospitalised or registered cases here restrict the validity of the results.

Trying to contribute to the question of specificity, we first examined the birth-date distribution of 2020 Mannheim inhabitants diagnosed as schizophrenics who had first been registered in the Cumulative Psychiatric Case Register in the period 1975–1980, and compared it to that of the population aged over 15 years from which they came and to that of a control group of 2020 persons living in Mannheim, matched for birth years and sex (Fig. 6).

There is a slight excess of births of schizophrenics in the months of March and April, reaching a maximum of 12% and a statistical significance of 0.05. In the other months of the year their birth pattern displayed nothing unusual.

To investigate the birth pattern of a group of mentally disordered people for whom the requirements of complete case finding and precise diagnoses were ful-

Table 5. Distribution of monthly births of schizophrenics in selected studied

Reference	n	Significance	Dec.	Jan.	Feb.	Mar.	Apr.	May	Jun.	Jul.	Aug.	Sep.	Oct.	Nov.
Northern hemisphere														
Tramer 1929	3 100	***												
De Sauvage 1934/1951/1954	4 679	***												
Hare and Price 1968	3 596	*												
Dalen 1968	16 238	***												
Hare et al. 1974	5 139	**												
Ødegard 1974	19 749	*												
Videbech et al. 1974	7 427	***												
Parker and Balza 1977	3 508	***												
Shimura et al. 1977	5 431	**												
Torrey et al. 1977	53 584	*												
O'Hare et al. 1980	4 855	***												
Watson et al. 1984	3 246	**												
Kendell and Kemp 1985	3 224	*												
Häfner et al. 1987	2 020	*												
Southern hemisphere														
Dalen 1975	2 947	*	(only females, $n = 1 506$)												
Parker and Neilson 1976	2 256	**	(only females, $n = 1 195$)												

Studies including fewer than 2000 cases are not listed

* $0.05 \geqq p > 0.01$
** $0.01 \geqq p > 0.001$
*** $0.001 \geqq p$

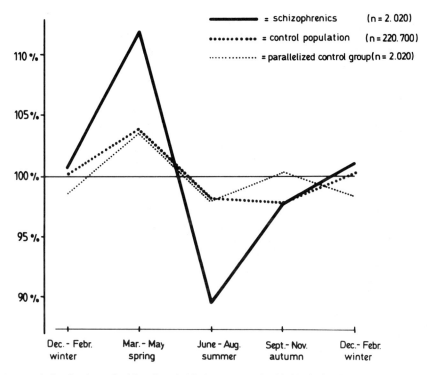

Fig. 6. Seasonal distribution of schizophrenic births compared with births in the control population and the control group in three decades and before 1920

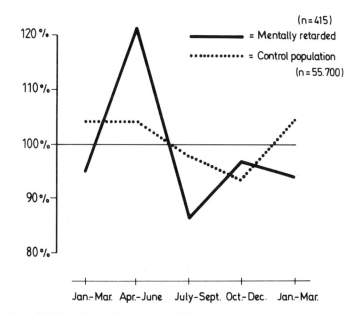

Fig. 7. Seasonal distribution of births of mentally retarded children

filled, B. Cooper provided us with the data of 415 children born in Mannheim in the period 1958–1971 (aged 7–16 years) with severe and moderately severe mental retardation (IQ ≤ 60). Compared to the population of Mannheim of the same birth years, we found a plus of about 20% in the second quarter (April to June), which is one month later than that of schizophrenics, and a minus of about 15% in the third, the summer quarter (Fig. 7).

The group of neuroses and personality disorders showed a significant excess of 10% for male births in spring when controlled for age and age group. These results do not yet prove a deviant birth seasonality in other diagnostic groups. The sample of mentally retarded children is small, and in neuroses and personality disorders the enormous shortcomings of sampling and diagnosing do not permit us to consider the findings as valid. Nevertheless they justify doubts about the specificity of the winter birth excesses in schizophrenics. It might be that an unknown noxious agent or a biological disadvantage – increasedly transmitted in winter births – are associated with a slightly increased unspecific risk of some severe mental disorder and thus also with the risk of schizophrenia. With a view to the procreational hypothesis, it might also be that a small proportion of the parents of schizophrenics, mentally retarded and other groups of mentally disordered people have a higher threshold of heterosexual mating behaviour which results in a minus of reproduction in the colder season and a plus in the warmer; the latter season would favour frequent and more intense erotic stimuli and better opportunities, as was assumed by Ødegard (1974). Indeed this is the most simple hypothesis for explaining the finding. Its plausibility is confirmed by the fact that the total population shows an analogous trend of seasonal reproduction behaviour. Births have a slight plus in the winter and spring months and a corresponding minus in summer and autumn. The birth distribution pattern of schizophrenics and of some other groups of mentally disordered people increases this trend in the same direction. These assumptions are vague; we are in need of sophisticated studies on the birth distribution of comparable mental and somatic diseases to test the specificity of the pattern to schizophrenia.

Sex Differences in Age at Onset of Schizophrenia

The cumulative expectancy of schizophrenia seems to be equal in males and females (Gottesman et al. 1982; Dohrenwend and Dohrenwend 1976; Strömgren 1935). However, the distribution of age at first admission almost consistently displays a marked sex difference (Huber et al. 1976; Munk-Jørgensen 1987; reviews, Lewine 1981; Angermeyer 1986).

The distribution of first admission rates of schizophrenia over 10-year age groups in the period 1975–1980 recorded by the Mannheim case register shows an earlier onset in males – reaching a peak in the 25–34 group – and an excess of females in the 35 and over group. The difference of the modal values is about 10 years and thus approximates the finding reported by Watt and Szulecka (1979). The numerous data on this subject obtained from various sources are consistent in their trend, but inconsistent in the age differences of the mean or modal values. We have compared our data with the age distribution of 658 first ad-

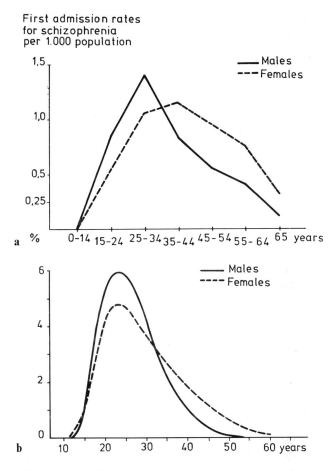

First admission rates
for schizophrenia
per 1.000 population

The amount of age (per percentage) with first admission
by males and females separately are together 100 % each

Fig. 8. a Annual incidence rates for schizophrenia by age and sex in Mannheim (1975–1980). **b** Age distribution of 658 first hospitalizations of schizophrenia in Bavaria, 1920–1925 (Strömgren 1935). Total percentage for males and females separately is 100 %

missions for schizophrenia in Bavaria in the period 1920–1925, which Strömgren (1935) related to the proportion of all first admissions by sex and age group (Fig. 8). In a preliminary evaluation of the "WHO Collaborative Study on Determinants of Outcome of Severe Mental Disorders", Sartorius et al. (1986) stated that higher incidence rates in males of younger age groups are also a fairly consistent cross-cultural finding.

In order to approach an explication, we should examine whether sex differences in the latency period between first onset and first contact with a treatment facility account for the difference in age at first hospitalisation (Fig. 9). This latency is due to delayed help-seeking behaviour, e.g. as a consequence of differing symptoms, self- and heteroperception, threshold of tolerance and social at-

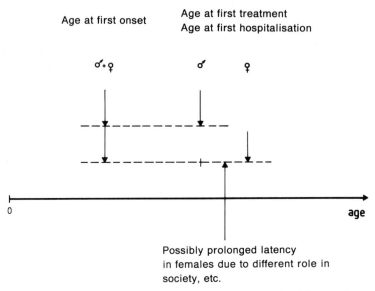

Fig. 9. Model description of the hypothesis of a sex-specific difference between first onset and first treatment

tribution of sickness role. The differing roles of males and females in most societies might effect differences in the latency period before the psychotic symptoms become conspicuous and help is sought. Variability in symptoms, such as an onset with more frequently uncharacteristic symptoms in females, might equally well have the same effect. The first data on this subject – besides the "WHO Collaborative Study on Determinants of Outcome of Severe Mental Disorders" – do not show considerable sex distinctions in latency periods (Lewine 1980).

Should a distinct sex difference in age at first onset really exist, it would have to be tested whether protective or risk factors confounded with sex, like the lower age of females at marriage or a higher work stress in young men, could explain part of the variances. Angermeyer (1985), who studied some of these questions on the basis of case records, found sex variation in age at first onset even when controlling for these factors.

Sex differences also seem to be evident in symptoms not corrected for age. Since age itself is an important predictor of symptoms and course, one should first investigate to what extent the variations in symptomatology, such as an accumulation of paranoid syndromes in females in the second half of life, are accounted for by differences in the age distribution of males and females.

When looking at the course of the disease, which was assessed by standardised instruments for the constructs of "productive symptoms" (PSE) and "impairment" (IMPS) in a prospective 5-year cohort of first-hospitalised schizophrenics (Biehl et al. 1986, in the frame of the WHO Disability Study), we may receive the impression that from the third year onwards the delayed first onset in females is followed by a catching-up with the previously more unfavourable course in males (Fig. 10).

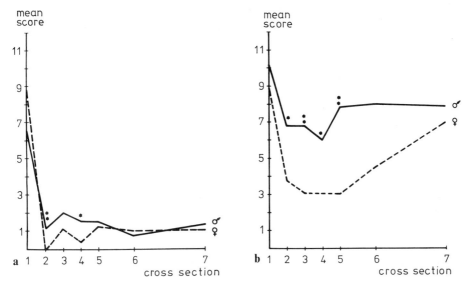

Fig. 10. a, b Sex-specific courses over a 5-year period in patients with first onset of schizophrenia (cross sections at points of time marked). **a** Productive symptoms (PSE); **b** social and psychological deficits (IMPS)

These preliminary results do not permit a generalised statement on the age-corrected, long-term differences in the course of schizophrenia among males and females. We have therefore started a study jointly with Strömgren, Dupont and Munk-Jørgensen, in which data from the Danish Case Register are included. The aim is to develop and test pathogenetic models for explaining the sex differences. This might also be a way to test the assumption that the threshold of vulnerability for schizophrenia is higher in females than in males because of the modulating effect of oestrogen on the dopamine metabolism (Lewine 1980, 1981; Seeman 1982) and that the protective effect may rapidly cease after the first episode due to an easier precipitation of the underlying processes in the transmitter metabolism.

Final Remarks

Aetiological models for explaining schizophrenia should be consistent with epidemiological data. This implies that aetiological hypotheses should reflect the peculiarities of the fairly homologous reaction pattern of schizophrenia which might be connected with uniform biochemical mechanisms of the brain, but also with heterogeneous aetiological factors. They should also allow for the environment-invariant morbid risk or vulnerability, which might result from an artificial cut at the extreme part of a behaviour dimension distributed almost evenly in all populations, like IQ (inversely). This assumption is more compatible with epidemiological data than a monocausal aetiology, especially specific environmental aetiologies such as viral infections or social conditions, which change with time and vary with the population under study. There is some probability that the minus symptoms and impairments influencing the social course are less specific to and less closely associated with the vulnerability for schizophrenia than are the productive symptoms or the psychotic episodes.

References

Angermeyer MC (1985) Zur Frage geschlechtsabhängiger Unterschiede im Verlauf schizophrener Krankheit. Vortrag am ZISG, Mannheim
Antonovsky A (1979) Health, stress and coping. Jossey-Bass, San Francisco
Astrup C (1956) Nervöse Erkrankungen und soziale Verhältnisse. Volk und Gesundheit, Berlin
Astrup C (1982) The increase of mental disorders. Unpublished manuscript from the National Case Register of Mental Disorder, Gaustad Hospital, Oslo
Babigian HM (1975) Schizophrenia: epidemiology. In: Freedman AM, Kaplan HI, Sadock BJ (eds) Comprehensive textbook of psychiatry: II. Williams and Wilkins, Baltimore
Berner P, Katschnig H, Lenz G (1986) The polydiagnostic approach in research on schizophrenia. In: Freedman AM, Brotman R, Silverman E, Hutson D (eds) Issues in psychiatric classification. Human Sciences Press, New York, pp 70–91
Bernsen AH (1976) Severe mental retardation among children in the county of Aarhus, Denmark. Acta Psychiatr Scand 54:43–66
Biehl H, Maurer K, Schubart C, Krumm B, Jung E (1986) Prediction of outcome and utilization of medical services in a prospective study of first onset schizophrenics – results of a prospective 5-year follow-up study. Eur Arch Psychiatr Neurol Sci 236:139–147
Biehl H, Maurer K, Schubart C (1987) Dimensionen der Psychopathologie und sozialen Anpassung im natürlichen Verlauf schizophrener Ersterkrankungen. In: Olbrich R (ed) Prospektive Verlaufsforschung in der Psychiatrie. Springer, Berlin Heidelberg Ney York Tokyo
Birch HG, Richardson SA, Baird D, Horobin G, Illsley R (1970) Mental subnormality in the community. Williams and Wilkins, Baltimore
Bleuler M (1972) Die schizophrenen Geistesstörungen im Lichte langjähriger Kranken- und Familiengeschichten. Thieme, Stuttgart
Boyd JH, Pulver AE, Stewart W (1986) Season of birth: schizophrenia and bipolar disorder. Schizophr Bull 12:173–186
Bradbury TN, Miller, GA (1985) Season of birth in schizophrenia: a review of evidence, methodology, and etiology. Psychol Bull 98:569–594
Brask BH (1972) Prevalence of mental retardation among children in the county of Aarhus, Denmark. Acta Psychiatr Scand 48:480–500
Ciompi L, Müller C (1976) Lebensweg und Alter der Schizophrenen. Monographien aus dem Gesamtgebiet der Psychiatrie, vol 12. Springer, Heidelberg Ney York Berlin
Cooper B (1978) Epidemiology. In: Wing JK (ed) Schizophrenia: towards a new synthesis. Grune & Stratton, New York
Cooper B, Lackus B (1984) The social-class background of mentally retarded children. A study in Mannheim. Soc Psychiatry 19:3–12
Crow TJ (1983) Is schizophrenia an infectious disease? Lancet 1:173–175
Crow TJ (1984) A re-evaluation of the viral hypothesis: is psychosis the result of a retroviral integration at a site close to the cerebral dominance gene? Br J Psychiatr 145:243–253
Dalen P (1968) Month of birth and schizophrenia. Acta Psychiatr Scand 203:55–60
Dalen P (1975) Season of birth: a study of schizophrenia and other mental disorders. North Holland, Amsterdam
de Sauvage NWJJ (1934) Verband tussen geboortemaand en schizophrene en manisch-depressieve geestesziekten. Ned Tijdschr Geneeskd 79:528
de Sauvage NWJJ (1951) Verband tussen geboortemaand en schizophrene en manisch-depressieve geestesziekten. Ned Tijdschr Genesskd 4:3855–3864

de Sauvage NWJJ (1954) Vitamin C and the schizophrenic syndrome. Folia Psychiatr Neerl 57:347–355

Dilling H, Weyerer S, Lisson H (1975) Zur ambulanten psychiatrischen Versorgung durch niedergelassene Nervenärzte. Soc Pschiatr 10:111–131

Dohrenwend BP, Dohrenwend BS (1976) Sex differences and psychiatric disorders. Am J Sociol 81:1447–1454

Dunham HW (1965) Community and schizophrenia: an epidemiological analysis. Wayne State University Press, Detroit

Dunham HW (1976) Society, culture and mental disorder. Arch Gen Psychiatry 32:147–156

Dupont A (1981) Definition and identification of severe mental retardation. In: Cooper B (ed) Assessing the handicaps and needs of mentally retarded children. Academic, London, pp 3–12

Eaton WW (1980) A formal theory of selection for schizophrenia. Am J Sociol 86:149–158

Eaton WW (1985) Epidemiology of schizophrenia. Epidemiol Rev 7:105–126

Essen-Möller E (1955) Individual traits and morbidity in a Swedish rural population. Acta Psychiatr Neurol Scand [Suppl] 100

Flynn MP (1970) Mental handicap in county Westmeath. J Irish Med Assoc 63:257–260

Gibbons JL, Jennings C, Wing JK (1983) Psychiatric care in 8 register areas. Statistics from eight psychiatric case registers in Great Britain 1976–1981. Southampton Psychiatric Case Register, University of Southampton, Southampton

Giel R, Sauer HC, Slooff CJ, Wiersma D (1980) Epidemiological observations on schizophrenia and disability in the Netherlands. Tijdschr Psychiatrie 11–12:710–722

Goldberg EM, Morrison SL (1963) Schizophrenia and social class. Br J Psychiatry 109:785–802

Goldhamer H, Marshall AW (1949) The frequency of mental disease: long-range trends and present status. Rand Corp, New York

Goodman MB, Gruenberg E, Downing JJ, Rogat E (1956) A prevalence study of mental retardation in a metropolitan area. Am J Public Health 46:702–707

Goodman N, Tizard J (1962) Prevalence of imbecility and idiocy among children. Br Med J 1:216–219

Gottesman I, Shields J, Hanson DR (1982) Schizophrenia: the epigenetic puzzle. Cambridge University Press, New York

Häfner H (1971) Der Einfluß von Umweltfaktoren auf das Erkrankungsrisiko für Schizophrenie. Nervenarzt 42:557–568

Häfner H, an der Heiden W (1986) The contribution of European case registers to research on schizophrenia. Schizophr Bull 12:26–50

Häfner H, Reimann H (1970) Spatial distribution of mental disorders in Mannheim 1965. In: Hare EH, Wing JK (eds) Psychiatric epidemiology. Oxford University Press, London, pp 341–354

Häfner H, Haas S, Pfeifer-Kurda M, Eichhorn S, Michitsuji S (1987) Abnormal seasonality of schizophrenic births – a specific finding? (to be published)

Hagnell O (1966) A prospective study of the incidence of mental disorder. Svenska Bokförlaget, Lund

Harding CM, Strauss JS (1985) The course of schizophrenia: an evolving concept. In: Alpert M (ed) Controversies in schizophrenia – changes and constancies. Guilford, New York, pp 339–350

Hare EH, Price JS (1968) Mental disorder and season of birth: comparison of psychoses with neuroses. Br J Psychiatry 115:533–540

Hare EH, Price JS, Slater E (1974) Mental disorder and season of birth: a national sample compared with the general population. Br J Psychiatry 124:81–86

Helgason L (1977) Psychiatric services and mental illness in Iceland. Acta Psychiatr Scand [Suppl] 268

Hogarty GE, Goldberg SC, Schooler NR, Ulrich RF (1974) Drug and sociotherapy in the aftercare of schizophrenic patients: II. Two-year relapse rates. Arch Gen Psychiatry 31:603–608

Hollingshead A, Redlich FC (1958) Social class and mental illness. Wiley, New York

Huber G (1966) Reine Defektsyndrome und Basis-Stadien endogener Psychosen. Fortschr Neurol Psychiatr 34:409–426

Huber G (1983) Das Konzept substratnaher Basissymptome und seine Bedeutung für Theorie und Therapie schizophrener Erkrankungen. Nervenarzt 54:23–32

Huber G, Gross G, Schüttler R (1976) Konsequenzen der Verlaufsuntersuchungen für Therapie und Rehabilitation der Schizophrenien. In: Huber G (ed) Therapie, Rehabilitation und Prävention schizophrener Erkrankungen. Schattauer, Stuttgart, pp 112–131

Huber G, Gross G, Schüttler R (1979) Schizophrenie. Eine Verlaufs- und sozialpsychiatrische Langzeitstudie. Springer, Berlin Heidelberg New York

Huber G, Gross G, Schüttler R (1980) Langzeitentwicklung schizophrener Erkrankungen („Bonn-Studie"). In: Schimmelpenning GW (ed) Psychiatrische Verlaufsforschung. Huber, Bern, pp 110–133

Imre PD (1967) The epidemiology of mental retardation in a S.E. rural U.S.A. community. In: Richards BW (ed) Proceedings of first congress of Int Assoc for Sc St of Ment Def, Montpellier, France. Michael Jackson, England

Innes G, Kidd C, Ross HS (1968) Mental subnormality in north east Scotland. Br J Psychiatry 114:35–41

Jablensky A (1984) Gli studi trans-culturali dell' organizzazione mondiale della sanita sulla schizofrenia: implicazioni teoriche e pratiche. In: Faccincani C, Fiorio R, Mignolli G, Tansella M (eds) Le psicosi schizofreniche. Patron, Bologna, pp 37–64

Janzarik W (1968) Schizophrene Verläufe. Springer, Berlin Heidelberg New York

Jaco E (1960) The social epidemiology of mental disorders. Russell Sage Foundation, New York

Kendell RE, Kemp IW (1985) Winter born vs summer born schizophrenics. Paper presented at the World Psychiatric Association Section Symposium "The Future of Psychiatric Epidemiology", Sept. 1985, Edinburgh, 23–26

Kramer M, Pollack ES, Redick RW (1967) Studies of the incidence and prevalence of hospitalized mental disorders in the United States: current status and future goals. In: Hoch PH, Zubin J (eds) Comparative epidemiology of the mental disorders. Grune & Stratton, New York, pp 56–93

Kretschmer E (1921) Körperbau und Charakter. Springer, Berlin

Krupinski J, Alexander L (1983) Patterns of psychiatric morbidity in Victoria, Australia, in relation to changes in diagnostic criteria 1848–1978. Soc Psychiatry 18:61–67

Kushlick A (1961) Subnormality in Salford. In: Susser MW, Kushlick A (eds) A report on the mental health service of the city of Salford for the year 1960. Salford Health Department

Lemkau P, Tietze C, Cooper M (1942) Mental hygiene problems in an urban district. Ment Hyg 26:100–119, 275–288

Lewine RJ (1980) Sex differences in age of symptom onset and first hospitalization in schizophrenia. Am J Orthopsychiatry 50:316–322

Lewine RJ (1981) Sex differences in schizophrenia: Timing or subtypes? Psychol Bull 90:432–444

Lewis EO (1929) Report on an investigation into the incidence of mental deficiency in six areas, 1925–1927. Report of the Mental Deficiency Commission, part IV. HMSO, London

Liepmann MC (1979) Geistig behinderte Kinder und Jugendliche. Eine epidemiologische, klinische und sozialpsychologische Studie in Mannheim. Huber, Bern

Martindale A (1977) A case register as an information system in a development project for the mentally handicapped. Br J Ment Sub XXII, Part 2 [43]

Maurer K, Biehl H (1986) Vergleich schizophrener Verlaufstypen bei Watt, Katz und Shepherd (1983) und der WHO Behinderungsstudie (Rhein-Neckar-Kohorte). Unpublished manuscript

Mishler EG, Scotch NA (1963) Sociocultural factors in the epidemiology of schizophrenia: a review. Psychiatry 26:315–351

Möller, H-J, v Zerssen D (1986) Der Verlauf schizophrener Psychosen unter den gegenwärtigen Behandlungsbedingungen. Springer, Berlin Heidelberg New York Tokyo

Munk-Jørgensen P (1987) Cumulated need for psychiatric service as shown in a community psychiatric project (to be published)

Murray RM, Reveley AM (1983) Schizophrenia as an infection. Lancet [March 12]:583

Ødegard Ø (1946) Marriage and mental disease. J Ment Sci 92: 35–49

Ødegard Ø (1953) Marriage and mental health. Acta Psychiatr Scand [Suppl] 80:153–161
Ødegard Ø (1971) Hospitalized psychoses in Norway: time trends 1926–1965. Soc Psychiatry 6:53–58
Ødegard Ø (1974) Season of birth in the general population and in patients with mental disorder in Norway. Br J Psychiatry 125:397–405
Ødegard Ø (1975) Social and ecological factors in the etiology, outcome, treatment, and prevention of mental disorders. In: Kisker KP, Meyer JE, Müller C, Strömgren E (eds) Psychiatrie der Gegenwart, vol III, 2nd edn. Springer, Berlin Heidelberg New York, pp 151–198
O'Hare A, Walsh D, Torrey F (1980) Seasonality of schizophrenic births in Ireland. Br J Psychiatry 137:74–77
Parker G, Balza B (1977) Season of birth and schizophrenia – an equatorial study. Acta Psychiatr Scand 56:143–146
Parker G, Neilson M (1976) Mental disorder and season of birth – a southern hemisphere study. Br J Psychiatry 129:355–361
Propping P, Hilger T, Haverkamp F (1982) Hat die Kinderzahl schizophrener Patienten zugenommen? Eine epidemiologische Studie in Nordbaden 1949–1950 und 1965–1967. In: Huber G (ed): Endogene Psychosen: Diagnostik, Basissymptome und biologische Parameter. Schattauer, Stuttgart, pp 133–142
Sanua V (1970) Immigration, migration, and mental illness: a review of the literature with special emphasis on schizophrenia. In: Brody EB (ed) Behavior in new environments. Sage, Beverly Hills
Sartorius N, Jablensky A, Shapiro R (1977) Two-year follow-up of the patients included in the WHO International Pilot Study of Schizophrenia. Psychol Med 7:529–541
Sartorius N, Jablensky A, Korten A, Ernberg G, Anker M, Cooper JE, Day R (1986) Early manifestations and first-contact incidence of schizophrenia in different cultures. Psychol Med 16:909–928
Scally B, McKay D (1964) Mental subnormality and its prevalence in Northern Ireland. Acta Psychiatr Neurol Scand 40:203–211
Schneider K (1950) Klinische Psychopathologie, 3rd edn. Thieme, Stuttgart
Schubart C, Schwarz R, Krumm B, Biehl H (1986) Schizophrenie und soziale Anpassung. Eine prospektive Längsschnittuntersuchung. Springer, Berlin Heidelberg New York Tokyo
Seeman M (1982) Gender differences in schizophrenia. Can J Psychiatry 27:107–112
Shapiro R, Shader R (1979) Selective review of results of previous studies of schizophrenia and other psychoses. In: World Health Organization (ed) Schizophrenia: an international follow-up study. Wiley, Chichester, pp 11–43
Shimura M, Nakamura I, Miura T (1977) Season of birth of schizophrenia in Tokyo, Japan. Acta Psychiatr Scand 55:225–232
Sorel FM (1974) Prevalence of mental retardation. Tilburg University Press, Netherlands
Stephens JH (1978) Long-term prognosis and follow-up in schizophrenia. Schizophr Bull 4:25–47
Strauss JS, Carpenter WT (1972) Prediction of outcome in schizophrenia: I. Characteristics of outcome. Arch Gen Psychiatry 27:739–746
Strauss JS, Carpenter WT (1974) Prediction of outcome in schizophrenia: II. Relationship between predictor and outcome variables: a report from the WHO International Pilot Study of Schizophrenia. Arch Gen Psychiatry 31:37–42
Strauss JS, Carpenter WT (1977) Prediction of outcome in schizophrenia. Arch Gen Psychiatry 34:159–163
Strauss JS, Carpenter WT (1981) Schizophrenia. Plenum Press, New York
Strauss JS, Carpenter WT (1978) The prognosis of schizophrenia: rationale for a multidimensional concept. Schizophr Bull 4 [1]:56–67
Strömgren E (1935) Zum Ersatz des Weinbergschen „abgekürzten Verfahrens". Zugleich ein Beitrag zur Frage von der Erblichkeit des Erkrankungsalters bei der Schizophrenie. Z Gesamte Neurol Psychiatr 153:784–797
Tansella M, Faccincani C, Mignolli G, Balestrieri M, Zimmermann-Tansella C (1985) Il registro psichiatrico di Verona-Sud. Epidemiologia per la valutazione dei nuovi servizi territoriali. In: Tansella M (ed) L'approcio epidemiologico in psichiatria. Boringhieri, Torino, pp 225–259

Thomas A (1978) A population study of children with severe mental handicap. MSc Thesis, University of Manchester

Thompson WD, Weissman MM (1981) Quantifying lifetime risk of psychiatric disorder. J Psychiatr Res 16:113–126

Torrey EF (1980) Schizophrenia and civilization. Aronson, New York

Torrey EF, Torrey BB, Peterson MR (1977) Seasonality of schizophrenic births in the United States. Arch Gen Psychiatry 34:1065–1070

Tramer M (1929) Über die biologische Bedeutung des Geburtsmonates, insbesondere für die Psychoseerkrankung. Schweiz Arch Neurol Psychiatr 24:17–24

Tsuang MT, Dempsey GM (1979) Long-term outcome of major psychoses: II. Schizoaffective disorder compared with schizophrenia, affective disorders, and a surgical control group. Arch Gen Psychiatry 36:1302–1304

Tsuang MT, Woolson RF, Fleming JA (1979) Long-term outcome of major psychoses: I. Schizophrenia and affective disorders compared with psychiatrically symptom-free surgical conditions. Arch Gen Psychiatry 36:1295–1301

Turner RJ, Wagenfeld MO (1967) Occupational mobility in schizophrenia. An assessment of the social causation and social selection hypothesis. Am Sociol Rev 32:104–113

Videbech T, Weeke A, Dupont A (1974) Endogenous psychoses and season of birth. Acta Psychiatr Scand 50:202–218

Warthen FJ, Klee GC, Bahn AK, Gorwitz K (1967) Diagnosed schizophrenia in Maryland. Psychiatric Research Report 22. American Psychiatric Association, Washington DC

Watson CG, Kucala T, Tilleskjor C, Jacobs L (1984) Schizophrenic birth seasonality in relation to the incidence of infectious diseases and temperature extremes. Arch Gen Psychiatry 41:85–90

Watt DC, Szulecka TK (1979) The effect of sex, marriage and age at first admission on the hospitalization of schizophrenics during 2 years following discharge. Psychol Med 9:529–539

Watt DC, Katz K, Shepherd M (1983) The natural history of schizophrenia: a 5-year prospektive follow-up of a representative sample of schizophrenics by means of a standardized clinical ard social assessment. Psychol Med 13:669–670

Wing JK (1975) Impairments in schizophrenia. In: Wist R, Winokur G, Roff M (eds) Life history research in psychopathology, vol IV. University of Minnesota Press, Minneapolis

Wing JK, Fryers T (eds) (1976) Psychiatric services in Camberwell and Salford. Statistics from the Camberwell and Salford psychiatric registers, 1964–1974. MRC Soc Psych Unit, London and Dept Comm Med, University of Manchester

Wing L (1971) Severely retarded children in a London area: prevalence and provision of services. Psychol Med 1:405–415

World Health Organization (ed) (1973) The international pilot study of schizophrenia, vol 1. WHO, Geneva

World Health Organization (ed) (1979) Schizophrenia. An international follow-up study. Wiley, Chichester

Yolles S, Kramer M (1969) Vital statistics. In: Bellak L, Loeb L (eds) The schizophrenic syndrome. Grune & Stratton, New York

Zubin J (1986) Mögliche Implikationen der Vulnerabilitätshypothese für das psychosoziale Management der Schizophrenie. In: Böker W, Brenner HD (eds) Bewältigung der Schizophrenie. Huber, Bern, pp 29–41

Zubin J, Spring B (1977) Vulnerability – a new view of schizophrenia. Abnorm Psychol 86:103–126

Processes of Healing and Chronicity in Schizophrenia *

J. S. STRAUSS

Psychiatry has made massive strides by using careful description of presenting symptomatology to define types of disorders [1] and to test these concepts [e.g., 2,3]. Just as a primary emphasis on cross-sectional description of symptoms has been the keystone for diagnostic progress, so a longitudinal descriptive approach could generate a clearer picture of the course of disorder. Such a picture might provide insight into the nature of longitudinal processes, the determinants of improvement and chronicity, and perhaps even supply a new orientation to the historically established practice of utilizing longitudinal principles for reconsidering diagnostic entities [4].

In this report, I will review recent data on the course of schizophrenia starting with the most established descriptive findings and moving progressively to the more speculative and theoretical. The review will start by noting data showing that an adequate longitudinal approach to understanding mental disorders requires a multidimensional description of symptomatology, social functioning, and other characteristics of the illness, the person, and the environment. Data will then be described showing that an adequate picture of course also requires repeated assessments of these characteristics over time. Then, considering these multidimensional and longitudinal complexities, I will describe systematic exploratory research suggesting patterns in the evolution of disorder and recovery in schizophrenia and some of the theoretical implications of these patterns for defining the underlying processes determining course. Specifically, I will suggest that the data indicate the existence of psychological control mechanisms in the patient that are a major determinant of the processes of healing and chronicity in schizophrenic disorders.

In the descriptive study of schizophrenia four types of findings suggest key characteristics in the nature and course of this disorder. These findings are: (1) outcome heterogeneity, (2) the importance of multiple interacting processes, (3) the active role of the patient, and (4) nonlinear patterns in the evolution of these characteristics. Together, these four findings provide clues to processes of healing and chronicity.

* This report was funded in part by NIMH grants MH00340 and MH34365 and by an award from the Scottish Rite Schizophrenia Research Program
Yale University, School of Medicine, Department of Psychiatry, 34 Park Street, New Haven, CT 06519, USA

Heterogeneity of Outcome. A number of investigations have built upon and revised some of the earlier valuable Kraepelinian notions about outcome in "dementia praecox" (schizophrenia). Kraepelin's utilization of prognosis for establishing a diagnostic entity provided a milestone in the history of psychiatry. But his notion that the vast majority of people with schizophrenia have a deteriorating course has now been challenged by studies carried out in a variety of settings. Results have shown a significant distribution of patients over a range of outcomes from recovery to chronicity [5–9].

Interacting Processes. Not only has the heterogeneity of the outcome of schizophrenia been demonstrated, but so has the fact that diverse areas of functioning – symptoms, work, social relationships, need for hospitalization – are involved in understanding outcome [10]. All these characteristics are related to each other, but they are also somewhat independent, each with a degree of continuity over time. The premorbid level of social relations, for example, is generally the best predictor of social relations level at follow-up. But to a lesser extent social relations predict follow-up symptom severity as well [11].

These findings have begun to demonstrate that the processes in the course of schizophrenia are multiple and interacting. To explain the findings in the correlation matrix involving work function, social relations, and symptoms over time, it appears most useful to conclude that the various areas of functioning represent open-linked systems [11]. Furthermore, analysis of the elements of these systems suggests that most, perhaps all, have foundations in both the person and the environment. For example, working involves the person's ability and motivation and the environment's providing an appropriate job opportunity and stimulus to be employed. Such combinations of person and environmental factors, for example related to work, interact with symptom severity.

The Active Role of the Patient. Beyond the various areas of functioning and their apparent interactions, recent studies suggest that the person is not merely the victim of a disease and of environmental factors, but takes an active role in dealing with the disorder and with his or her life situation [12–15]. The person may take action to control symptoms, to select stresses or supports, and to collaborate with treatment – all together probably impacting on the ultimate outcome of disorder.

Nonlinearity in the Course of Disorder. When, as part of recent developments in longitudinal research, repeated sequential follow-up assessments of these different characteristics are made, they demonstrate that the paths to the heterogeneous outcome of patients with schizophrenia probably never follow a straight line [16]. Prospective short-term study thus agrees with impressions from retrospective long-term follow-up investigations regarding the multiple patterns in the course of disorder that lead to the various points traditionally considered as "outcome" [7, 8].

Longitudinal Processes

How can these complexities in the course and outcome of schizophrenia be under-stood? Recent studies suggest that the variations in the course of disorder over time may not be merely random fluctuations but may reflect definable longitudinal processes in the various open-linked systems of functioning, systems involving the disorder itself, the person more generally, and the environment [16]. For example, the level of demand from society that a person be employed, the person's own ability to work, and the level of symptoms each appears to some extent to have its own temporal pattern. In the environment, families often give a recently discharged patient a few months before they put increasing pressure on him or her to resume responsibility for self-support. Some patients have a period of temporary social withdrawal for a few weeks or months after hospital discharge before taking on a more active life. And symptoms may evolve from florid psychotic manifestations to more pervasive affective and behavioral characteristics such as anxiety and withdrawal [17].

Thus, interestingly, the progression of research has brought conceptualization back to the Kraepelinian-like notion of longitudinal processes, perhaps with a significant endogenous component. But now, from a broader perspective, these longitudinal processes appear to involve not only the disorder but the person's social functioning, certain environmental characteristics, and the interactions among these factors.

Is it possible to specify more precisely the nature of these processes? Given the complexities of the phenomena involved, traditional studies of one or two variables, while valuable, can provide only a very incomplete and sometimes even a misleading perspective. Systematic exploratory research employing pattern-recognition techniques is required as well [18]. Such an approach involves empirical studies focusing on an overview of the phenomena involved to search systematically for patterns of relationships and the description of potentially important variables at various levels of abstraction. Utilizing such an approach, clues to the nature of the longitudinal processes in schizophrenia have recently become available.

Phases

To begin with, these clues involve the possibility of phases existing in the course of disorder. Data from patients interviewed repeatedly at regular intervals about symptoms, personal functioning, and environmental shifts have suggested that there are certain phases that may be identified in the period following an exacerbation in the course of schizophrenia. The phases include a symptomatic and functioning plateau with minor shifts that we have called "woodshedding" during which time small, barely measurable increments of skills and self-esteem occur. There are other periods with rather sudden shifts in symptoms and functioning status that we have called "change points." At a change point, many new situations may arise at once even though only one change had been planned. When a patient takes a job, for example, not only is a new work experience involved, but new relationships (with supervisor and coworkers), new family roles, new abilities to transport oneself to and from work, and new expectations are generated. Such phases help to characterize the nonlinear evolution of disorder and recovery processes [16].

Beyond these simple phases reflecting only global functioning, we have described complex phases such as "mountain climbing" in which a plateau of function in one area such as work is accompanied by an increase of functioning in another such as social relationships.

Toward a Theoretical Synthesis

It is important to reach beyond these beginning descriptions. Several possibilities present themselves. For example, the phases can be considered in relation to developmental phenomena [19], or a more detailed demonstration of the descriptive validity of the phases can be undertaken [20]. But in this report I would like to take a third approach – the characterization of broader processes of course by more detailed but more speculative analysis of the phases and then by attempting to synthesize theoretically the range of empirically based descriptions.

We have reviewed data related to heterogeneity and multidimensionality of outcome in schizophrenia, the likelihood that these dimensions constitute open-linked systems, the active role of the patient in course of disorder, the nonlinearity of course, and the possibility that phases exist in the evolution of personal functioning, symptoms, and environmental features. These are still relatively isolated notions not following or reflecting any general principles. To understand how these might suggest more general processes, a greater degree of speculation in the goal of pattern recognition is required. It is important to take this step in order to develop hypotheses and to begin the ultimately essential task of synthesis.

In order to take such a step from an empirical base and thus utilize the data that are available to harness the speculations as much as possible, we return again to the findings from our intensive follow-up studies, the research of other investigators, and some examples from clinical experience as well. Two kinds of information are particularly useful: a more detailed analysis of certain phases and phase transitions, and a broader overview of patterns in the course of disorder.

Some Details of Phases and Phase Transitions

Ongoing, more focused investigations with a new series of subjects have developed further some of the earlier hypotheses regarding characteristics of the phases. In preliminary work, Aronson and I have suggested that the mountain-climbing pattern may be the path that leads most often to sustained improvement. In contrast, simultaneous upward shifts in several areas of functioning may eventually lead more often to failure. In other studies, Ownbey and I have suggested that following hospital discharge there is a woodshedding period with special characteristics of a refractory period. In this period following discharge, the person is minimally responsive to new demands and acts to avoid them. Finally,

Lieberman and I have suggested certain kinds of psychological changes in cognitive functioning, self-esteem, and perception of others that patients may go through during hospitalization which underlie these phases and, for example, permit patients to be discharged from the hospital and be strong enough even to have a refractory period [21]. Together, these observations indicate that certain processes may be operating that limit the suddenness of change and require functional improvements before productive changes can occur. Although these tentative findings are still isolated, they begin to suggest an outline that needs another piece to provide a more substantial picture.

Patterns

From a broad perspective, what does the course of schizophrenia look like? If the course is heterogeneous and if it is nonlinear, then a major question is that of what patterns can be found in the vicissitudes. Reviewing our data from a point of view still broader and more speculative than that reported above, as well as the reports of others, such as Bleuler [6], Ciompi [7], and Huber et al. [8], who have retrospectively described the evolution of schizophrenia, suggests several clues that might help us move further towards a speculative synthesis.

In spite of the difficulties with recall problems in data from retrospective studies and the shortcomings in definitively establishing sequences in our subjects, certain patterns are found in both kinds of research and in clinical reports that may provide data to help interpret findings on the course of schizophrenia. Four patterns may be particularly important. The first is that of a relatively sudden recovery after a long chronic or deteriorating course. In such instances patients report waking up and just feeling different or, adding a causal attribution, they say such things as "I just saw the other patients around me and decided I had to pull myself together, that I had sunk as low as I could go." Hospital staff will report: "One day he was just better," or "I came back to work after the weekend and he had really changed." As likely as such reports are to generate skepticism in those of us used to thinking in a more linear and mechanistic fashion, their clarity and frequency emanating from a variety of sources is such that they are ignored at the risk of avoiding data in order to satisfy skepticism.

And the skepticism itself may arise more from bias than do the data. Although attributions of cause must be viewed with caution in such instances, sudden changes occurring after a prolonged phase are not at all rare in illness, human functioning, or in nature more generally. Especially if one is dealing with complex systems rather than additive processes, sudden change may be the rule rather than the exception. A longstanding fever may resolve suddenly. Long plateaus of motor function may be followed by sudden surges in skill level, and insight learning occurs suddenly after extended periods of minimal apparent cognitive improvement [22]. Possible mechanisms of such change have been suggested in many areas and demonstrated in the field of biochemistry [23] and psychopharmacology [24].

A second pattern in the evolution of disorders is that in which variations in some aspects of the person's symptoms, functioning, or environment change but the totality or other parts remain the same. This is almost the antithesis of the first pattern. Rather than a sudden major state change occurring, minor or moderate shifts take place that have almost no impact on other aspects of functioning or on the person generally. One subject in our study, a young woman with persistent hallucinations lasting for over a year, was hospitalized after decompensating to the point where she could not work and could only barely relate socially. Following discharge she took a job and worked adequately, but the hallucinations and limited social relations persisted over the 2-year follow-up period.

A third pattern is the helical progress towards recovery described by McCrory (personal communication). This pattern is characterized by slow improvement followed by slight relapse followed by further improvement and another slight relapse.

A fourth pattern is one characterized by what we have called a ceiling [16]. A patient improves to a certain level but then finds it extremely difficult to penetrate that level, perhaps relapsing, reaching it again, staying there or relapsing once more. One subject in our study tried three times over a 6-year period to attend college. Although he had improved in many areas such as autonomous living, relating, and work, each time he returned to college he became psychotic again.

Control Mechanisms as Contributors to Healing and Chronicity: Three Hypotheses

The data from detailed and overview perspectives on the course of schizophrenia indicate that patterns in the course of disorder might be nonrandom, and suggest mechanisms that might determine those patterns. Although arguments could be made for psychodynamic hypotheses or for deciding that not enough information was available even to speculate, I would like to suggest three hypotheses. Considered together, the totality of information now available suggests that: (1) We are dealing with systems whose changes are governed by control mechanisms. (2) These mechanisms are conscious and unconscious psychological regulatory processes that modulate change during the course of disorder and recovery through compensatory shifts in the organism. Although these mechanisms may be best understood at a psychological rather than a social or biological level of explanation, the latter are certainly relevant. (3) Finally, because of the complexity of these processes there is considerable variability in their operation, making it difficult to identify them reliably.

In the patterns, for example – sudden recovery, consistency in spite of change in one area, the helix, and ceilings – the occurrence or absence of changes in the processes of healing and chronicity may take place because of compensatory operations that permit or prevent major system shifts. Perhaps, for instance, after an episode of disorder certain amounts of energy, self-esteem, and skills are needed before an effort at a higher level of functioning and engagement can succeed. In such a case, a psychological control mechanism may serve to keep the person in a woodshedding phase until an increased level of these characteristics is attained to make survival of a change point likely or even a possibility. Such a control mechanism generating a woodshedding phase could be essential to providing a chance for survival through the many new demands at coping and adaptation that even a relatively common change point such as starting a job involves. A phasic process of this kind involving control mechanisms to help modulate the timing of shifts might be an essential part of the healing process.

Before developing these hypotheses further, some comments about control theory are necessary. Control theory has many foundations in the work of Claude Bernard [25], in cybernetics [26], and in systems theory [27–29]. It emphasizes that for complex systems, regulatory processes exist that provide both for constancy ("homeostasis") and for the maintenance of certain aspects of constancy while also generating change in the course of adaptation and development. Although of demonstrated value in understanding such biological processes as neuroendocrine functioning and ecological systems, control theory, especially when applied to more speculative fields, has often been used as a panacea to explain all things and has added little while giving the impression of providing answers. In spite of this hazard, control theory is used here to suggest a foundation for understanding processes of healing and chronicity in schizophrenia because so many of the clues from the data reviewed seem to point in that direction. This is not to say that control mechanisms account entirely for the evolution of schizophrenia and recovery or that other causal processes are not important as well.

Thus in reviewing a wide range of available data, we have arrived at a way of organizing their complexity [30] that may serve as an explanation for them. This organization allows for the inclusion not only of results from large sample studies and systematic intensive research, but also of clinical reports and observations that have been systematically ignored because they were too anecdotal to be in keeping with the methods, concepts, and metaphors dominant in this area of inquiry [31].

Why have regulatory processes in severe psychiatric disorders been proposed only infrequently [32]? Why have they been explored so rarely from an empirical base? To some extent these questions can be approached by noting the conceptual foundation often viewed currently as the only legitimate basis for scientific inquiry. Aristotle described four kinds of causality, among them efficient cause, focusing on the immediate precursor of an event, and final cause, the goal toward which a process leads. Modern science is often believed to be valid if it focuses on only efficient cause. This focus is particularly effective in learning about simple, linear processes. Perhaps the more vigorously a field attempts to be scientific, the more uncompromisingly it strives to limit itself to this type of causality. But if control processes are involved in the course of schizophrenia and other severe mental disorders, a focus on final cause may be particularly important in spite of the problems of teleology and method involved. Traditional research methods that homogenize data from large samples and define variables concretely rather than in terms of function may be useful to detect efficient causes in linear systems, but may render it difficult, perhaps impossible, to define the causal processes in complex systems governed by control mechanisms. Attention to the functional equivalences of concrete variables, to the feedback processes and sequences of events and states in an individual may be essential to detect control mechanisms.

The basic notion of the course of schizophrenia which I am suggesting is that it is arrived at by the juggling of several interacting systems under the guidance of control mechanisms. These control mechanisms are most readily viewed as psychological in nature and as "seeking" certain psychological state properties required for the organism to function. Furthermore, the specific variables central to reaching the psychological states may vary for different individuals, depending on the functional roles of those variables for that person.

What are these control processes that tend to generate certain states or goals? What do they involve? To offer a possible answer, it is best to review the phenomena of course from the vantage point that such mechanisms might exist. We will begin with the phases in the course of disorder. One way of viewing these is in terms of their implications for governing rate of change. It is possible to view the process of mountain climbing, for example, as using stability in one area of function to balance change occurring in another, i.e., to limit the maximum amount of change occurring during a period of time. It is possible to view the combination of a woodshedding phase plus the following change point as limiting the total change that can occur in a temporal period. In these instances the phases may be longitudinal mechanisms for limiting the amount of change the organism will have to traverse in a given time, a limit related perhaps to the amount of change the person is psychologically and/or biologically capable of managing in that period.

Moving to the phase transitions observed in more detail, as noted earlier, we have suggested that at the time of certain environmental shifts such as hospital discharge, many patients pass through a kind of refractory – or mini-hibernation – period. Originally, when considering the question of how patients change, Ownbey and I decided that change points in the person might be most likely to occur around major environmental shifts. Viewing hospital discharge as an excellent, relatively standard and predictable environmental shift, Ownbey conducted a series of interviews of patients just before and just after hospital discharge. Our first reaction was one of disappointment; the patients did not seem to change at all. After discharge, they often sat apathetically at home watching television for long periods and rarely engaged in any activity. They seemed listless at the follow-up interview and had little to report. Then we speculated that perhaps they were telling us something, that what was being reflected by such patients was a reduction in their energy output and activity, perhaps as a compensation for the major environmental shift through which they were passing.

The possibility that regulatory processes are involved in the course of severe mental illness is further supported by reviewing earlier work [13] on mechanisms patients use to control their symptoms. Withdrawal, increased activity, self-instruction: all can be viewed, especially when amplified by patients' more detailed descriptions, as ways of modulating pressures and changes through the use of compensatory mechanisms.

Perceptual processes and affect as well as cognition and behavior may be essential to the control mechanisms. In all instances – the phases, the patterns, the more detailed observations of mountain climbing and hospital discharge, and the self-help studies – patients' perceptions and feelings about their situation as potentially overwhelming or too blandly neutral may be important, influencing their reactions and activating various mechanisms they use consciously and unconsciously to regulate their situation.

But a major problem, even at this early level of conceptualization, remains. In what sense is it meaningful to talk about control processes in people with severe mental disorders? Control specifically of what? Although the concept of "level of stimulation" used in some of the research cited earlier might be an answer, this notion is somewhat like "stress," in that it seems to be specific, but when one looks at it carefully major complexities appear. Academic psychology learned long ago that the concept of stimulus level as it relates to organism behavior was far more elusive than had been imagined – even for lower organisms [39]. The volume of a tone, the temperature of water, or other such simple notions of stimulus level are of little value for understanding behavior in many instances and certainly in the complex situations of everyday human life.

Unfortunately, any simple definition of what is controlled seems likely to be inaccurate and perhaps even harmfully misleading. It is not possible to generalize from the decibel levels of a tone to the amount of stimulus a person is dealing with in his or her life in any direct way. Patients with schizophrenia are supposed to be vulnerable to high levels of stimulation but certainly this is not just noise level or its equivalent – many patients with schizophrenia appeared at least as able to tolerate the old noisy back wards as did staff. And in terms of even broader notions of stimulus, there are many instances of catatonic patients who had been immobile providing major assistance or even leadership for ward staff at the extremely high "stimulus level" generated by a fire or flood.

It appears that the best way of considering what is being controlled is to use a complex but tentative answer. What is being controlled may best be considered at two levels.

The Most Basic Level of what Is Controlled

Perhaps the "final cause" that is the goal of regulatory behavior is to modulate the demand for functioning to fit the person's adaptive capacity available. If adaptive capacity must be utilized for dealing with increased demands from environmental change, for example, the person may reduce functioning in other areas such as improvement in social relations or work. This hypothesis is offered because it provides a general orientation to key processes that seem to operate. It is proposed in spite of the problems involved in arriving at operational definitions of key variables such as "demand for functioning" and "adaptive capacity available."

A major source of these problems is the difficulty in defining these variables by descriptors rather than by individualized functional criteria. Environmental changes are one example of this problem. For some people, certain environmental changes involve major efforts at adjustment. For other people, the same "objective" environmental changes are not associated with increased adaptive demands but actually supply components essential for psychological functioning such as optimal levels of structure, self-esteem, social contacts, or involvement in purposeful activity [40]. One subject in our study who was chronically delusional became less symptomatic on leaving the hospital in order to return to work. The work setting she said was far better than the hospital for "organizing" her.

An Intermediate Level of what Is Controlled

The problem of definition is reduced significantly by description of a second level more specific than modulating "demand for functioning" to fit "adaptive capacity available." Among the more specific factors of what gets controlled appear to be the components – structure, self-esteem, social contacts, and involvement in purposeful activity – mentioned above. These characteristics are relatively definable indicators of what is likely to be a demand for functioning or a level of adaptive capacity. For example, when a patient has disorganized thinking, low levels of environmental structure are likely to place an extreme demand on this aspect of adaptive capacity. Such a lack of fit between person and environment is likely to generate attempts to adapt, perhaps by one of the self-control mechanisms described earlier, and/or decompensation in terms of increased psychotic symptoms. But even at this intermediate level the individualized functional implications of a situation are crucial. A particularly routine job, for example, appears to be structuring for a disorganized patient, contributing to a reduction in hallucinations. But the same job may be boring to a better organized patient, contributing to distraction and worsening of hallucinations.

Modulating Variables

At both levels of what is controlled, the functional impact of a given environmental situation seems to be modulated by perceptual and interpretational proclivities of the person, and perhaps by that person's own sense of vulnerability, goals, and behavioral options. Trying to exclude the patient as a person from the equation for some kind of supposed scientific neatness seems unwise and inaccurate. For example, the capacity of a person to "pull myself together" is influenced by his or her state of fragmentation, motivation, perception of social supports, seeing sick people around, length of disability, and perhaps also by some endogenous characteristics of symptomatology and premorbid social function.

Although the complexity generated by considering the two levels of control and the modulating variables is immense, research may be facilitated by intensive study of individual patients over time. Such an approach controls some of the variability for research analogous to what clinicians face and attempt to deal with in practice.

Relation of the Control Hypotheses to Other Theories

Pathology or Health?

One might view the control mechanisms as related to problems in management of incoming information, connecting our hypotheses to several long-standing theories focusing on the etiology of mental illness, especially of schizophrenia [33–35]. The notion of control mechanisms might similarly be viewed as relating to certain theories of symptom formation. Delusions, for example [37], are often viewed as a way of attempting to compensate for being overwhelmed by painful ideas or by cognitive disorganization. Our work has implications for such theories about the etiology of disorder, but its major focus at present is on the course of disorders suggesting that control processes are important especially for healing and recovery. In fact, our findings suggest that control processes are some of the major mechanisms governing recovery.

Lower or Higher Mechanisms of Functioning?

In another related area, investigators have conducted research focusing on the roles of families and phenothiazines as influencing symptomatology through their effects on "arousal levels" [36, 38]. These studies have contributed to understanding problems that people with schizophrenia may have in dealing with certain kinds of experiences, but in their theoretical framework the investigators have focused on lower biological mechanisms such as arousal and on patients as more or less passive recipients of environmental stimuli. I am suggesting that there is a higher, more complex, but perhaps related level at which patients are best viewed as active participants in person/illness/environment interactions. In their activity patients appear to use control mechanisms involving the highest levels of psychological functioning. What has been almost universally left out of the arousal studies, based probably on the use of a relatively narrow and mechanistic interpretation of the medical model, is the impact of the patient as a person on the processes influencing course of disorder.

Diagnostic Specificity

Certain theories of psychopathology, especially of schizophrenia, hypothesize the existence of specific underlying problems and view the removal or amelioration of these problems as the basic goal of treatment. The various control processes described in this report do not appear to be diagnostically specific. The data currently available suggest that there may be some similarity of control efforts and problems within a diagnostic group but that in many aspects – the phases and self-help methods, for example – similar control mechanisms are used across several diagnostic entities.

Thus, reviewing all these considerations, the three hypotheses stated earlier can be elaborated further. First, control mechanisms appear crucial in the course of disorder, influencing improvement as well as relapse. Second, these mechanisms involve conscious and unconscious psychological processes that focus on regulating the amount of demand faced to fit the adaptive capacity available. This is accomplished by dealing with stresses, supports, and life changes and their impact on the patient through complex perceptual, interpretive, and behavioral means. Finally, I suggest that because people may attempt to use various kinds of mechanisms to deal with different kinds of problems arising from a range of environmental, psychological, and neurophysiological sources, there is considerable variation by person and perhaps by diagnosis regarding the kind of regulation required and the best mechanism for accomplishing that regulation. There seems likely to be no universal solution based on diagnosis alone. However, intensive study of the coping styles and vulnerabilities of individuals over time might reveal a finite number of person-diagnosis patterns [4].

The implications of such mechanisms for research and treatment are immense. Research on patients during their course, whether focused on clarifying an aspect of psychopathology or on treatment impact, would require consideration of these control mechanisms. Determining when a patient should return home, to work, or to school following a psychotic episode would depend on understanding and assessing these processes.

What these findings and this conceptualization suggest then is that in the course of schizophrenia and other severe mental disorders we are dealing with complex interacting processes, that these processes, among other things, involve conscious and unconscious psychological control mechanisms the person uses, and that these in turn are constituted not only of simple stimulus/response reflex arcs or arousal mechanisms, but involve a wide range of individualized "person" characteristics such as perceptual style, meaning, affect, and goals. Thus, to understand and treat schizophrenia and ameliorate its course it seems most likely that we must attend in research and treatment to these psychological control mechanisms, the related person variables, and the ways in which the control mechanisms influence interactions between the illness, the person, and the environment over time.

Acknowledgements. The author wishes to thank Drs. Hisham Hafez, Courtenay Harding, and Paul Lieberman and also Mr Carrie Clark for their helpful suggestions.

References

1. American Psychiatric Association (1980) Diagnostic and statistical manual III. APA Press, Washington DC
2. Strauss JS, Gabriel KR, Kokes RF, Ritzler BA, VanOrd A, Tarana E (1979) Do psychiatric patients fit their diagnoses? Patterns of symptomatology as described with the biplot. J Nerv Ment Dis 167:105–113
3. Berrios GE (1984) Descriptive psychopathology: conceptual and historical aspects. Psychol Med 14:303–313
4. Strauss JS (1986) Psychiatric diagnosis: a reconsideration based on longitudinal principles. In: Klerman G, Millon T (eds) Contemporary issues in psychopathology. Guilford Press, New York
5. Strauss JS, Carpenter WT Jr (1974) Characteristic symptoms and outcome in schizophrenia. Arch Gen Psychiatry 30:429–434
6. Bleuler M (1972) Die schizophrenen Geistesstörungen im Lichte langjähriger Kranken- und Familiengeschichten. Thieme, Stuttgart. (English 1978) The schizophrenic disorders: long-term patient and family studies. Yale University Press, New Haven
7. Ciompi L (1980) Catamnestic long-term study on the course of life and aging of schizophrenics. Schizophr Bull 6(4):606–618
8. Huber G, Gross G, Schuttler C, Linz M (1980) Longitudinal studies of schizophrenic patients. Schizophr Bull 6(4):592–605
9. Harding CM, Zubin J, Strauss JS (in press) Chronicity in schizophrenia: fact, partial fact, or artifact? Hosp Community Psychiatry

10. Strauss JS, Carpenter WT Jr (1972) Prediction of outcome in schizophrenia. I. Characteristics of outcome. Arch Gen Psychiatry 27:739–746
11. Strauss JS, Carpenter WT Jr (1974) Prediction of outcome in schizophrenia. II. Relationships between predictor and outcome variables. Arch Gen Psychiatry 31:37–42
12. Falloon IRH, Talbot RE (1981) Persistent auditory hallucinations: coping mechanisms and implications for management. Psychol Med 11:329–339
13. Breier A, Strauss JS (1983) Self-control in psychotic disorders. Arch Gen Psychiatry 40(10):1141–1145
14. Cohen CI, Berke LA (1985) Personal coping styles of schizophrenic outpatients. Hosp Community Psychiatry 36:407–410
15. Boeker W (in press) On self-help among schizophrenics: problem analysis and empirical studies. In: Huber G (ed) The psychosocial treatment of schizophrenia
16. Strauss JS, Hafez H, Lieberman P, Harding CM (1985) The course of psychiatric disorder: III. Longitudinal principles. Am J Psychiatry 142(3):289–296
17. Cheadle AJ, Freeman HL, Korer J (1978) Chronic schizophrenic patients in the community. Br J Psychiatry 132:221–227
18. Strauss JS, Hafez H, Harding CM, Liebermann P (in preparation) Clinical questions and real research: II. Systematic exploratory research in psychiatry (submitted for publication)
19. Strauss JS, Harding CM (in press) The impact of adult development on the course of psychiatric disorder. In: Rolf J, Master A, Cicchetti D, Nuechterlein K, Weintraub S (eds) Risk and protective factors in the development of psychopathology. Cambridge University Press, New York
20. Harding CM, Strauss JS, Liebermann P, Hafez H (in preparation) Phases in the course of severe psychiatric disorder: reliability and validity
21. Liebermann P, Strauss JS (in press) Brief hospitalization: what are its effects? Am J Psychiatry
22. Kohler W (1925) The mentality of apes. Routledge & Kegan Paul, London
23. Prigogine I, Allen PM, Herman R (1977) The evolution of complexity and the laws of nature. In: Laszlo M, Bierman S (eds) Goals of mankind, vol 1. Pergamon, New York
24. Bunney BS, Grace AA, Meltzer LP (1974) Midbrain dopaminergic neurons: a new model of their functioning. Clin Neuropharmacol 7 [Suppl 1]:92–93
25. Bernard C (1957) An introduction to the study of experimental medicine. Dover, New York
26. Wiener N (1948) Cybernetics. Wiley, New York
27. Von Bertalanffy L (1968) General system theory. Braziller, New York
28. Miller JG (1978) Living systems. McGraw-Hill, New York
29. deRosnay J (1975) Le macroscope. Editions du Seuil, Paris
30. Simon HA (1973) The organization of complex systems. In: Pattee HH, Brazilier G (eds) Hierarchy theory. The challenge of complex systems. New York
31. Lakoff G, Johnson M (1980) Metaphors we live by. University of Chicago Press, Chicago
32. Melges F, Freeman AM (1975) Persecutory delusions: a cybernetic model: Am J Psychiatry 132(10):1038–1044
33. Silverman J (1967) Variations in cognitive control and psychophysiological defense in the schizophrenias. Psychosom Med 29(3):225–251
34. Nuechterlein KH, Edell WS, Norris M, Dawson ME (1986) Attentional vulnerability indicators, thought disorder and negative symptoms. Schizophr Bull 12:408–426
35. Freud S (1955) Beyond the pleasure principle. In: The complete works of Sigmund Freud, standard edition. Hogarth, London, pp 7–64
36. Wing JK (1975) Impairments in schizophrenia: a rational basis for social treatment. In: Wirt RD, Winokur G, Roff M (eds) Life history research in psychopathology, vol 4. University of Minnesota Press, Minneapolis
37. Oltmanns TF, Maher BA (eds) (in press) Delusional beliefs: interdisciplinary perspectives. Wiley, New York
38. Tarrier N, Vaughn C, Lader MH, Leff JP (1979) Bodily reactions to people and events in schizophrenics. Arch Gen Psychiatry 36:311–315
39. Tolman EC (1932) Purposive behavior in animals and men. Century, New York
40. Strauss JS, Loevsky L, Glazer W, Leaf P (1981) Organizing the complexities of schizophrenia. J Nerv Ment Dis 169(2):120–126

Long-Term Outcome of Schizophrenia and Other Psychoses

M. T. TSUANG and J. A. FLEMING

Introduction

Long-term outcome has been used extensively for the purpose of validation and refinement of psychiatric disorders. Outcome data is also essential for the assessment of psychiatric illness because the cross-sectional presentation of a disorder may vary over time and because long-term outcome is one of the distinguishing characteristics of these illnesses. The classification of psychiatric illness according to outcome and other factors such as genetic and biochemical measures have implications in terms of treatment and prognosis.

Over the years a large number of outcome studies concerning schizophrenia have been published (Hawk et al. 1975; Bland and Orn 1978; Carpenter et al. 1981; May et al. 1981; Bland 1982; Knesevich et al. 1983; Cloninger et al. 1985). The results have varied greatly along with the methods of assessing outcome. A well-designed follow-up and outcome study should consider the following factors: (a) diagnostic practices (criteria used to define study groups); (b) length of follow-up; (c) definition of outcome; (d) systematic data collection; (e) use of independent raters to assess outcome; (f) testing of interrater reliability; (g) use of control conditions for comparison purposes and blindness; and (h) use of appropriate statistical techniques.

The results reported here are from an outcome study based on 30- to 40-year field follow-up. We applied specific research criteria for the selection of our psychiatric study subjects; included a surgical control group for comparison purposes and to maintain blindness; used operational criteria to assess outcome on four variables; rated outcome without knowledge of the original diagnoses; and performed interrater reliability studies.

The above standards have previously been applied to our long-term outcome study of schizophrenia and affective disorders (Tsuang et al. 1979). Outcome was determined from a 30- to 40-year follow-up of 685 patients with schizophrenia, affective disorders, and surgical conditions (controls). outcome was analyzed in terms of the patient's marital, residential, occupational, and psychiatric status. The results indicated that psychiatric patients showed a significantly poorer outcome than the surgical controls and that schizophrenia showed a significantly poorer outcome than affective disorders. There was no significant difference between mania and depression. Based on research criteria used to select schizophre-

---

Harvard Schools of Medicine and Public Health; Brockton-West Roxbury VA Medical Center, 940 Belmont Street, Brockton, MA 02401, USA

nia and affective disorders, long-term outcome separated the mentally ill from the healthy control group and also separated the two illnesses.

The aim of this paper is to compare the long-term outcome of the patients with a clinical diagnosis of schizophrenia that were excluded from the original study sample with that of the typical groups of schizophrenia and affective disorder. Exclusion had been on grounds of failure to meet the research criteria (Feighner et al. 1972; Morrison et al. 1972) by reason of short duration of symptoms, episodic course, or the presence of affective symptoms. Since patients in this group received an original (clinical) diagnosis of schizophrenia but failed to meet research criteria we have labeled them "atypical schizophrenics." This study allows us to examine the long-term outcome of all consecutive cases diagnosed as schizophrenia who were admitted to a psychiatric hospital between 1934 and 1944. By comparing the outcome of atypical schizophrenia with that of the typical cases we hope to clarify our understanding of the disorder and its relationship to schizophrenia and affective disorders.

As part of a preliminary study we compared a subsample of the atypical schizophrenics with schizophrenia, affective disorder, and a control group (Tsuang and Dempsey 1979). Eighty-five patients with both schizophrenic and affective features (schizoaffective disorder) at the time of admission were compared with 200 schizophrenic, 325 affective disorder, and 160 control (surgical) patients on the basis of 30- to 40-year outcome. Again patients were assessed on the basis of marital, residential, occupational, and psychiatric status. Patients with schizoaffective disorders had an outcome significantly better than those with schizophrenia but significantly poorer than those with affective disorders and surgical conditions (controls). Overall, schizoaffective disorder fell somewhere between the schizophrenia and the mania group. Therefore, based on long-term outcome, schizoaffective disorder seemed to be different from schizophrenia and affective disorder.

Subjects and Methods

Sample Selection

Samples for this study were chosen from 3800 consecutively admissions to the University of Iowa Psychiatric Hospital between 1934 and 1945. The psychiatric charts were reviewed, and based on research criteria (Feighner et al. 1972; Morrison et al. 1972) we selected 200 cases of schizophrenia, 100 of mania, and 225 of depression. There were 310 patients who had a chart diagnosis of schizophrenia but did not meet the research criteria for schizophrenia (atypical schizophrenia). The controls consisted of 336 appendectomy and herniorrhaphy patients admitted to the surgical department of the University of Iowa's general hospital between 1938 and 1948. The control group is a stratified random sample proportionate to the psychiatric groups in terms of age range at admission, sex ratio, and mode of payment (public or private) as a measure of socioeconomic status.

Mean age at admission for schizophrenia was 28.6 years; atypical schizophrenia, 27.7 mania, 34.2; depression 43.8; and the control group 29.8 years. One-hundred and three (52%) of the schizophrenics were male; 147 (47%) of the atypical schizophrenics; 38 (38%) of the manics; 100 (44%) of the depressives; and 148 (44%) of the controls.

Field Work (Outcome)

The follow-up field work for these subjects was initiated in 1972 and the data collection was completed by the end of 1980. Medical records, which included extensive psychiatric histories, detailed family histories, past medical histories, mental status reports, consultations, progress and treatment notes, and reports on discharge formed the basis for our special search to locate the study subjects. Supplementing these records were complete social histories and reports from physicians at the other four Iowa State Mental Health Institutes.

We first conducted telephone interviews with the surviving subjects and with surviving first-degree relatives of the deceased subjects. For this purpose, we designed a special telephone interview form. If the study subject was dead, we located and talked with another informant from among the study subject's first-degree relatives. Additional information was obtained from public records, churches, school records, and other organizations. After these initial telephone interviews, personal interviews with the living patients were arranged. Interviews of index patients (probands and controls) were conducted using the Iowa Structured Psychiatric Interview (Tsuang et al. 1980). The interview form was rigorously tested for validity and interrater reliability and designed for accurate and efficient administration by trained interviewers. Use of the interview form allowed us not only unbiased and consistent ratings of the subjects, but also the inclusion of a large number of subjects, since the assessments could be performed by well-trained nonpsychiatrists.

Table 1 presents a description of the study groups in terms of follow-up information. All available material up to the time of death or of follow-up, for the

Table 1. Rating and follow-up information for study subjects

	Proband group				
	S	AS	M	D	C
n	200	310	100	225	336
No. traced	195	304	92	223	321
(% n)	(98)	(98)	(92)	(99)	(96)
No. rated	186	291	86	212	307
(% traced)	(95)	(96)	(94)	(95)	(96)
No. deceased	78	115	54	162	101
(% traced)	(40)	(38)	(59)	(73)	(31)
No. living	117	189	38	61	220
(% traced)	(60)	(62)	(41)	(27)	(69)
Personal interview	93	133	25	35	155
(% living)	(79)	(70)	(66)	(57)	(70)

S, schizophrenia; AS, atypical schizophrenia; M, mantia; D, depression; C, control

living, was used to rate the outcome. We were able to trace successfully, to death or current address, 98% of the schizohrenic, 98% of the atypical schizophrenic, 92% of the manic, 99% of the depressive, and 96% of the control subjects. Among the patients traced we obtained adequate information to rate all four outcome variables in 95% of the schizophrenic, 96% of the atypical schizophrenic, 94% of the manic, 95% of the depressive, and 96% of the control subjects. Table 1 also shows the number and percent of the deceased and living along with the percent living who were personally interviewed.

Four outcome variables were rated: marital, residential, and occupational status and the presence of psychiatric symptoms at follow-up. Ratings were made on the basis of all follow-up material collected in addition to the personal interview. A three-point scale was used in which good, fair, and poor were ratings for each outcome variable. The fair category can be analyzed separately or combined with good or poor ratings. Operational criteria for each variable have been defined and presented elsewhere (Tsuang et al. 1979), but for the purpose of this paper the criteria will also be repeated here. The four different outcomes were rated according to the following criteria: (a) For marital status, married or widowed was good, divorced or separated was fair, and being single was poor. (b) For residential status, living in own home or with relatives was good, living at a nursing or county home was fair, and confinement to a mental hospital was poor. (c) For occupational status, being employed, retired, a housewife, or a student was good, being unable to work due to physical incapacity was fair, and being unable to work due to mental illness was poor. (d) For psychiatric status, the absence of symptoms was good, presence of some symptoms was fair, and presence of incapacitating symptoms was poor.

Statistical Analysis

Previously we have compared the long-term outcome of our schizophrenics with that of manic-depressives and controls. For the purpose of this paper, we were interested in comparing atypical schizophrenia with schizophrenia, mania, depression, and the control group. To do this the fair and poor categories were combined which resulted in a comparison of the distribution of cases falling into the good and fair/poor categories for atypical schizophrenia versus the other study groups. This analysis was performed by using a χ^2 statistic to test independence between diagnostic groups. Significant differences are reported at both the $p < 0.05$ and $p < 0.01$ levels, but because of the number of pairwise comparisons performed care should be taken in interpreting those results at the usual 0.05 level.

Results

Table 2 presents the distribution of outcome status by diagnostic group. Shown are the actual numbers and percentages of individuals falling into the good, fair, and poor categories for each outcome variable (marital, residential, occupational,

Table 2. Long-term outcome of atypical schizophrenia (AS) compared with schizophrenia (S), mania (M), depression (D), and a matched control group (C)

Outcome status	Diagnostic group				
	AS $(n=291)$	S $(n=186)$	M $(n=86)$	D $(n=212)$	C $(n=307)$
Marital					
Good	121 (42)	39 (21)[a]	60 (70)[a]	172 (81)[a]	265 (86)[a]
Fair	46 (16)	22 (12)	7 (8)	20 (9)	24 (8)
Poor	124 (43)	125 (67)	19 (22)	20 (9)	18 (6)
Residential					
Good	155 (53)	64 (34)[a]	59 (69)[a]	148 (70)[a]	284 (93)[a]
Fair	107 (37)	89 (48)	15 (17)	39 (18)	21 (7)
Poor	29 (10)	33 (18)	12 (14)	25 (12)	2 (1)
Occupational					
Good	127 (44)	65 (35)	58 (67)[a]	142 (67)[a]	258 (84)[a]
Fair	21 (7)	14 (8)	7 (8)	33 (16)	43 (14)
Poor	143 (49)	107 (58)	21 (24)	37 (17)	6 (2)
Psychiatric					
Good	98 (34)	38 (20)[a]	43 (50)[a]	129 (61)[a]	255 (83)[a]
Fair	71 (24)	48 (26)	18 (21)	37 (18)	39 (13)
Poor	122 (42)	100 (54)	25 (29)	46 (22)	13 (4)

Values in parentheses are percentages
[a] $p<0.01$; [b] $p<0.05$ (comparison with AS for Good vs Fair/Poor)

psychiatric), for atypical schizophrenia, schizophrenia, mania, depression, and a matched control group. Contrasts were made between atypical schizophrenia and the other diagnostic groups by comparing the numbers falling into the good category. Note that in Table 2 atypical schizophrenia is located in the first column with the four comparison groups following in colums 2–5.

For marital status, schizophrenia has the lowest percentage (21%) of good ratings while the control group had the highest (86%). The percentage of good marital status in atypical schizophrenia (42%) is significantly different ($p<0.01$) from schizophrenia, mania (70%), depression (81%), and the control group. Over half of the schizophrenics (67%) and close to half of the atypical schizophrenics (43%) have a poor rating for marital status. In contrast, the affective disorders and controls have a much lower rate of poor outcome.

The distribution of ratings for residential status is similar to that for marital status, with schizophrenia having the lowest percentage (34%) of good ratings and the control group the highest (93%). The percentage of good residential status for atypical schizophrenia (53%) is significantly ($p<0.01$) higher than that for schizophrenia and significantly lower than that for mania (69%), depression (70%), and the control group. The comparison with mania is significant at the $p<0.05$ level, whereas the comparisons with depression and the control group are significant at the $p<0.01$ level. Schizophrenia had the highest percentage of poor ratings (18%), while the percentages of poor ratings in atypical schizophrenia

(10%), mania (14%), and depression (12%) were lower. Only two cases (1%) were rated as poor residential status for the control group.

For occupational status there is no significant difference between atypical schizophrenia (44%) and schizophrenia (35%) for good ratings. However, the percentage of good occupational status in atypical schizophrenia did differ significantly ($p<0.01$) from those in mania (67%), depression (67%), and the control group (84%). Again, schizophrenia had the lowest percentage while the control group had the highest percentage with good occupational status. Almost 60% of the schizophrenics received a poor rating, compared to 49% for atypical schizophrenia, 24% for mania, 17% for depression, and 2% for the control group.

Psychiatric status presents a very clear distinction between the atypical schizophrenia group and the other diagnostic categories. The percentage of good psychiatric status in atypical schizophrenia (34%) is significantly higher ($p<0.01$) than that found in schizophrenia (20%) and significantly lower ($p<0.01$) than those found in mania (50%), depression (61%), and the control group (83%). The schizophrenia group has the largest percentage of poor ratings (54%), compared to 42% in atypical schizophrenia, 29% in mania, 22% in depression, and 4% in control group.

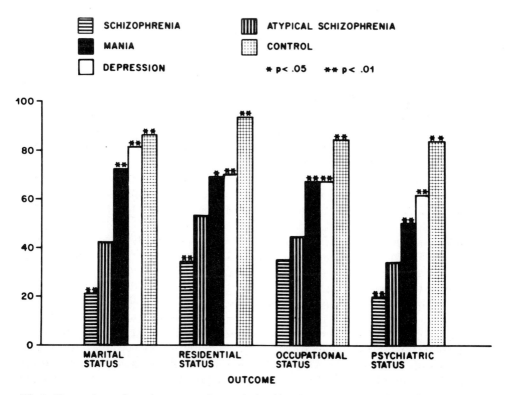

Fig. 1. Comparison of good outcomes in atypical schizophrenia with those in schizophrenia, mania, depression, and a matched control group

The results from Table 2 are presented graphically in Fig. 1. Histograms shown for each outcome variable and diagnostic group represent the percentage of patients with good outcome. For each outcome variable the percentage of good ratings increases by diagnostic group, with schizophrenia having the lowest percentage followed by atypical schizophrenia, mania, depression, and the control group. This becomes most evident on observing the histograms for psychiatric status, where the percentage of good ratings increases progressively through the five study groups. It is clear from Fig. 1 that for all outcomes atypical schizophrenia falls between schizophrenia and affective disorder (mania, depression), and has a significantly poor outcome compared with the controls.

Discussion

Four outcome variables were selected for a comparative study of schizophrenia, atypical schizophrenia, mania, depression, and a matched control group. Marital, residential, occupational, and psychiatric status were rated independently on a three-point scale representing good, fair, and poor outcome in each area. In our categorical analysis presented here, we compared the good category between atypical schizophrenia and each of the other diagnostic groups. This study incorporated important methodology which included: specific research criteria for the selection of our psychiatric study subjects; a surgical control group for comparison purposes; operational criteria to assess outcome on the four variables; a blind study to rate outcome; and a categorical data analysis.

Our results indicate that long-term outcome in atypical schizophrenia is significantly better than that in schizophrenia and significantly poorer than that in mania, depression, and a matched control group. We have previously shown (Tsuang et al. 1979) that the research criteria used to select schizophrenia, mania, and depression separates these disorders on the basis of long-term outcome. The findings presented here show that atypical schizophrenia can also be separated on this basis. Therefore, even though the schizophrenics and atypical schizophrenics all had original clinical diagnoses of schizophrenia, we were able to distinguish the two groups according to 30- to 40-year follow-up information. Research criteria seem to have divided clinical schizophrenia into two categories which differ in prognosis.

Additional work is now being completed to verify these results using multivariate statistical techniques. Since patients vary according to their status at admission, a multivariate analysis of covariance (Morrison 1976) will be performed in order to adjust for differences in the initial assessment. Using this method, not only will we compare atypical schizophrenia with schizophrenia, mania, depression, and the control group for each outcome variable, we will also make simultaneous comparisons of the diagnostic groups across all outcome variables. In our previous work comparing the outcome of four study groups (schizophrenia, mania, depression, and control), we found that the results of the categorical analysis were the same as those of multivariate analysis of covariance. We would also expect in the present analysis, where we are now comparing atypical schizophrenia to these four diagnostic groups, that the results using the multivariate techniques will be very similar to those we have reported here. In addition, inter-active effects between outcome measures and diagnostic categories are being tested using log-linear models (Fienberg 1981). Using this methodology we will also be able to stratify on other variables of interest such as age and sex in order to measure their effect.

Our results suggest, on the basis of long-term outcome, that atypical schizo-phrenia is neither a form of schizophrenia nor a form of major affective disorder, but rather a distinct and possibly heterogeneous diagnostic category. Since it is highly likely that homogeneous subgroups exist within atypical schizophrenia, we have developed a method for subtyping the disorder. Using our four outcome variables (marital, residential, occupational, psychiatric) we made comparisons among the subgroups, and also between the subgroups and the typical groups of schizophrenia and affective disorder, as a means of validating the subtypes ac-cording to prognosis.

The subtyping procedures have been published elsewhere (Tsuang et al. 1986) but will be summarized for the purpose of this paper. Logistic regression tech-niques (Engelman 1981) were used to break down the 310 atypical schizophrenics into three subtypes. Because we felt that there would be a subtype resembling schizophrenia and one resembling affective disorder, we used admission data from the schizophrenia and affective disorder groups to accomplish the analysis. At admission each of the patients was rated according to variables categorized as either demographic or clinical. From this information we isolated individual vari-ables that would be useful in separating the atypical schizophrenia patients into homogeneous subgroups. In selecting a discriminating set of variables, two prin-ciples were kept in mind. First, a variable had to reflect substantial variability within the atypical schizophrenia group, or else it would have no discriminating power when applied to subtyping. Secondly, to distinguish subtypes a set of vari-ables must be chosen that separate schizophrenia from affective disorder. Eleven variables met both criteria and were used for the subtyping analysis. If a subject was not rated on all 11 variables he/she was omitted from the analysis.

A logistic regression equation was generated where the admission data were independent variables and the dependent variable was defined according to whether the patient was schizophrenic or affective. This equation, when applied to the atypical schizophrenia data acts as a means of prediction by calculating the probability that an individual patient belongs to the schizophrenia population. When calculated for each atypical schizophrenic, the probabilities ranged from 0.0027 [closest to affective disorder (0.0)] to [most resembling schizophrenia (1.0)]. Cutoff probabilities which yielded maximum discrimination between sub-groups were determined, resulting in three distinct subgroups. An examination of the probability distribution indicated that the selected cutoff points coincided with natural breaks in the frequency distribution. One group ($n = 111$) resembled schizophrenia (schizophrenic subtype, probability > 0.75)), one group ($n = 103$) resembled affective disorder (affective subtype, probability < 0.5), and a third group ($n = 57$) fell in between the schizophrenic and affective subtypes (undiffer-entiated subtype, probability 0.5–0.75).

Diagnostic categories can be verified in a number of ways, including the ex-amination of family history, biochemical measurements, and long-term outcome (prognosis). Using the same outcome rating described previously we compared schizophrenic, affective, and undifferentiated subtypes on the basis of marital, residential, occupational and psychiatric status at follow-up. The comparisons among the three subgroups across the four outcomes suggest an initial validation of subtypes. For all four variables the schizophrenia subtype had the poorest outcome and the affective subtype had the best outcome, the undifferentiated subtype falling between them.

To carry the validation process one step further we compared the outcome in each atypical schizophrenic subtype with the corresponding outcome in the typical groups of schizophrenia and affective disorder. For each of the outcome variables there was no significant difference between the schizophrenic subtype and the schizophrenia group; in fact their rates of good outcome were very similar. When we compared the schizophrenic subtype and the affective disorder group, we found that the rate of good outcome status was significantly ($p < 0.01$) lower in the schizophrenic subtype for all four measures. The opposite was found when the affective subtype was examined. The affective subtype had a significantly ($p < 0.01$) higher rate of good outcome for all four variables when compared with schizophrenia, but only one difference was found when it was compared with the affective disorder group, namely the rate of good marital status in affective disorder was significantly higher than that found in the affective subtype.

As expected, there was no clear pattern with the undifferentiated subtype. For marital status the undifferentiated subtype had a signficantly higher percentage of good rating than schizophrenia and a significantly lower rate of good status than the affective disorder group. The undifferentiated subgroup had a significantly higher percentage of good ratings than schizophrenia for residential status, but did not differ from affective disorder. Conversely, for occupational status the undifferentiated subtype differed from affective disorder but not from schizophrenia. Finally, for psychiatric status the undifferentiated subtype did not differ from schizophrenia but had a significantly lower percentage of good ratings than affective disorder.

We have examined the long-term follow-up data of 510 consecutive admissions, all of whom received a clinical diagnosis of schizophrenia. Based on a review of all chart material 200 of these cases met research criteria for schizophrenia. The remaining 310 cases who had a clinical diagnosis of schizophrenia on admission but did not meet research criteria for schizophrenia were labeled "atypical schizophrenia." Based on four outcome variables measured at follow-up, the atypical schizophrenia group seems to be a separate but heterogeneous disorder when compared with schizophrenia and affective disorder. We have defined three subtypes of atypical schizophrenia; one which behaves like schizophrenia, one which resembles affective disorder, and one which falls between these two subtypes (undifferentiated). These results have implications for the treatment of psychiatric disorders falling in between schizophrenia and affective disorder and also for the definition of homogeneous subgroups for future biological and genetic research.

References

Bland RC (1982) Predicting the outcome in schizophrenia. Can J Psychiatry 27:52–62

Bland RC, Orn H (1978) 14-year outcome in early schizophrenia. Acta Psychiatr Scand 58:327–338

Carpenter WT, Heinrichs DW, HanLon TE (1981) Methodologic standards for treatment outcome research in schizophrenia. Am J Psychiatry 138:(4):465–471

Cloninger RC, Martin RL, Guze SB, Clayton PJ (1985) Diagnosis and prognosis in schizophrenia. Arch Gen Psychiatry 42:15–25

Engelman L (1981) Stepwise logistic regression. In: Dixon W (ed) BMDP statistical software. University of California Press, Berkeley, pp 330–344

Feighner JP, Robins E, Guze SB, Woodraff RA, Winokur G, Munoz R (1972) Diagnostic criteria for use in psychiatric research. Arch Gen Psychiatry 26:57–63

Fienberg SE (1981) The analysis of cross-classified categorical data, 2nd edn. Wiley, New York

Hawk AB, Carpenter WT, Strauss JS (1975) Diagnostic criteria and five-year outcome in schizophrenia. Arch Gen Psychiatry 32:343–347

Knesevich JW, Zalcman SJ, Clayton PJ (1983) Six-year follow-up of patients with carefully diagnosed good- and poor-prognosis schizophrenia. Am J Psychiatry 140(11):1507–1510

May Pr, Tuma AH, Dixon WJ (1981) Schizophrenia: a follow-up study of the results of five forms of treatment. Arch Gen Psychiatry 38:776–784

Morrison DF (1976) Multivariate analysis of covariance. In: Morrinson DF: Multivariate statistical methods, 2nd edn. McGraw-Hill, New York, pp 193–204

Morrison J, Clancy J, Crowe R, Winokur G (1972) The Iowa 500: I. Diagnostic validity in mania, depression and schizophrenia. Arch Gen Psychiatry 27:457–461

Tsuang MT, Dempsey GM (1979) Long-term outcome of major psychoses: II. Schizoaffective disorder compared with schizophrenia, affective disorders, and a surgical control group. Arch Gen Psychiatry 36:1302–1304

Tsuang MT, Woolson RF, Fleming JA (1979) Long-term outcome of major psychoses: I. Schizophrenia and affective disorders compared with psychiatrically symptom-free surgical conditions. Arch Gen Psychiatry 36:1295–1301

Tsuang MT, Woolson RF, Simpson JC (1980) The Iowa Structure Psychiatric Interview: rationale, reliability and validity. Acta Psychiatr Scand [Suppl 283]:1–38

Tsuang MT, Simpson JC, Fleming JA (1986) Diagnostic criteria for subtyping schizoaffective disorder. In: Marneros A, Tsuang MT (eds) Schizoaffective psychoses. Springer, Berlin Heidelberg New York Tokyo, pp 50–62

Factors Influencing the Course and Outcome of Symptomatology and Social Adjustment in First-Onset Schizophrenics

C. Schubart, B. Krumm, H. Biehl, K. Maurer, and E. Jung

Introduction

The increasing knowledge accumulated in recent years concerning relevant social factors and psychological variables in course and outcome of schizophrenia has emphasized the variability of schizophrenic patterns of course. As a consequence, there has been an increasing interest in long-term studies to define clinically relevant risk groups that should be provided with special care. Predictors should help to identify patients facing a special risk of relapse at an early point of time.

Theoretical Background and Methodological Problems

In recent studies (Bleuler 1972; Ciompi and Müller 1976; Strauss and Carpenter 1977; Huber et al. 1979; Andreasen 1982; Crow et al. 1982; Möller and v. Zerssen 1986) a set of biological, psychopathological, and psychological variables have been identified as relevant prognostic factors in schizophrenia. Concerning psychopathological variables, the prognostic relevance of the acute psychotic symptomatology could not be confirmed, whereas the presence of "negative symptoms," the chronicity of illness, and the type of onset were found to be significant predictors. Concerning biological variables, anatomical abnormalities of the cerebral ventricles were reported to be the most relevant prognostic factor. Additionally, premorbid adjustment and personality, some sociodemographic factors, and life events at the beginning of psychotic episodes were reported to be significant predictors, with high agreement between the different long-term studies.

Nevertheless, there are still many equivocal results. What are the reasons for these inconsistencies? One possible explanation is insufficient comparability between the studies:

1. The criteria for the definition of outcome are different: outcome is assessed by psychopathological variables (e.g., duration and extent of psychotic symptomatology), by social adjustment, or, in some cases, by a mixture of both.

2. Even if the criteria are precisely defined, they are operationalized and assessed in different ways.

3. The cohorts under study differ in many respects, e.g., they consist of varying proportions of chronic and first-hospitalization schizophrenics.

Central Institute of Mental Health, J5, P.O. Box 5970, 6800 Mannheim, Federal Republic of Germany

4. The studies are based on varying time periods between initial assessment and outcome.

One common aim of all long-term studies – the identification of clinically relevant risk groups – was not achieved. Therefore, many results do not permit general statements which are of practical relevance for psychiatrists working with schizophrenic patients, nor do they enlarge our knowledge on the process of illness.

Questions concerning the different relative weight of predictors and their significance for the course of illness remain more or less open. One reason for this may be that former studies paid too little attention to certain theoretical considerations and methodological problems:

1. The predictors were related singly to course and outcome without investigating possible interactions of these variables.

2. The association between predictors and outcome may be biased by the influence of confounding variables. For example, it was possible to demonstrate that the association between sex and severity of illness is affected by the different patterns of utilization of mental health care facilities (Salokangas 1983). Analyzing sex as a predictor of outcome, one can conclude that men are more likely to show a worse outcome than women which might have implications for their treatment. It is possible, however, that the correlation between sex and outcome is produced by a correlation between age and sex. If this is so, one would, for example, consider only the younger male schizophrenics as a poor-prognosis group. Ignoring existing confounding variables and interactions may lead to wrong conclusions.

3. Predictors assessed immediately after onset of psychosis may change during the course of the investigation. Changes may occur in occupational status, living situation or in variables concerning the expressed emotions (EE) of the key figure (the person with whom the patient spent most time). As a consequence, the associations between predictors and outcome may vary at different cross sections during the course of illness.

Based upon these considerations, we formulated the following list of formal requirements for an "ideal" predictor:

– Early assessment: it should be possible to assess the predictor immediately after onset of psychosis; longitudinal data, for example duration of treatment, do not meet this criterion.
– Reliability: it should be possible to assess the predictor in a reliable way.
– Vector of association: characteristics predictive for a good outcome at one time point should remain predictive for a good outcome over time, and vice versa.
– Exclusion of confoundation: it has to be excluded that the predictor-outcome association is attributable to confounding variables; if there is such an influence, variables which change these results must be taken into consideration.
– Stability of association: the predictor-outcome association should remain stable over time; inconsistency of results must be explained.

We will now present data from a prospective 5-year follow-up study of schizophrenic patients with recent onset of illness with special reference to these theoretical considerations, which will be illustrated by examples.

The WHO Collaborative Study on the Assessment and Reduction of Psychiatric Disability

Definition of Outcome and Measuring Scales

Psychopathology was assessed separately for the acute psychotic symptomatology and the observed "minus signs" (behavior). The acute symptomatology was operationalized by the reported symptoms in the Present State Examination (PSE). This instrument only takes into account 4 weeks preceding each examination. Therefore, it is necessary to record the presence of psychotic symptoms for the periods in between, in order to obtain longitudinal information on time spent in acute psychotic episodes. This was done by summing up the number of months during the past year in which the patient had had productive symptoms, such as delusion, hallucinations and/or thought disorders. The minus signs were rated by means of observed behavior with the Psychological Impairment Rating Scale (PIRS); the single items of the different sections (slowness, loss of initiative, reduced gesture, flatness of affect) are then added to give a global score.

In the context of this study, deficits in "social adjustment" are called (social) "disability," a term used by WHO in the *International Classification of Impairments, Disabilities and Handicaps* (ICIDH; WHO 1980). Disability is defined as a disturbance of social functions or roles (in family, social group, work, etc.) expected by the social group of the index person and assessed by the Disability Assessment Scale (DAS), which measures the actual social role performance during the last 4 weeks and developed within the framework of this study (Jablensky et al. 1980).

Description of the Cohort

The following analyses are based on the WHO collaborative study on the assessment and reduction of psychiatric disability, which has been carried out since 1978 in seven different centers. The investigation at the Central Institute of Mental Health in Mannheim – one of the seven centers – included seven assessments over 5 years in an epidemiologically defined sample of 70 first-onset schizophrenics of the Mannheim-Heidelberg area.

We included patients aged between 15 and 44 years who suffered from hallucinations, delusions of nonaffective type, and/or thought and speech disorder, and whose onset of illness – defined by these criteria – was not more than 1 year previously.

The exclusion criteria were gross organic brain disease, serious mental or sensory disability, and alcohol or drug addiction.

Sixty-two patients participated in all seven interviews, which is a high follow-up rate, with nearly 95% of data sets completed. At the 5-year follow-up, all 67 surviving patients could be located and contacted (three patients had committed suicide). More details on this study have been reported elsewhere (Schwarz et al. 1980; Schubart et al. 1986a, b; Biehl et al. 1986).

The following report will demonstrate the correlation between a set of predictors and four different dimensions of outcome:
- Disability
- Time in psychotic episodes during the year preceding follow-up
- Productive psychotic symptoms at time of follow-up
- Observed minus signs (impairments)

The predictors were taken from earlier investigations and from clinical experience, and were expected to be especially important and influential in the course of schizophrenic disorders. The following groups of potential predictors were taken into the analysis:
- Sociodemographic variables
- Symptomatology at initial assessment
- Observed minus signs, observed plus signs (impairments) and the disability score 6 months after initial assessment
- Variables concerning home atmosphere (the EE of the key figure) at initial assessment.

A further step will be to test whether any given predictor fulfills the five formal requirements listed above.

Method and Results

The cohort was divided in two or more subgroups on the basis of the scores of the different predictors at the time of the first or second cross section. First, these groups were compared by one-way analysis of variance, with regard to mean values of the different criteria of outcome. Different mean values in the subgroups were regarded as indicators for an association between predictor and the respective dimension of outcome. The p values provided by the analysis of variance are used as descriptive measures of association.

In a second step (to control for confoundation) two- and three-way analyses of variance were carried out with the outcome criteria as dependent, and the predictor and certain confounding variables as independent variables. We postulate a predictor to be unconfounded, if an association found in step one is maintained in step two as main effect and is not attributable to an interaction effect.

Table 1 gives these findings at 1, 2, 3, and 5 years after initial assessment for the trend or significant associations, which were found. The best predictors were observed minus and plus signs and the disability score 6 months after initial assessment. These variables (especially the negative symptoms and the disability score) predict the outcome at each follow-up at a high level of significance.

The symptomatology at initial assessment did not influence the outcome of illness. Concerning sociodemographic variables as well as home atmosphere variables (EE type), no systematic associations with outcome were found in the total group except for the predictors key figure and criticism, which are partly associated with the disability score, whereas warmth predicted a shorter stay in rehabilitation institutions over the 5 years.

Table 1. Associations between predictors and dimensions of outcome 1, 2, 3, and 5 years after onset of illness

Predictors	Disability score				Duration of psychotic episodes during preceding year				Productive psychotic symptoms at follow-up				Observed minus signs (impairments)		
	1	2	3	5	1	2	3	5	1	2	3	5	1	2	5
Living situation		t	**			*									
Sex	*				**	t									
Age															
Educational level	*			t	*	*	*								
Occupation			*							**					
Marital status		t	t		t				**	*					
Parental social class	*														
ICD diagnosis (psychiatrist)				t											
ICD diagnosis (Catego)															
Type of onset															
Minus signs	*	**	**	**	*	**	**	t		*	t		**	**	**
Plus signs (second cross section)	**	*	**	**	**	**		t	**				t		**
Disability score (second cross section)	**	**	**	**	**	**	**	*					*	**	**
Key figure		t	*						t						
Face-to-face contact (hours per week)	t										t				t
Emotional involvement (key figure)										t					
Control and demand			*												
Rejection		t	*												
Premorbid sexual adjustment															

**, $p \leq 0.01$; *, $p \leq 0.05$; t, $p \leq 0.1$

Regarding only variables which predict at least two of the four cross sections, the sociodemographic variables living situation (alone, with parents, with partner or else), marital status, and educational level correlate with the disability score at two different cross sections; the duration of time in psychotic episodes is best predicted by sex and educational level, the acute psychotic symptoms 1 and 2 years after initial assessment by the marital status of the patients. Concerning observed minus signs as outcome measure, no significant association with the sociodemographic variables could be found.

Generally, there was a clear decrease of predictive accuracy over time; the most significant correlations between predictors and outcome appear 1 year after initial assessment.

In a next step, the sociodemographic variables will be discussed exemplarily with regard to our five criteria for an ideal predictor. Concerning the first two cri-

Table 2. Mean disability scores in different living situations

Living situation	Disability	
	Two-year follow-up	Three-year follow-up
Alone	3.4	3.7
With parents	3.8	3.9
With spouse	2.9	2.6
Sheltered apartment	2.5	2.5

teria, it is possible to assess sociodemographic variables at an early time stage in a reliable way.

In order to check the third criterion the predictor-outcome relation has to be analyzed, i.e., it has to be examined whether the association between the living situation of the patients and the disability 2 years after initial assessment is in the same direction as after 3 years; the appropriate statistical procedure is a comparison of mean values. As to our data, this is actually the case. It can be demonstrated at all follow-ups that patients living alone or with their parents are more disabled than patients living with their spouse or in a sheltered apartment (Table 2).

The two predictors sex and educational level serve to illustrate the fourth criterion. We looked for confounding variables that may bias the associations between predictors and outcome.

Concerning sex, such confounding variables may be, for example, age, marital status, or utilization of mental health care facilities; concerning educational level, the influences of parental social class and age have to be taken into account. This point is to be examined by using a statistical procedure analyzing the corresponding variables (i.e., the confounding variables together with the predictor) simultaneously and by looking for interactions; this will again be done by means of analysis of variance.

For the predictor to meet the fourth criterion, the results of Table 1 have to remain unchanged, i.e., no interactions between the variables should occur.

Table 3 gives data about additional significant results considering the bias caused by the confounding variables. The table demonstrates that especially the acute psychotic symptoms 1, 2, and 3 years after initial assessment are predicted by patient's sex only if corrected for differences in age, in marital status, and in utilization of mental health care facilities; when ignoring these differences, no significant sex effect could be found.

Concerning the predictor educational level, a similar influence is revealed by the confounding variables of parental social class and age. In this analysis, additional correlations with the acute psychotic symptomatology at 2- and at 3-year follow-up can be demonstrated. Additionally, the parental social class proved to be prognostically relevant. Therefore, when considering the interactions between parental social class, age, and educational level, there are many more significant correlations with outcome than are found on analyzing one of the three predictors separately.

Table 3. Additional significant associations of the predictors sex and educational level, controlling for age, marital status, and parental social class

Predictors	Disability score				Duration of psychotic episodes during preceding year				Productive psychotic symptoms at follow-up				Observed minus signs (impairments)			
	1	2	3	5	1	2	3	5	1	2	3	5	1	2	3	5
Sex								t	**	*		t				
Age		t			*								t			
Educational level							t		t	*						
Marital status							t			t						
Parental social class					t	*			*	t						

**, $p \leq 0.01$; *, $p \leq 0.05$; t, $p \leq 0.1$

Table 4. Additional significant associations of the predictors living situation and occupation, considering only those patients with no changes in the course of 5 years

Predictors	Disability score				Duration of psychotic episodes during preceding year				Productive psychotic symptoms at follow-up				Observed minus signs (impairments)			
	1	2	3	5	1	2	3	5	1	2	3	5	1	2	3	5
Living situation																
Occupation	**	**			*	t										

**, $p \leq 0.01$; *, $p \leq 0.05$; t, $p \leq 0.1$

The fifth and last criterion relates to the frequency of significant correlations between predictor and outcome at the different time stages in the course of illness. Regarding the results in Table 1, it can be noticed that the predictive power of the sociodemographic variables decreases in the course of time: the 5-year follow-ups cannot be predicted by these variables. One could explain this result by the fact that some predictors may have changed meanwhile; for example, some patients may have changed their occupation or their living situation. Therefore, we have analyzed in a further step whether the later follow-ups can be predicted more precisely if changes of the predictor are taken into account.

In this case, too, we have confined ourselves to the sociodemographic variables and have investigated whether the predictive power of the living situation and the occupation increases by considering only those patients in whom no changes occur in the course of 5 years compared with their starting value (Table 4). The results can be summarized as follows: Concerning living situation, no further significant associations were found. Concerning occupation, some additional correlations were found which, however, never persisted until the 3-year follow-up.

This illustration of the five criteria referred only to the sociodemographic variables, similar procedures with the other groups of predictors will be reported by the authors elsewhere.

Summary and Conclusions

Summing up, the following general statements can be made:

1. In a critical test of potential predictors, the extent of observed early minus and plus behavior signs (impairments) as well as the disability score 6 months after initial assessment (which coincides for most of our patients with the discharge from their first admission or their first assessment outside hospital) turned out to be the best prognostic variables for all dimensions of outcome.

2. Of the four dimensions of outcome, the presence of later observed minus signs (impairments) is most difficult to predict by other variables (i.e., other than PIRS or DAS scores).

3. As to the other three dimensions of outcome, the 1-year follow-up can be predicted best, whereas by the 5-year follow-up many predictors fail, even if changes which may occur over time have been controlled. It is apparent that over longer periods, other variables influencing the course of illness gain increasing importance – possibly the utilization of mental health care facilities, the efficacy of psychiatric treatment, etc.

With regard to the form to be taken by future research in this field, the following conclusions can be drawn:

1. The standardization of research methods is an essential prerequisite for comparability of the data. Without identical instruments and screening criteria, findings concerning the prognostic value of predictors will continue to be inconsistent.

2. When looking for prognostic factors in the course of schizophrenia, the influence of confounding variables, which may either weaken or strengthen the association between predictor and outcome, is to be taken into account. It can be imagined that some risk factors exert an additive effect which may only be uncovered when analyzing the predictors simultaneously.

In order to investigate the reciprocal influences among the predictors, it is necessary to develop a prognostic model which includes interactions of the relevant dimensions based on theoretical considerations and empirical results. First attempts in this direction were made by Strauss and Carpenter in 1981 with their interactive developmental systems model. In their paper "Organizing the Complexities of Schizophrenia," Strauss et al., 1981 write:

The accumulated evidence that diverse factors constitute and influence onset, course, and treatment response reflects the amount of knowledge acquired in recent years. It also suggests the complexity of the issues involved, and the need for a conceptional framework to understand this complexity, generate further hypotheses, and provide the basis for more rational prevention and treatment.

References

Andreasen NC (1982) Negative symptoms in schizophrenia. Arch Gen Psychiatry 39:784–788

Biehl H, Maurer K, Schubart C, Krumm B, Jung E (1986) Prediction of outcome and utilization of medical services in a prospective study of first onset schizophrenics. Results of a prospective 5-year follow-up-study. Eur Arch Psychiatr Neurol Sci 236:139–147

Bleuler M (1972) Die schizophrenen Geistesstörungen im Lichte langjähriger Kranken- und Familiengeschichten. Thieme, Stuttgart

Ciompi L, Müller C (1976) Lebensweg und Alter der Schizophrenen. Eine katamnestische Langzeitstudie bis ins Senium. Springer, Berlin Heidelberg New York

Crow TJ, Cross AJ, Johnstone E, Owen F (1982) Two syndromes in schizophrenia and their pathogenesis. In: Henn F, Nasrallah HA (eds) Schizophrenia as a brain disease. Oxford University Press, New York

Huber G, Gross G, Schüttler R (1979) Schizophrenie. Eine Verlaufs- und sozialpsychiatrische Langzeitstudie. Springer, Berlin Heidelberg New York

Jablensky A, Schwarz R, Tomov T (1980) WHO collaborative study on impairments and disabilities associated with schizophrenic disorders. A preliminary communication: objectives and methods. Acta Psychiatr Scand [Suppl 285] 62:152–163

Möller HJ, v Zerssen D (1986) Der Verlauf schizophrener Psychosen unter den gegenwärtigen Behandlungsbedingungen. Springer, Berlin Heidelberg New York Tokyo

Salokangas RKR (1983) Prognostic implications of the sex of schizophrenic patients. Br J Psychiatry 142:145–151

Schubart C, Krumm B, Biehl H, Schwarz R (1986a) Measurement of social disability in a schizophrenic patient group – definition, assessment and outcome over 2 years in a cohort of schizophrenic patients of recent onset. Soc Psychiatry 21:1–9

Schubart C, Schwarz R, Krumm B, Biehl H (1986b) Schizophrenie und soziale Anpassung – eine prospektive Längsschnittuntersuchung. Springer, Berlin Heidelberg New York Tokyo

Schwarz R, Biehl H, Krumm B, Schubart C (1980) Case-finding and characteristics of schizophrenic patients of recent onset in Mannheim. In: Strömgren E, Dupont A, Nielsen JA (eds) Epidemiological research as basis for the organization of extramural psychiatry. Acta Psychiatr Scand [Suppl 285]:212–219

Strauss JS, Carpenter WT (1977) Prediction of outcome in schizophrenia. III. Five-year outcome and its predictors. Arch Gen Psychiatry 34:159–163

Strauss JS, Carpenter WT (1981) Schizophrenia. Plenum, New York

Strauss JS, Loevsky L, Glazer W, Leaf P (1981) Organizing the complexities of schizophrenia. J Nerv Ment Dis 169:120–126

WHO (1980) International classification of impairments, disabilities and handicaps. WHO, Geneva

Course of Schizophrenia in Different Countries: Some Results of a WHO International Comparative 5-Year Follow-up Study *

N. Sartorius[1], A. Jablensky[2], G. Ernberg[3], J. Leff[4], A. Korten[5], and W. Gulbinat[6] on behalf of the collaborating investigators[7]

Nearly 20 years ago, the World Health Organization embarked on an ambitious programme in social and epidemiological psychiatry. This programme included a component that dealt with the standardisation of psychiatric diagnosis of classification and statistics, a component directed towards the exploration of specific mental disorders in different cultures, a component concerned with the assessment of incidence and prevalence of mental disorders in geographically defined populations, and a component dealing with the training of psychiatrists in public health, with particular emphasis on epidemiology [1, 2].

The programme has been rich in scientific rewards over the years and has produced results which have influenced psychiatric research, education and practice in many countries. The component which concentrated on the standardisation of psychiatric diagnosis and classification resulted in the ninth revision of the International Classification of Diseases, the glossary accompanying the classification, a series of publications with recommendations to governments and in the establishment of a network of individuals and centres involved in WHO's efforts in this field. Methods which were produced and tested in this programme are widely used in many countries.

The component concerned with training has also been well-developed, and a series of training courses and fellowship training programmes have been carried out [2]. The components dealing with research on specific mental disorders and with the epidemiological studies of mental disorders in geographically defined populations had as their flagship and forerunner the International Pilot Study on Schizophrenia (IPSS) [3–7].

* This paper presents some of the points and data incorporated in the comprehensive report of the 5-year follow-up of patients included in the International Pilot Study of Schizophrenia (to be published)
[1] Director, Division of Mental Health, World Health Organization, Geneva
[2] Associate Professor of Psychiatry, Medical Academy, Sofia
[3] Technical Officer, Division of Mental Health, World Health Organization, Geneva
[4] Head, MRC Social Psychiatry Unit, Friern Hospital, London
[5] Statistician, WHO Collaborating Centre for the Epidemiology of Mental Disorders, Canberra
[6] Senior Scientist, Division of Mental Health, World Health Organization, Geneva
[7] The collaborating investigators in this study were: E. Strömgren, A. Bertelsen, M. Fischer, C. Flach, N. Juel-Nielsen (Aarhus); K. C. Dube, B. S. Yadav (Agra); C. León, G. Calderon, E. Zambrano (Cali); T. A. Lambo, T. Asuni, M. O. Olatawura (Ibadan); J. K. Wing, J. Birley, J. P. Leff (London); R. A. Nadzharov, N. M. Zharikov (Moscow); L. Hanzlicek, C. Skoda (Prague); C. C. Chen, M. T. Tsuang (Taipei); L. Wynne, J. Strauss, W. Carpenter, J. Bartko (Washington)

This major international study brought together researchers from nine different countries and created a new model of international cooperation in psychiatry. The study set out to explore whether international scientific collaboration in the field of psychiatry was feasible; it proved that it was. It aimed at producing instruments that would be transculturally applicable and developed them. It also set as its goal to answer the question of whether schizophrenia as defined by European psychiatrists around the turn of the century, exists in different cultures.

The answer to this question is now well known. Patients with a characteristic clinical syndrome closely corresponding to classical descriptions of schizophrenia were found in each of the settings studied. Although there were symptomatological differences between patient groups from different centres, the similarities overshadowed the differences. This was true for all the variables examined, which were many (over 450), since a whole range of instruments were used to elicit a large amount of information in a standardised way in each centre.

The most puzzling result of the IPSS was that 2 years after the initial examination there were significant differences in the course and outcome of schizophrenia among the centres. Both the course and outcome of groups of schizophrenic patients were significantly better in centres in developing countries than in those in the developed world. This was true for all the clinically relevant characteristics which were examined – including variables such as percentage of follow-up time during which patients showed psychotic symptoms, social impairment, quality of remission and the overall rating on pattern of course.

Although some earlier studies had indicated that such a difference in outcome may exist, these results were puzzling and contrary to expectations. The standardisation of instruments and the meticulous training of investigators which characterised the IPSS made it highly probable that these results were not an artefact resulting from an invalid manner of data collection.

Two possible explanations come easily to mind. The first is that the results reflected some kind of systematic bias in the selection of patients (e.g. that in the groups of patients recruited for the study) in developing countries there was an overrepresentation of patients with a good prognosis); and the second is that such course and outcome differences are only observable in the first few years of the disease and disappear in its later phase.

To answer the first question, WHO launched a new study entitled the Determinants of Outcome of Severe Mental Disorder [8]. This study included 12 research sites in ten countries, which encompassed all agencies likely to be in contact with schizophrenic patients, including traditional healers, religious institutions, social and health services. A comprehensive ongoing monitoring of contact points of schizophrenic patients in the catchment areas was achieved. It thus became possible to obtain information about the first contact incidence of schizophrenia and to recruit patient groups which allowed the exploration of differences in outcome without an undue sampling bias. The patients were examined with a battery of research instruments developed on the basis of previous experience of the IPSS or other current research. The core study design envisaged an initial assessment and a 2-year follow-up of all patients included in the study. The results are being analysed and will be published in full in 1987. Preliminary impressions indicate that the course and outcome differences found in the IPSS are replicated even when a sampling bias is avoided.

The Determinants of Outcome Study also explored some other explanations of the difference in outcome. Various explorations, which involved different subgroups of the centres, aimed to assess:

(a) whether there are differences in the numbers and types of stressful life events in patients in different cultures, and whether such factors are significantly associated with the onset of schizophrenia;

(b) whether the pattern of emotional interaction in families in the developing countries differs from that in the developed world, and if so what impact this has on relapse rates;

(c) whether the difference between developed and developing countries can be explained by the differences in "social processing" of impairment (e.g. in terms of specialisation of labour, type of social networks)

(d) whether there is reason to suspect that the pattern of morbidity in schizophrenics differs from the normal population;

(e) whether the perception of mental disease in the immediate social network of the patient in different countries can explain some of the variance observed.

Results of these studies are in press now, and it can be stated that in spite of their intrinsically interesting results, none alone explains the difference in outcome to a sufficient and satisfactory degree.

The second possibility mentioned above was that the differences found in IPSS patients were only transitory and disappeared subsequently. To explore this question, the follow-up study was extended to cover a 5-year period. (The centres in Cali [9] and Prague carried out a 10-year follow-up study and the centre in Agra, a 13–14-year follow-up study.) Special schedules were developed paying particular attention to the nature of episodes of illness which the patients experienced between the 2- and the 5-year follow-up point. A full description of the results of this study is being published elsewhere, and only some of the data from this follow-up study will be used to raise issues for discussion.

Feasibility

A first important finding of this study revealed that it was possible to account for some 90% of the 1065 patients who had full psychiatric assessment on initial evaluation. (Excluding the patients from the centre in Taipei, who were included in the IPSS but for whom follow-up data are not available.) In no centre was the proportion lower than 77% of the original sample, and in two all patients could be traced. Full information was obtained on approximately 75% of the patients, ranging from over 90% in Aarhus and Cali to 59% in Ibadan and 53% in Washington.

With regard to the feasibility of tracing and assessing psychiatric patients 5 years after the inclusion, there is no major difference between the centres in developing and developed countries. Furthermore, the 5-year follow-up period decreased the cohort attrition rate in five of the eight centres. This finding is of particular importance for future studies in developing countries, which can obviously ensure adequate medium-term follow-up of patients with psychiatric disorders.

The patients who could not be assessed in full were compared with those in the fully assessed group. There was no evidence of any differences in age and sex distribution. Some variability between the groups existed but it was minor, centre-specific and on the whole not surprising. In London, for example, patients of a lower socio-economic status were more often lost to follow-up than others. In Moscow, female patients could be traced more easily than males, and those followed up were significantly older than those who were not. In developing countries, urban follow-up was somewhat easier. Those who were married or had been married previously were more often followed up than those who were single, particularly as regards the Moscow and London centres. If data from all centres are combined, patients at higher socio-economic levels were more often traced and followed up. This trend is present in most of the centres but does not reach statistically significant levels.

Survival of Patients in the Different Centres

Of the 1065 patients who were assessed originally, 22 died of various causes between initial evaluation and the 2-year follow-up, and a further 30 died between the 2-year and 5-year follow-up examinations. This constitutes 52 patients, or 4.9% of the initial cohort. In two of the centres (Ibadan and Agra), both in developing countries, the percentages of patients who died were considerable, 9.7 and 7.1 respectively. The centre with the lowest percentage of deaths (0.8%) was surprisingly not in a developed country but in Cali.

Schizophrenic patients appear to have a slightly higher mortality rate than patients with other diagnoses included in the study: as they made up 71% of the total study population, schizophrenics constitute 80% of the fatalities. Suicide (ascertained and suspected) was the leading single cause of death, accounting for 38%. This was particularly marked in some of the centres, and in one (London) there was no other cause of death. Suicides occurred also in centres in developing countries (Agra and Cali), and the impressions of the investigators suggest that the cause of death in some of the 14 patients who died in Ibadan might have been suicide. Of the 19 cases of ascertained or suspected suicide, 14 were patients with a diagnosis of schizophrenia, showing that the risk of suicide in schizophrenia is as great, if not greater, than the risk of suicide associated with affective disorders.

Mental State

Another issue which was examined was the mental state of patients on 5-year follow-up. Patients were divided into three groups according to qualitative distinctions between the patterns of symptomatology. The three groups are: (a) psychotic (i.e. presence of symptoms such as delusions, hallucinations, qualitative disorder of thought, etc.); (b) non-psychotic (including presence of affective, neurotic and other symptoms but none of the psychotic symptoms); and (c) non-symptomatic (i.e. practically symptom-free). The operational criteria designed for assigning patients to each of these three groups on the basis of Present State Examination data have been described in detail elsewhere [4].

Table 1. Percentage of time spent in psychotic episodes by number of schizophrenic patients: 5-year follow-up

	>15%	16%–45%	46%–100%
Developed countries	50	16	34
Developing countries	68	10	22

It could be seen that a higher proportion of schizophrenic patients in developed countries was in a psychotic episode both at the time of the 2-year follow-up and the 5-year follow-up, in comparison with patients in developing countries. This difference had increased by the time of the 5-year follow-up. The proportions of patients who were found to be in psychotic episodes on two or on all three occasions were also different in the two groups of centres, being consistently higher in the centres in developed countries (Table 1). Inverse relationships were observed with regard to the proportions of patients who were symptomatic but nonpsychotic at first examination and symptom-free at the follow-up examinations. Although the "cross section" of the mental state at defined points in the follow-up period is a partial and limited measure of the course and outcome of groups of patients, the differences described are consistent with other differences in the measures of the longitudinal aspects of course and outcome.

Pattern of Course

The generally more favourable course of the disease in developing countries was clearly observable in the 5-year follow-up (Table 2). Over one-quarter of the patients in developing countries had one single episode followed by full remission, compared with only 8% of patients in the developed countries. There were 50% of patients in the developing countries who had full remission between episodes (as compared with 17% of the patients in developed countries). Some 14% and 24% of patients, respectively, had a continuing episode of illness over the 5 follow-up years.

Table 2. Pattern of course (in percentages of cases) in schizophrenia: 5-year follow-up. *1*, only one episode with full remission; *2*, only one episode with incomplete remission; *3*, several episodes with full remissions; *4*, several episodes with incomplete remission; *5*, continuous illness

	1	2	3	4	5
Developed countries (297 cases)	8	17	9	41	24
Developing countries (235 cases)	27	12	23	23	14

Impairments of Social Functioning

The 5-year follow-up assessment included several specific measures of social functioning (e.g. self-care, occupational adjustment, sexual adjustment, interpersonal functioning in the community) and a global rating of social functioning, which was made by the investigators on the basis of all information available.

In Table 3, the same pattern as before can be seen. Patients with schizophrenia in the developing countries experienced no or mild impairment in social functioning in 65% of the cases, nearly one-third more than patients in the developed countries. It is remarkable, however, that a relatively high percentage of patients in the developed countries did not experience a significant disturbance in social functioning.

The overall outcome figures further confirm these findings (Table 4). Overall outcome was calculated on the basis of percentage of time spent on psychotic episodes, impairment in social functioning and the type of course. Comparing the 2-year and the 5-year follow-up data, the mildest type of overall outcome showed

Table 3. Impairment in social functions (by percentage of cases) in schizophrenia: 5-year follow-up

	Number of cases	None or mild	Moderate or severe
Developed countries	297	43	56
Developing countries	235	65	33

Table 4. Comparison of percentage distribution and overall outcome in schizophrenia (by centre): 2-year and 5-year follow-up

	Aarhus		London		Moscow		Washington	
	$n=48$ 2-year	$n=50$ 5-year	$n=58$ 2-year	$n=63$ 5-year	$n=66$ 2-year	$n=65$ 5-year	$n=31$ 2-year	$n=51$ 5-year
Type 1+2 (best)	35.5	30.0	36.2	52.4	48.5	61.5	38.7	60.8
Type 5 (worst)	31.3	38.0	31.0	20.6	10.6	18.5	19.4	19.6

	Prague		Agra		Cali		Ibadan	
	$n=44$ 2-year	$n=60$ 5-year	$n=88$ 2-year	$n=71$ 5-year	$n=72$ 2-year	$n=86$ 5-year	$n=58$ 2-year	$n=67$ 5-year
Type 1+2 (best)	34.1	54.0	65.9	77.5	52.7	64.0	86.2	79.1
Type 5 (worst)	29.5	25.4	14.8	11.3	15.3	12.8	5.2	13.4

an increase in most of the centres (six of eight), the group with poorest outcome increased in four centres, and the in-between groups decreased in numbers.

Conclusion

Information obtained in the 5-year follow-up assessments of the patients included in the IPSS suggests that the important trend which emerged in the analysis of the 2-year follow-up data is, on the whole, confirmed. Patients with an initial clinical diagnosis of schizophrenia in the centres in developing countries had a more favourable course and outcome than their counterparts in the developed world. This was so for practically all course and outcome measures, including symptomatic state at the time of follow-up, pattern of course, proportion of the follow-up period during which the patients were in psychotic episodes and social functioning. However, in both developed and developing countries there are patients with a poor prognosis who deserve special attention.

The results of the 2-year follow-up in the Determinants of Outcome Study have not yet been analysed, but a preliminary review of the data seems to indicate that the same trend is present for most of the course and outcome measures applied. This second study avoided sampling bias and used more sophisticated techniques for patient assessment developed on the basis of experience of years of work on cross-cultural studies.

References

1. Sartorius N (1974) The programme of the World Health Organization on the epidemiology of the mental disorders. In: Proceedings of the Vth World Congress of Psychiatry, Mexico, 1971. Excerpta Medica, Amsterdam
2. Sartorius N (1985) Gli usi dell'epidemiologia nei programmi per la salute mentale dell'Organizzazione mondiale della Sanità. In: Tansella M (ed) L'approccio epidemiologico in psichiatria: programme di psicologia psichiatria psicoterapia. Boringhieri, Turin, pp 105–135
3. Sartorius N (1980) The research component of the WHO mental health programme. Psychol Med 10:175–185
4. World Health Organization (1979) Schizophrenia: an international follow-up study. World Health Organization, Geneva and Wiley, Chichester
5. World Health Organization (1975) Schizophrenia: a multinational study. Public Health Pap 63. World Health Organization, Geneva
6. World Health Organization (1973) The international pilot study of schizophrenia. Vol 1. Results of the initial evaluation phase. WHO Offset Publication no 2. World Health Organization, Geneva
7. Jablenski A (1984) Gli studi trans-culturali dell' Organizzazione Mondiale della Sanità sulla schizofrenia: implicazioni teoriche e pratiche. In: Faccineani C. et al. (eds) Le psicosi schizofreniche dalla ricerca alla pratica clinica. Pàtron Edifore, Bologna, pp 36–64
8. Sartorius N, Jablensky A, Korten A, Ernberg G, Anker M, Cooper JE, Day R (1986) Early manifestations and first-contact incidence of schizophrenia in different cultures. Psychol Med 16:909–928
9. Leon C (1986) Curso clinico y evolución de la esquizofrenia en Cali, un estudio de seguimiento de diez años. Acta Psiquiát Amér Lat 32:95–136

Epidemiology and Course of Schizophrenia: Discussion

Both Professor Häfner and Dr. Sartorius, the initial and final contributors to this session point out the tremendous progress that has occurred in the field of schizophrenia. From my own vantage point, since the 1930s, I agree heartily. I am, however, reminded of what Szent Györgyi once said regarding the science of biochemistry. When he entered the field as a young man, there were few facts but many theories; now we have a plethora of facts but meaning still escapes us. The same seems to apply to psychopathology. However, the search for truth seems to be the shifting residue of competition in ideas, as Justice Oliver Wendell Holmes Jr. once said, and it is in this spirit that I propose to present my remarks.

Perhaps the most exciting finding reported in Professor Häfner's paper is the constancy of the rate of incidence of schizophrenia across the 10 different countries and cultures, and the most challenging conclusion is that this constancy may be interpreted as signaling the absence of causality in the social cultural forces.

The constancy of the expectancy rate, reputed to be about 1% of the general population has been heralded ever since I can remember. Furthermore, while many of us have for a long time leaned in the direction of believing that internal factors are more important in the causation of schizophrenia than external factors, this is the first time that I have heard this claim to be based on such reliable epidemiological evidence. For this reason it behooves us to examine carefully both the evidence as well as the cogency of the conclusion.

Let us first lay aside the question of whether the S + category really represents „echte" schizophrenia.

Are there any other ways of interpreting the data? I believe that any other plausible, even though unproven, interpretation cannot yet be dismissed.

First, there is no other disorder, to my knowledge, which has a constant incidence rate across the world. This would put schizophrenia into a class all by itself and raise the question of whether indeed it is a disorder. We would have to add the incidence of schizophrenia to such other natural constants as the speed of light.

Second, the incidence rate of schizophrenia represents the phenotypic expression of an underlying causal agent. For example, under the genetic hypothesis of causality and under a monogenic hypothesis it can be demonstrated that the degree of penetrance is about 0.26, and a similar figure can be calculated under

VA Medical Center, Highland Drive, Pittsburgh, PA 15206, USA, and Department of Psychiatry, University of Pittsburgh School of Medicine, Pittsburgh, Pennsylvania, USA

certain assumptions for polygenic causation. Let us assume that the genetic hypothesis is tenable and analyze the various possibilities that might give rise to a constant incidence rate.

One possible alternative explanation is that though the phenotypic rate is constant, the genotypic rate is *not* constant but that the degree of penetrance, which is postulated to explain the discrepancy between phenotype and genotype, varies inversely with the genotypic rate. That is, if r is the phenotypic incidence rate, $r = pg$ where p is the degree of penetrance and g is the genotypic rate. As the genotypic rate rises, the penetrance drops correspondingly so as to keep the incidence rate constant and vice versa when the genotypic rate drops. Is there a rationale for this assumption? The appeal can be made here to a perceptual threshold for the conspicuousness of symptoms. The assumption is that the community has a threshold for the perception of deviance. If the frequency of deviance rises above a certain level of tolerance, only the most conspicuous are categorized as truly deviant and milder deviance is ignored. On the other hand, as the frequency of deviance falls below a certain level, even the milder deviances become conspicuous. In this way, the incidence rate may remain constant even though the genotypic rate varies. Is this explanation plausible?

A careful reading of the original report on the WHO study supplied by Dr. Sartorius indicates that the source of the patients was not a survey of the total population in a given catchment area, but of those who "had made a first contact with any 'helping' agency because of problems suggesting the presence of a psychotic illness." The authors admit that patients "who never contact any agency would still be missed." Whether these missing cases reflect the tolerance threshold for deviancy which I suggested remains an open question and can be answered only by a complete sampling survey of the populations discussed. But even such a survey may not entirely remove the effect of community tolerance for deviance. In other words, as long as the incidence rate is phenotypic, there is always a possibility that culture gets its licks in somehow.

I wonder whether mortality plays a part in incidence rates? Would the more severe cases tend to die off in all cultures and in this way make the rate more constant, if the severity is proportional to the basic rate? That is, if the basic rate is low there would be fewer deaths of severe cases and mutatis mutandis when the basic rate is high.

Only when we develop objective markers for the presence of vulnerability for schizophrenia can this question be finally settled. The markers must be either the genetic alleles themselves or linkage markers, but not pathophysiological markers, since the latter may already represent the emergence of the phenotype.

It seems highly plausible that the same argument will hold true for other etiological models beside the genetic, but this topic needs further elaboration. The parallel that Häfner draws between mental retardation and schizophrenia may also reflect ceiling and floor effects with regard to tolerance of deviant behavior in the community. As the author points out, perhaps the perceived threshold for tolerance may vary with incidence.

Regarding differences between males and females in age of onset, one wonders whether the closer ties of the female to the family in most cultures prevent earlier perception on the part of the family of the deviant behavior in the daughter. Perhaps protective attitudes toward the female and the warmth of her social network postpone the emergence of the psychosis.

To summarize, Häfner maintains that both transculturally and transtemporally, the constancy of the incidence rate would suggest that incidence of schizophrenia, like Avogadro's number, is a natural constant independent of time and place. This would put schizophrenia in a class by itself, a maverick among all the other disorders of mankind.

Dr. Strauss' paper came as a surprise in this session, since it deals primarily with the course of illness in individual cases – a far cry from the usual epidemiological concerns. Strauss wishes to discover the particular mechanism which determines the circuitous path that recovery takes in the single individual, although he probably hopes to find groups of like-minded individuals that cohere in these paths. The latter might bring him into the epidemiological fold. The most striking factor he focuses on is the person himself as a controlling agent, a factor which epidemiologists often lose sight of. Rene Dubos has called attention to this neglect in a dramatic way. According to Dubos, the biological approach assumes that "all the constituents and processes found in living things, including man, obey the laws of inanimate matter," something which the early Freud, before he became involved in psychoanalysis, also believed.

Dubos (1971) goes on to explain:

We know a great deal concerning the physiochemical phenomena that make life possible, and we can formulate reasonable hypotheses concerning their origin and evolution. We can imagine, even though we do not completely understand, how each particular living thing is shaped by genetic constitution, experiences and environment ... the physiochemical forces provide [however] only the props and stage machinery.

The etiologic models are described by Dubos as blind forces which control man's destiny and to some extent, given the current scene, this is a true picture. For the ecological niche in which man finds himself does determine his wellbeing, his genetic make-up does limit his potential, his internal environment and neuropsychologic make-up control his behavior. In fact, we might agree with Dubos that all of these forces are merely the props for the drama that man is to enact on the stage of life. However, we have omitted perhaps the most important determinant of man's stage behavior – his ability to be a self-starter, to alter developmental trends, to modify the internal environment as well as his neurophysiologic equipment. Unlike other organisms, which are shaped by their environment through eons of gradual evolutionary developments, man can shape his own environment if he chooses to do so and has developed the know-how to apply changes not only to the exogenous but also to the endogenous environment. It is in these directions that the future of man's normal development, as well as the containment and improvement of abnormal development, lies.

I have been impressed with Dr. Strauss' appeal to the process of healing in his title. I may be putting words in his mouth, but it strikes me that we have forgotten that man is not only a self-determiner but also a self-healer. Much of what therapists do may be regarded as removing the obstacle from the path of natural healing which nature provides us with. It is often said that in order to prove the efficacy of a treatment we must beat the spontaneous improvement rate. But what is spontaneous improvement if not natural self-healing? Perhaps Dr. Strauss should concentrate on finding his mechanisms in spontaneous recoveries and discovering how nature brings them about. For this, of course, he would have to conduct an epidemiological experiment by monitoring a catchment area for individuals who develop episodes that spontaneously heal and identifying the mechanisms involved in such healing.

Tsuang and Fleming have presented another study in the famous Iowa series and this time devoted themselves to the problem of atypical schizophrenia.

Four outcome variables were considered: marital status, residential status, occupational status, and psychopathological status.

One wonders whether marital status can really be regarded as an outcome variable, but it seems to serve as a differentiator between atypical schizophrenia and the comparison groups. In general, establishing the authenticity of a diagnostic category on the basis of the variables chosen reminds me of Squires' attempt after World War II to classify patients on the basis of outcome of treatment, which in those days consisted of insulin, ECT, and psychosurgery. The classification system did not outlast the therapies!

I also wonder whether the isolated treatment of the four outcome variables is a satisfactory procedure. The authors indicate that they are planning a multivariate attack and maybe that will help us understand the results better. In the proposed analysis linear relationships of the regression variety are contemplated. I wonder whether a pattern analysis by means of a clustering procedure might be helpful. Thus, a divorced man, not working and living alone with little or no psychopathology present, may represent an outcome which is quite different in quality of life from the same individual living with his family. In other words, the regression analysis may crush all the possible nonlinear relationships out of existence.

All in all, Tsuang and Fleming have made a valiant effort to establish the category of atypical schizophrenia on a more certain footing, and if the proposed multivariate analysis they promise bears out their previous conclusions, they will have made a considerable contribution to the category of atypical schizophrenia.

Their paper seems to present the very antithesis of the Strauss' paper, since it deals with specifically identifiable factors like marital, occupational, residential, and psychopathological status in relation to outcome on follow up of a specifically delimited group of patients. The individual's course of outcome with regard to these variables is completely ignored and the statistical product of an equation is used to indicate whether the outcome was good or poor in each factor. This study fits well into the epidemiological mold.

In contrasting the epidemiological approach as represented by Tsuang and Fleming with the individual approach of Strauss, we might note that *both* these approaches have led to well-known fallacies. The epidemiological-statistical approach has sometimes suffered from the ecological fallacy, while the individual approach has sometimes given rise to the clinical fallacy. The ecological fallacy has been illustrated by the Faris and Dunham claim that low socioeconomic level, as measured by average rent in an area, is negatively related to rate of schizophrenia. A more individual analysis by Edward Hare in Bristol found that living alone was the differential factor, regardless of socioeconomic status.

On the other hand, the clinical fallacy is well illustrated by the claim that Buergher's disease was a Jewish disease until the King of England developed it.

The essential problem of these two fallacies inheres in the fact that the total covariance between factors x and y is divisible into two portions, the covariance between the means of the subgroups in the population and the covariance within the subgroup $r_{xy} = r_{\bar{x}\bar{y}} + \bar{r}_{x_i y_i}$. The ecological fallacy results when only the covariance between the means is attended to, while the clinical fallacy results when only the covariance within the groups is considered. By harnessing together a keen individual clinician like Strauss and ingenious epidemiologists like Tsuang and Fleming we might be able to avoid both types of fallacies.

The study by Schubart and colleagues is an investigation of a prospective 5-year follow-up study of schizophrenic patients with recent onset of illness based on the WHO Collaborative Study on the assessment and reduction of psychiatric disability. The focus of this paper is on the influence of risk factors on the course and outcome of symptomatology (psychopathology) and social adjustment in long-term follow up. I must admit that either because I am unacquainted with their work, or because of language difficulty in the presentation, my comments may be beside the point.

The outcome variables were: (1) disability at time of final assessment on 5-year follow-up; (2) time in psychotic episodes during follow-up; (3) acute psychotic symptoms (positive symptoms) at time of follow-up; (4) negative symptoms at time of follow-up. The predictors of outcome were sociodemographic variables; symptomatology at initial assessment; negative symptoms, positive symptoms, and the disability score 6 months after initial assessment; and variables concerning expressed emotions of the key figure (most important relative?) at initial assessment. (Note that predictors are earlier estimates of outcome variables.)

The results indicated that the 1-year outcome can be predicted best. The 5-year outcome can *not* be predicted. Proximity in time between the measures which are used initially as predictors and later as criteria of outcome may explain the results. For example, correlation between initial symptomatology (the predictor) with symptomatology at 6 months (outcome) may reflect the effect of self-correlation. That is why the correlation is high when the 6-month outcome is predicted but quite low when the 5-year outcome is predicted. I hope that the final version of the paper may clarify these issues.

Norman Sartorius had not let me have the benefit of previewing his paper but he did send me two of his recent papers on which he built his presentation. The magnificent scope of the systematic studies of WHO into the problems of schizophrenia which he describes cannot help but arouse our admiration. He focused on the advances in this field stemming from the WHO effort to the exclusion of some of the other contributions to the common goal. One of the predecessors of the WHO effort in which he himself participated, to my great satisfaction, was the US-UK Project which laid the foundation for cross-*national* if not cross-*cultural* studies.

The three most striking results which he reported are first, the constancy of the incidence rate of the S+ category, second, the better outcome of the developing countries, and third, the replication of the Brown and Birley findings on the importance of life events in the 3 weeks preceding an episode as triggers of episodes on a cross-cultural basis. Regarding the constancy of the incidence rate for nuclear schizophrenia (S+), I have already discussed some of the possible interpretations in the context of Professor Häfner's paper. It should be noted that in a forthcoming paper Sartorius regards the "first contact" incidence rate as only an approximation to the "true" rate and in need of replication.

Here all I would like to point out is that because of the importance of that finding, the exact method for computing the χ^2 value should be described for the uninitiated. Would it have clarified matters if a multiple-contingency analysis, including the sex differences, had been undertaken and the total χ^2 decomposed into the sex differential component and the center differential component? Freed from the sex component, which is not really germane here, the constancy of the rate could be more purely examined. The value of the first-rank symptoms as measures of severity is a noteworthy added feature, since there is such a strong demand for overall measures of severity. Perhaps also the speculation regarding the effect of the drop in size of the sample on the outcome when the restricted S+ category is used could be resolved simply by computing the coefficient of variation for the total group and the restricted group.

There are three findings that seem to need further explanation – the better outcome for developing countries, the delay in onset in females, and the better outcome for females. Is there a common link here? Is it possible that the social network and family relations in developing countries, and similarly the social network and family relations of the females, serve as buffers to ameliorate outcome and by the same token delay the onset of episodes in females?

There seems to be a tendency for the developing countries to show a higher frequency of positive symptoms. Is there a corresponding gain for negative symptoms in developed countries? If so, is this balancing of symptoms partly responsible for the constancy in the apparent incidence?

Regarding the replication of the Brown and Birley findings of the relation between life events during the 3 weeks preceding an episode and the occurrence of the episode, it should be pointed out that though Brown and Birley did not regard life events as important in the triggering of an episode, the cross-cultural replication seems to enhance the value of the finding. Furthermore, though life events seem to have come into prominence only since the work of Holmes and Rahe, it should be pointed out that precipitating events have a long history in schizophrenia. Furthermore, the importance of the concept dates back to Burton, who in his *Anatomy of Melancholy* listed a series of life events in the "causes" of mental disorders.

In general, the evidence presented in Sartorius' paper does not give any weight to causality for the psychosocial variable of culture, season of birth, and age of onset (delayed in females), but it does lend support to the notion that psychosocial factors may be important in determining time of onset, maintenance of the episode, relapse, and recovery.

Reference

Dubos R (1971) The despairing optimist. American Scholar 41:16–26

Part III
The Genetics of Schizophrenia

Contributions of Genetic Studies on Schizophrenia

E. Kringlen

The study of schizophrenia illustrates in a special way how ideas within psychiatry have changed and how psychiatric thought is determined by the zeitgeist. Until recently the psychiatric establishment held the view that schizophrenia was a genetic disease. In the mid-1960s this view changed, partly because of new twin studies that de-emphasized the genetic component. But more important was perhaps the influence of the humanistic existential movement, the new family hypotheses and the emphasis on social processes in general, which grew out of a liberal reformist ideology created by the economic growth that followed the postwar period in the United States and Western Europe. During recent years, in an age of economic stagnation, the pendulum has swung back to a more conservative and biological point of view.

The first systematic genetically-oriented epidemiological studies of schizophrenia were carried out by Ernst Rüdin and his pupils in Munich before World War I. Investigations from Germany and other countries confirmed that schizophrenia ran in the family – a fact that without further ado was cited in support of a hereditary predisposition. The problem for these research psychiatrists was in fact not whether schizophrenia was inherited or not, but how the genetic transmission took place.

However, in mental disorder, family incidence is no proof of a hereditary disposition, because environmental influences might be confounded with genetic factors. In order to throw light on the complicated problems of heredity and environment, one has to employ strategic populations. In this review, the main emphasis will therefore be on twin and adoption studies, because these studies contain the most important etiological information that we possess about the disorder.

Twin Studies

Twin research might in principle be able to shed some light on the following questions:
- Are genetic factors present in the disorder under discussion (concordance studies)?
- Are various traits or syndromes genetically related, and is it possible to discover vulnerability factors in the non-affected co-twin (nosological research)?

Department of Psychiatry, University of Oslo, 85 Vinderen 0319 Oslo 3, Norway

– Is it possible to identify certain environmental factors that discriminate between disturbed twins in affected and non-affected monozygotic pairs (studies of discordance)?

Concordance Figures

By and large, previous investigations of twins have shown much higher concordance figures for monozygotic (MZ) than for dizygotic (DZ) twins with respect to schizophrenia. This difference was most conspicuous in Kallmann's (1946, 1950) extensive samples; he reported concordance of 86% in MZ and 15% in DZ twins.

With regard to Kallmann's studies, the high concordance rates in MZ twins can be ascribed to shortcomings in sampling, with the disproportionately large inclusion of concordant pairs, but also the etablishment of zygosity, the statistical handling of the data and the psychiatric diagnostics are disputable (see e.g. Rosenthal 1970).

In more recent studies by Inouye (1961), Tienari (1963), Kringlen (1967), Gottesman and Shields (1966) and Fischer (1973), the difference in concordance rates between MZ and DZ is considerably less marked.

Kringlen's 1967 study, which has the largest sample, included both same-sex and opposite-sex DZ pairs. A national twin register for the period 1901–1930 was established, based on birth lists from the Norwegian Central Bureau of Statistics. This twin register – comprising 25 588 pairs – was subsequently matched with the National Register of Psychoses, yielding a sample of 342 pairs of twins. These twins were in the age group 35–64, and one or both of each pair had at some time in their lives been hospitalized in Norway for functional psychosis, i.e. schizophrenia, manic-depressive illness or reactive psychosis. The majority of the families of the MZ pairs, including the parents and the siblings, were personally investigated. Forty-two pairs of DZ twins of the same sex were also personally investigated, but not their families.

The concordance figures for strictly defined schizophrenia plus the group with schizophreniform psychoses (Langfeldt's criteria), are presented in Table 1.

Table 2 shows the concordance figures when a rather wide concept of concordance is being used, based on personal investigation as well as hospitalization. A

Table 1. Concordance for schizophrenia and schizophreniform psychoses: hospitalized and registered cases (based on Kringlen 1967)

	Number of pairs	Concordant pairs	Discordant pairs	Concordance (%)
MZ	55	14	41	25
DZ (same sex)	90	6	84	7
Unknown zygosity (same sex)	6	0	6	0
DZ (opposite sex)	82	8	74	10
Total pairs	233	28	205	12

Table 2. Concordance for schizophrenia and schizophreniform psychoses: further personal investigation (based on Kringlen 1967)

	Number on pairs	Concordant pairs	Disordant pairs	Concordance (%)
MZ	55	21	34	38
DZ (same sex)	90	9	81	10
Total pairs	145	30	115	21

Table 3. Concordance in MZ and DZ twins with respect to schizophrenia in four studies

Investigator(s)	Year	Country	n	MZ Concordance (%)[a]	n	DZ Concordance (%)[a]
Gottesman and Shields	1966	England	24	42	33	9
Kringlen	1967	Norway	55	25–38	172	8–12
Fischer	1973	Denmark	21	24–48	41	10–19
Tienari	1975[b]	Finland	20	15	42	7

[a] Values for concordance are percentages. The lower figures usually refer to concordance when a strict concept of schizophrenia is employed (hospitalization). The higher figures refer to concordance when a broad concept is used – for instance, designating a pair concordant if the index twin is typically schizophrenic and the co-twin is a borderline case (by follow-up).
[b] Tienari's 1975 study is based upon follow-ups of his 1963 study with a few additional pairs of twins included.

pair is grouped as concordant if one twin has a diagnosis of schizophrenia or schizophreniform psychosis and the co-twin has either the same diagnosis or a diagnosis of reactive psychosis or borderline.

Based on a summary of recent studies, concordance is on average around 30% for MZ and around 10% for DZ twins, with regard to schizophrenia (Table 3). The difference between MZ and DZ is in fact lower if founded on the studies from the Nordic countries (Tienari, Kringlen, Fischer) that are based upon population samples. To quarrel about the true concordance rate is a waste of time, but to maintain, as several reviews do nowadays, that concordance in schizophrenia for MZ is 50% is simply wrong.

Table 4 gives the concordance with respect to schizophrenia for the two sexes separately, based on several investigations. The literature clearly shows a trend toward higher concordance rates for females, both in MZ and in DZ same-sex twins. This is apparent in the studies of Luxemburger, Rosanoff et al. and Slater. Kallmann and Inouye did not give breakdowns of their concordant and discordant pairs by sex. Tienari studied only male pairs. Furthermore, there is a higher concordance rate for same-sex DZ twins than for opposite-sex DZ twins in the studies for which such figures are available. The differences, however, seem to disappear in more recent studies; this is particularly so in the Kringlen study.

Table 4. Concordance (%) with respect to schizophrenia in male and female MZ and DZ twins

Investigator(s)	MZ		DZ (same sex)		DZ (opposite sex)
	Female	Male	Female	Male	
Luxenburger (1928)	88	67	–	–	–
Rosanoff et al. (1934)	78	42	14	9	6
Slater and Shields (1953)	73	45	16	10	5
Inouye (1961)	62	58	–	–	–
Gottesman and Shields (1966)	45	38	12	6	–
Kringlen (1967)[a]	29	23	9	6	10
	33	42	–	–	–

Kallmann (1946) did not break down the figures according to sex, but from his figures for same-sex and opposite-sex pairs one can compute that the ratio is 17.6 to 11.5
[a] Schizophreniform psychoses included. First row based on hospitalized registered cases, second row on personal investigation.

It is unlikely that differential sampling techniques can explain this tendency (Rosenthal 1961). A more plausible hypothesis seems to be that girls were formerly brought up more strictly with less opportunity than boys for social contacts outside the home, and thus were less able to escape a disturbed family milieu. Increasing female emancipation may offer an explanation as to the disappearance of the higher female concordance rates in more recent studies.

Concordance in Twins and Ordinary Siblings

Table 5 summarizes the results obtained in various studies as regards the morbidity figures for twins compared with those in ordinary siblings. As the table shows,

Table 5. Morbidity risk in siblings of schizophrenics, based on twin populations in per cent

Studies compared		Relation to index case		
		MZ co-twins	DZ co-twins	Full sibs
Luxenburger	1935 Germany	54.0	14.0	11.8
Kallmann	1946 USA	69.0	10.3	10.2
		(85.8)	(14.7)	(14.3)
Slater and Shields	1953 England	68.3	11.3	4.6
		(76.3)	(14.4)	(5.4)
Kringlen	1967 Norway	25.4	8.1	3.0
		(38.2)	(12.0)	(–)
Fischer	1973 Denmark	56.0	26.6	10.0

The percentages in parenthesis refer to age-corrected figures with respect to the studies by Kallmann and Slater and Shields. The figures in parenthesis with respect to Kringlen's study refer to percentages based on personal investigation and employment of a wide concept of concordance (the first figures are based on hospitalized cases). The figures in Fischer's study refer to schizophrenia and schizophrenic-like psychosis.

there is first of all a clear difference in morbidity rates (concordance) between MZ co-twins and the other groups. One should note, however, that there is also a difference in concordance between DZ twins and ordinary siblings, the rates for DZ being higher. Clear-cut differences are observed especially in the studies of Slater and Shields (1953), Kringlen (1967) and Fischer (1973). Tienari (1963) and Gottesman and Shields (1966) did not investigate siblings. These findings are rather consistent. One reservation must be made, namely that it is theoretically possible that the twins in the various samples were investigated more carefully than the siblings, although Fischer denies this possibility with regard to her sample.

It is natural to attach some importance to these observed differences, and to ascribe the higher morbidity figure in co-twins of DZ twins than in ordinary siblings to the twinship itself. From a genetical point of view one should expect to find the same rate for DZ twins as for siblings.

The Co-twin of MZ Schizophrenics

The pronounced discordance for schizophrenia in MZ twins proves that environmental factors play a significant role in the etiology. One could argue, however, that it is not schizophrenia as such that is inherited, but a kind of borderline condition or a certain personality structure which predisposes to development of schizophrenia. If most of the nonschizophrenic co-twins were more or less schizophrenic, borderline or schizoid, this would suggest a relationship between schizophrenia and such states. However, a greater variability of clinical pictures in the non-schizophrenic co-twin would not constitute adequate support for such a hypothesis.

The variability of psychiatric symptoms within MZ pairs was noted by Luxenburger (1928) and Rosanoff et al. (1934). Essen-Møller (1941), Slater and Shields (1953), Tienari (1963), Kringlen (1967), Fischer (1973) and Gottesman and Shields (1972) all report considerable disparity in the clinical picture of MZ pairs when the index case is schizophrenic. All these authors have also described co-twins of MZ schizophrenics who are quite normal. The main results are set out in Table 6.

Kringlen (1967) observed that in 31% of cases both twins showed the same psychopathology. In another 9% the co-twins of schizophrenics had either been affected with a reactive psychosis or could be described as borderline cases. According to DSM-III, these borderline cases would most likely be classified as schizotypal personality disorders (Table 7).

In a group of neurotic co-twins, we find a broad spectrum of clinical symptoms, namely character disorders (personality disorders), anxiety states, depressive neuroses, somatic neuroses and one case where alcohol was the main problem. In the group of "normal" co-twins, the deviances or symptoms have all been of a trivial nature, not warranting a clinical diagnosis.

In a series of 11 pairs, later enlarged to 17 pairs, especially selected because they were discordant for schizophrenia, Pollin and coworkers (1965) observed that although many of the co-twins had obsessive compulsive traits, they were less disturbed, and none were schizoid.

Table 6. Co-twins of definite schizophrenic MZ twins in systematic studies (schizophreniform psychosis excluded)

Study	No. of pairs	Schizophrenia	Possible schizophrenia, reactive psychosis, borderline states	Neurotic-like disorder	Clinically normal
Essen-Møller (1941)	6	–	4	1	1
Slater and Shields (1953)	34	18	8	2	6
Tienari (1963)	14	–	–	6	8
Kringlen (1967)	45	14	4	13	14
Gottesman and Shields (1972)	22	8	3	6	5
Fischer (1973)	21	5	5	2	9
Total	142	45 (32%)	24 (17%)	30 (21%)	43 (30%)

Table 7. Classification of the MZ co-twins of index cases with typical schizophrenia, excluding schizophreniform disorders. (Based on Kringlen 1967)

Type of psychopathology	n	%
Typical schizophrenia	14	31
Reactive psychosis	1	2
Borderline	3	7
Neurosis	13	29
Normality	14	31
Total	45	100

The existence of a normal co-twin of a clear-cut schizophrenic MZ is remarkable both from a genetic and an environmental point of view. If the genes play a significant role, one would expect to observe, if not identical clinical syndromes, at least some deviance in a schizophrenic direction (schizophrenic spectrum) in the co-twins. If environmental factors such as family conflicts might predispose to schizophrenia, one would expect that both twins in the MZ pairs should be affected in one way or another.

One might wonder if all the so-called normal or neurotic co-twins are more or less randomly paired with various subtypes of schizophrenia and the various degrees of severity this disorder presents. Would, for instance, a case of malignant schizophrenia – believed by many to be of genetic origin – be more aptly paired with a psychotic who shows either the same type of psychosis or a borderline type with marked schizoid traits, whereas a case of benign schizophrenia – believed to be non-genetic in origin – ought to be paired with a merely neurotic co-twin or even with a normal co-twin? The data show that the normal co-twin may be paired with any type of schizophrenia. Furthermore, the normal co-twin may be paired not only with moderately severe cases of schizophrenia, but even with extremely deteriorated partners (Kringlen 1967; Gottesman and Shields 1972).

In conclusion, several twin studies clearly show that the clinical picture found in the non-schizophrenic MZ co-twin is rather variable, ranging from a duplication of the schizophrenic psychosis to neurosis, or even clinical normalcy. The findings lend no support to the idea that some subtypes of schizophrenia are considerably more genetically determined than others; furthermore, there is no clear evidence of hereditary factors influencing the course and outcome.

Environmental Factors

One of the main aims of the twin studies reviewed above has been to study the relative contribution of heredity and environment in schizophrenia. It ought to be stressed, however, that the twin method is also one of the best milieu methods, because here the genetic factor is under control and each difference encountered in MZ twins can be ascribed to environmental influences. How this opportunity is utilized is shown in *The Genain Quadruplets*, edited by Rosenthal (1963). Here one was able to show that different life experiences were related to different clinical states and furthermore that severity and outcome were also clearly related to premorbid personality.

Pollin and coworkers (1965, 1966) have clearly shown that there is a consistent tendency of a number of interacting features to differentiate the life course of the schizophrenic twin from that of the co-twin. The most remarkable finding – at variance with most of the literature – was that each one of the 11 index twins was smaller at birth. The sampling method employed may perhaps explain the contrasting findings of this study. The authors noted that the parents, particularly the mother, had regarded the schizophrenic twin as more vulnerable in childhood than the non-schizophrenic twin. He had been the recipient of more anxious care and attention. His early development was slower, he was more passive and dependent, and he performed less successfully in school. The same research group also observed that the disturbed twin of the discordantly affected MZ pairs had usually identified with the parent with the more deviant personality (Mosher et al. 1971). Similar observations have recently been done in an on-going study in my department (Onstad and Kringlen).

Slater and Shields (1953), Tienari (1963) and Kringlen (1967) all found that in discordant MZ pairs, the more submissive, dependent and neurotic twin tends to be the one who develops schizophrenia. Kringlen also observed that MZ discordant schizophrenic twins had been exposed to a more variable milieu than concordant pairs. Concordant pairs tended to have had less social contact with other children and thus less varied social experience, had been closer to each other in childhood, more overprotected and more often brought up alike by their parents. Discordant pairs, on the other hand, had been separated more often in childhood and for longer periods of time, and had more frequently received differential treatment and affection from their fathers. In general the concordant pairs seemed to have faced a more stressful as well as more similar environment. They tended to come from a lower social class and a worse economic situation than their discordant counterparts, and appeared to be more socially isolated. Thus the life history of schizophrenics and their non-schizophrenic co-twins displays consistent early differences in personality and parental treatment (Wahl 1976).

In the main, the results from the larger twin studies show that birth order, birth weight, difficulties during birth, physical strength in early childhood and psychomotoric development during the first years of life are of practically no significance for later development of schizophrenia. On the other hand, there is a clear coprrelation between some personality factors in childhood and later schizophrenia.

In both MZ and DZ groups, the schizophrenic twin has significantly more often been submissive, reserved, lonely, obsessive and more dependent than the other twin. The same tendency is present with such traits as sensitivity and obedience. Furthermore, in both MZ and DZ twins, the schizophrenics have significantly more often been more mentally disturbed in childhood. Premorbidly, the schizophrenic twin had fewer friends of both sexes and was more passive sexually than the non-schizophrenic twin, and also more often unmarried. The schizophrenic twin also had a lower social status than the non-schizophrenic twin. These differences in personality can be ascribed to environmental factors, because they are present not only in DZ twins, but also in MZ twins.

MZ Twins Reared Apart

As mentioned above, one of the problems in twin research is related to the fact that MZ twins usually have a more similar environment than DZ twins. The best method is therefore to study MZ twins separated in early childhood and reared apart. It goes without saying that it is hard to find such pairs.

The literature comprises only seven descriptions of schizophrenic MZ pairs separated in early childhood and brought up apart. Four of these were concordant and three discordant for schizophrenia (Table 8). Some of the concordant

Table 8. MZ twins with schizophrenia or schizophrenic-like psychosis separated in early childhood and brought up apart

Investigator	Diagnosis	
	Twin A	Twin B
Kallmann (1938)	Schizophrenia	Schizophrenia
Craike and Slater (1945)	Schizophrenia (paranoid?), sensitiver Beziehungswahn	Reactive psychosis, depressive-paranoid (schizophrenia?)
Kallmann and Roth (1956)	Schizophrenia	Schizophrenia
Shields (1962)	Schizophrenia (paranoid-catatonic)	Schizophrenia
Tienari (1963)	Schizophrenia (hebephrenic)	Normal, introverted
Kringlen (1964)	Schizophrenia (catatonic)	Normal
Kringlen (1967)	Schizophreniform (catatonic)	Schizophreniform (paranoid-depressive)

pairs are to some extent subject to the same criticism as case histories of twins in general, namely that the pairs were chosen for publication just because they were concordant. Secondly, one observes on examining the case histories in detail that in most cases the childhood conditions were extremely miserable and stressful and quite similar for both twins (Kringlen 1967).

Offspring of MZ Twins Discordant for Schizophrenia

By studying offspring of MZ twins discordant for schizophrenia one should be able to get an impression of the magnitude of the genetic contribution. Some of these children have a biological mother or father who has been schizophrenic, the others have biological parents who are both clinically normal (non-schizophrenic) although one of them has the same genes as a psychotic index twin. A genetic hypothesis would predict that the children of discordant MZ twins develop psychopathology to the same degree, since both have the same genetic disposition. An environmental hypothesis, i.e., one stressing rearing in a psychotic milieu, would predict that the children of the co-twins develop psychoses less frequently.

In a recent study by Kringlen and Cramer (1986), 155 offspring of MZ and DZ twins were investigated clinically using a structured interview (SCID). As one can observe from Table 9, the number of schizophrenic subjects is higher in the offspring of MZ probands than in the offspring of co-twins, although the difference is not statistically significant.

According to family, twin and adoption studies, there is a preponderance of odd, eccentric, paranoid or schizotypal personalities in the biological relatives of schizophrenics. As can be seen from Table 10, there are also relatively more such cases in the offspring of probands than in the offspring of co-twins in the MZ group. Although the difference is not statistically significant, it tends to indicate that also these "spectrum cases" have a strong environmental component.

Table 9. Offspring of index and co-twins in MZ pairs discordant for schizophrenia

Diagnosis DSM-III axis I	Offspring of index		Offspring of co-twins	
Normal	15	60.0%	24	60.0%
Adjustment disorder	2		4	
Simple phobia	–		2	
Panic disorder	–		1	
Posttraumatic stress disorder	–	28.0%	1	37.5%
Dysthymia	–		2	
Cyclothymia	1		1	
Major depression	3		2	
Substance abuse	1		2	
Schizophrenia	2	12.5%	1	2.5%
Total	25	100%	40	100%

Table 10. "Schizophrenic spectrum" in offspring of index and co-twins in MZ pairs discordant for schizophrenia

Diagnosis (DSM-III axes I and II)	Offspring of index twins		Offspring of co-twins	
Schizophrenia I	3 ⎫		1 ⎫	
Paranoid II	2 ⎬ 20.0%		(1) ⎬ 5.0% (7.5%)	
Schizotypal II	– ⎭		1 ⎭	
Total	25		40	

Adoption Studies

By studying adopted children, it is theoretically possible to distinguish the effects of an environment from the effects of genes. The transmitters of heredity and social experience can be separated because the biological parents are not the parents who rear the children. If schizophrenia is mainly genetically determined, one should expect that adopted children of schizophrenic biological parents will suffer from schizophrenia as frequently as children who grow up with their schizophrenic parents. On the other hand, if schizophrenia is largely socially transmitted, one would expect that the frequency of schizophrenia in adopted offspring of schizophrenics would go down.

Three strategies have been employed in the adoption studies. First, one can examine the adopted-away offspring of biological parents known to be affected by schizophrenia. This method was used by Heston, Rosenthal and now by Tienari. In the second method, one starts with adoptees known to be schizophrenic and then investigates their biological and adoptive families. This design was used by Kety. A third method employed by Wender should also be mentioned, namely the study of children of normals "crossfostered" to adoptive parents who later became schizophrenic.

Adopted Offspring of Schizophrenics

Heston (1966) compared the psychosocial adjustment of 47 adults born to schizophrenic mothers with 50 matched controls of non-schizophrenic mothers. Five of the 47 persons born to schizophrenic mothers developed schizophrenia versus none in the control group, thus strongly supporting a genetic hypothesis. However, not only schizophrenics but sociopathic, neurotic as well as mentally deficient and artistically gifted persons were found in greater numbers than usual in the offspring born to schizophrenic mothers. Thus, the experimental group showed considerably more variability in personality and behaviour than did the control group.

A few questions may be raised in connection with this study. First, how far are the two groups of adoptive parents comparable? Because the adoptive parents evidently received information about the child's biological parents, one might

Table 11. Schizophrenic-like disorders in adopted-away children of schizophrenic and normal parents in Rosenthal's study: records and interview data

Category	Total offspring	Definite schizophrenia		Borderline condition		Total affected	
		n	%	n	%	n	%
Offspring of schizophrenics (adopted-away index)	52	3	5.8	11	21.1	14	26.9
Offspring of normals (adopted-away control)	67	0	0.0	12	17.9	12	17.9

wonder who would adopt such a child. Such questions are important in view of the fact that the author found a high incidence not only of schizophrenic but also of neurotic and sociopathic behaviour, as well as cases of mental deficiency, in the experimental group.

Rosenthal and coworkers obtained a pool of 5483 adopted Copenhagen children and matched the biological parents against the Danish psychosis register in order to obtain psychotic parents who had given their children up for adoption. Of the 76 parents originally selected, we are left with 52 parents with the diagnosis of schizophrenia (including four cases of reactive schizophrenia and four of borderline schizophrenia). A summary of the clinical data is shown in Table 11.

Although the difference in psychopathology between adopted offspring of schizophrenics and of normal controls is not statistically significant at the 5% level, the figures are in accordance with a genetic hypothesis. Three offspring of schizophrenic parents as opposed to none of the offspring of controls were diagnosed as schizophrenics, although only one had been hospitalized with such a diagnosis. There are also more offspring with borderline conditions in the schizophrenic group than in the control group, although the difference here is less conspicuous.

The rate of 17.9% of borderline conditions in the adopted offspring of normals is remarkably high. The uncorrected rate of 1.3% for hospitalized schizophrenia among the index adoptees is remarkably low when compared with the rates reported for offspring of schizophrenics in general. In different studies, these rates have varied around 10%. If one considers only the offspring of the definitely schizophrenic parents, one does not find a single hospitalized schizophrenic among the 30 offspring. Rosenthal (1971) suggests that adoptive rearing may reduce the expected rate of schizophrenia, because it is difficult to see how such a low rate could be explained by sampling bias.

During the last decade, a sample of 288 adopted-away offspring of schizophrenic mothers have been investigated by Tienari and coworkers. These high-risk subjects have been compared with matched adopted controls, i.e. adoptees of non-schizophrenic biological parents (Tienari et al. 1981). Whereas Rosenthal et al. (1968) studied the adoptive parents indirectly, Tienari et al. have investigated the adoptive families directly with family and individual interviews and psychological tests.

Table 12. The mental health ratings of 91 index adoptees and matched controls[a]

Adopted offspring	Schizophrenic parent	Non-schizophrenic controls
Healthy	1	9
Mild disturbance	43	37
Neurotic	23	31
Character disorder	9	8
Borderline	8	5
Psychotic	7	1
Total	91	91
Mean mental health rating[b]	3.01	2.63

[a] Modified after Tienari et al. (1984).
[b] Index and control offspring were rated from 1 (healthy) to 6 (psychotic).

Preliminary data from this comprehensive study support the hypothesis of an *interaction* of genetic and environmental rearing factors in schizophrenia. First of all, more subjects with severe mental disorders were observed in the offspring of schizophrenic mothers than in the offspring of non-schizophrenic mothers. Among 91 index offspring and 91 matched controls, Tienari et al. observed six schizophrenic and one manic-depressive offspring in the first group as opposed to one psychotic (schizophrenic?) subject in the second group. The total proportion of subjects with a spectrum diagnosis (schizophrenia, borderline, character disorder) is 27% in the index group and 15% in the control group. Of considerable interest is the observation that severely disturbed adoptive families produce a large number of seriously disturbed individuals if these are offspring of schizophrenic mothers. In both experimental and control groups, the mean rating of the offspring increases if the disturbande in the adoptive family becomes more severe. In other words, there is a clear-cut interaction effect, and notably it would appear that subjects with a genetic predisposition are particularly vulnerable to a noxious family environment. The offspring of schizophrenic mothers who had been brought up in a severely disturbed adoptive family, received the gravest rating in 63% of cases and only 6% have been rated healthy, in contrast to the control cases, where 37% received the most severe rating and 23% were rated healthy (Tienari et al. 1983, 1984).

Biological Relatives of Adopted Schizophrenics

Like Rosenthal, Kety and coworkers obtained a national sample of adoptees from Denmark. Most of the published reports deal with a Copenhagen sample of 5483 adoptees of whom 507 had been hospitalized for psychiatric reasons. On the basis of case summaries, the diagnosis of schizophrenia was established for 34, of whom 17 were chronic schizophrenics. Thirty-four controls consisted of

Table 13. Schizophrenic-like disorders in biological and adoptive relatives of schizophrenic and normal adoptees in Kety's study: records and interview data

Category	Total	Definite or uncertain schizophrenia	
		n	%
Biological parents of schizophrenic adoptees	66	8	12.1
Biological parents of control adoptees	65	4	6.2
Adoptive parents of schizophrenic adoptees	63	1	1.6
Adoptive parents of control adoptees	68	3	4.4
Biological half-sibs of schizophrenic adoptees	104	19	18.3
Biological half-sibs of control adoptees	104	3	2.9

carefully matched adoptees who were not reported to the central psychiatric register (Kety et al. 1968, 1975).

A genetic hypothesis would predict higher prevalence of schizophrenia in the biological relatives of schizophrenic adoptees than in the biological relatives of normal adoptees. At first sight, the hypothesis was confirmed. Biological relatives of the schizophrenic adoptees contained an excees of schizophrenic spectrum disorders as opposed to both the biological relatives of normal adoptees and the adoptive relatives who reared these adoptees. More specifically, when the 21 relatives with schizophrenic spectrum disorder were broken down into the various groups, 13 were biologically related to the schizophrenic adoptees and only three were biologically related to the control adoptees.

The problem with this result, however, is that the clear-cut difference is due to a very high frequency of schizophrenic spectrum disorder in the half-sibs (second-degree relatives). Nine of the 13 biological relatives of the schizophrenic adoptees with a spectrum disorder were in fact half-sibs. If one compares only first-degree relatives in the groups of biological relatives of schizophrenics and biological relatives of normals, there are, true enough, more schizophrenic spectrum disorders in the index group (9/69 or 13%) than in the control group (5/70 or 7%), but the difference is not statistically significant. With regard to definite chronic schizophrenia there is no difference at all, with one case in each group. This result is not remarkable, since the majority of first-degree relatives are parents, where the prevalence is expected to be low, but it does weaken the genetic hypothesis. From a scientific point of view, it is regrettable that there are so few ordinary sibs in the sample, only three compared with the 73 half-sibs.

In order to strengthen the validity of these findings, psychiatric interviews of these biological and adoptive relatives were carried out by a Danish psychiatrist who did not know to which group they belonged. A significantly greater frequency of schizophrenic spectrum disorders occurred among the biological than among the adoptive relatives of the schizophrenic adoptees (Kety et al. 1975). Of the biological relatives of the 173 index cases, 37 (21.4%) received a schizophrenia spectrum diagnosis, compared with 19 (10.98%) of the 174 controls. In the initial report by Kety et al. (1968) less than 5% of the relatives received a schizophrenia spectrum diagnosis, whereas in the more recent reports approximately 20% of the relatives were so diagnosed.

Crossfostering Studies

Wender and coworkers (1974) were able to study offspring of normal parents who for various reasons had given their child for adoption to parents who later developed schizophrenia. Compared with children of schizophrenics adopted by normals, the children of normals adopted by future schizophrenics were less often schizophrenic. In fact the children of normals adopted by future schizophrenics had no more schizophrenia-like disorders than the adopted controls (10.7% vs 10.1%). Again, the number of cases is low and the difference between the groups is not statistically significant. Furthermore, it turned out that half of the biological parents of the adopted controls were so-called schizophrenia spectrum subjects. Nor can one be certain that the hypothesized environmental schizophrenogenic factor was permitted to manifest itself in the future schizophrenic group. Obviously the parents had been healthy enough to have been accepted as adoptive parents in the first place.

General Discussion

Both theoretical criticism and empirical studies have clearly documented that earlier twin studies, owing to various sources of error, yielded results overestimating the genetic factor. More recent investigations that have attempted to avoid the pitfalls of unrepresentative sampling and uncertain zygosity diagnosis have arrived at considerably lower concordance rates in MZ twins with respect to schizophrenia. In the investigations so far, this pattern seems rather consistent: the more accurate and careful the sampling, the lower the concordance figures for MZ twins.

What are then the representative concordance figures with respect to schizophrenia? If one uses direct pairwise concordance, which is simple and reasonable when comparing MZ and DZ twins, the four recent twin studies based on systematic sampling yield average concordance rates for MZ twins of around 30%–40% or less; for DZ twins 10%–12%. These are maximum figures, however, because of shortcomings in the sampling even in these studies.

The total difference in concordance rate between MZ and DZ twins cannot be ascribed to genetic factors only. A series of studies of both normal and abnormal twins show that the environment of the MZ twin pairs is more similar than the environment of the DZ twin pairs.

One should also note that there is a difference in concordance rates between DZ twins and ordinary siblings. In the study by Kringlen (1967), the rates for strict schizophrenia are 8%–9% for DZ co-twins and 3% for siblings (of MZ twins). Similar differences are also to be found in the studies by Slater and Shields (1953) and Fischer (1973).

In the main, the adoption studies support the findings of the twin studies. Whereas the twin studies prove the significance of the environment and indicate that genes are also of importance, the adoption studies prove the existence of genetic factors and suggest the importance of the environment.

Having said this, one ought to add that the Danish-American adoption studies are surrounded by methodological uncertainties. With regard to sampling, only definite parents were permitted to give their children up for legal adoption. Furthermore, the adopting parents represented, as in most western countries, a restricted range of environment for the child. In addition, as in most of the previous adoption studies, a strong correlation was observed between the socioeconomic status of the biological parents and that of the adopting parents. Finally, the spouses of schizophrenics whose offspring are adopted tended to be sicker than such spouses in general. It would appear that these weaknesses with regard to sampling probably lead to an overestimation of genetic factors.

A recurring problem in adoption studies, as in twin research, is the small size of the sample. The differences reported between experimental and control groups are usually small, and mostly not statistically significant, except for the Tienari study. The more pronounced differences are usually arrived at by enlarging the concept of schizophrenia to a so-called schizophrenia spectrum of doubtful heuristic value.

In the studies by Heston, Rosenthal and Tienari, the starting point was schizophrenic parents, in most cases mothers who had given their child up for adoption. Based on family studies of schizophrenia, it is known that the risk of schizophrenia in offspring of schizophrenic parents is about 10%. The adoptive method makes it possible to discover whether the same risk persists when the children are separated from their schizophrenic parents and reared in another milieu. If such is the case, the genetic hypothesis is strongly corroborated. One might ask, however, if these schizophrenic parents are representative of the general population of schizophrenics. Ninety per cent of schizophrenics are born to nonschizophrenic parents, although some in addition have parents who are mentally disturbed. In this connection it is of interest to note that children of schizophrenic parents, as a group, show more thought disturbance than normal controls, i.e. children of non-schizophrenic parents (Kendler and Hays 1982; Walker and Shaye 1982). Could it be that the genetic contribution to schizophrenia is higher in that special group of schizophrenia? This would follow from a hypothesis of polygenic inheritance. If such is the case, the adoptive method as used by Heston, Rosenthal and Tienari overestimates the genetic contribution to schizophrenia in general.

Much of the debate regarding Kety's studies has focused on the biological half-silbings (see e.g. Gottesman and Shields 1966; Grove 1983; Kety 1983; Lidz and Blatt 1983 a, b). The different studies of morbidity of schizophrenia in the families of schizophrenics have revealed that approximately 4% of the parents, 7%–8% of siblings and 3% of half-sibs develop schizophrenia. In the Kety study the number of half-sibs with schizophrenic spectrum disorders far exceeds what one would expect. The extensive psychopathology in the half-sibs cannot be ascribed to genetic factors, but must be due to environmental influences, most likely adverse rearing and unstable care, for instance in institutions. Thus the interpretation of the findings of Kety's studies is far from easy. A conservative view would hold that the findings indicate some role for genetic factors in the etiology of schizophrenia, but do not prove it.

The Borderline of Schizophrenia

There are patients with both a schizophrenic and an affective symptomatology, usually labelled schizoaffective disorder. No twin or adoption studies have addressed themselves specifically to this group. One must therefore, rely on family studies that can only be suggestive.

In the main, the recent studies by Tsuang (1979), Baron et al. (1982) and Gershon et al. (1982) do not support the hypothesis that schizoaffective disorder is transmitted as a separate and specific diagnostic entity. Obviously, there is a familiar overlap between affective disorder and schizophrenia in the transmission of the schizoaffective syndrome.

During the last decade, clinicians and research workers have increasingly been discussing a group of conditions which do not meet any clear-cut criteria for schizophrenia, manic-depressive disorder or neurosis. Labels such as borderline state, schizophrenic borderline, borderline personality and narcissistic personality have been given to these conditions. The DSM-III has grouped these patients into schizotypal and borderline personality disorders.

No schizophrenic cases are observed in the co-twins of MZ with borderline conditions (Torgersen 1984). And although Kendler and Greuenberg (1984) confirmed previous results with a higher incidence of schizotypal personality disorders in the biological relatives of adopted-away chronic schizophrenics, the Danish-American adoption studies do not observe a single person with chronic schizophrenia in the biological relatives of adoptees with borderline schizophrenia.

A possibility might be as Siever and Gunderson (1979) have suggested that a subgroup of patients with schizotypal characteristics might have a stronger relationship to chronic schizophrenia. However, this needs to be demonstrated. Furthermore, a relationship does not necessarily mean a genetical relationship.

What Is Inherited and How Is the Genetic Transmission?

That the genes contribute to the etiology of schizophrenia has been established by twin and adoption studies. However, views differ with regard to the magnitude of the genetic contribution, nor do we know what is inherited and how specific the genetic liability is.

Obviously, the genes are not sufficient to produce the schizophrenic disorder. The number of discordantly affected MZ twins shows this. However, we do not know whether the genes are a necessary precondition. In some cases the genetic predisposition may be relatively strong, in other cases absent. Neither twin nor adoption studies have, however, been able to identify subgroups that are particularly genetically loaded.

The schizophrenic symptoms and functioning are evidently not inherited, but acquired by social learning and human interaction. Could it be that a certain potential for response patterns in the perceptual and cognitive field is inherited or that a genetic vulnerability predisposes to ego weakness with a certain risk of schizophrenic development?

Opinions among research workers also vary with regard to the specific genetical liability of schizophrenia. In a study of dual mating, Kringlen (1978) observed a positive correlation between various types of functional psychoses (schizophrenia, manic-depressive illness or reactive psychosis) in parent and child, although no relationship among subtypes of schizophrenia in parents and offspring was observed.

In the adoption study by Rosenthal and coworkers (1968, 1971), seven parents diagnosed as probably manic-depressive were included by the investigators. It is of interest for our discussion that these affectively ill parents contributed several cases to the schizophrenic spectrum, a finding which throws doubt upon the assumption that schizophrenia and manic-depressive illness are distinct from a genetic point of view.

In the adoption study by Tienari et al. (1984) six of the psychotic adoptees of schizophrenic parents were diagnosed schizophrenic, as opposed to only one case of manic-depressive illness. The same tendency is apparent in Kety's studies, where the majority of the biological relatives of schizophrenic adoptees were found to be in the schizophrenic spectrum (Kendler et al. 1984). Thus, it would appear that there is a moderately strong genetic specificity in schizophrenia.

Schizophrenia does not follow a single abnormal gene model. If recessivity or dominance was the case, one would expect higher concordance in MZ twins with regard to schizophrenia, and a higher frequency of disturbed offspring of dual mating pairs (Rosenthal 1966; Kringlen 1978).

The genetic hypothesis most widely favoured by research workers today is the multifactorial or polygenic model. The polygenic hypothesis is implicit in the view according to which schizophrenic illnesses are to be considered as extremes of a continuum which extends from clinical normalcy to schizophrenia. A polygenic model would give a range of dysfunction from mild to severe, severely ill probands usually having more affected relatives than do borderline cases. The risk when it comes to relatives would increase as the number of affected members of the family increases, and the risk would drop as one goes from close relatives to distant ones. A polygenic inheritance can best explain the gliding transition from normality to severe mental illness found in twin partners and siblings and in parents of schizophrenics. This hypothesis also explains the fact that these illnesses occur rather frequently. Single-gene diseases are extremely rare.

The polygenic model might be divided into continuous and quasi-continuous (threshold) ones. The continuous model might be applied to traits such as height, blood pressure and intelligence, whereas the quasi-continuous model might be useful in theorizing on diseases such as diabetes and piloric stenosis and mental disorders such as schizophrenia. The distribution of this liability might be visualized by a normal bell-shaped curve, at one end of which is a point called the threshold which discriminates the individuals affected.

Future Prospects

At the Department of Psychiatry of the University of Oslo, we have now embarked on a comprehensive study of the co-twins of first-admission MZ twins with all types of functional psychosis, as well as borderline states. Hopefully this will bring us closer to understanding the factors that predispose to psychotic development. It goes without saying that such studies could also contribute to a more valid classification of mental disorder. With regard to discordance, our aim is to focus attention on the years prior to the outbreak of psychosis. First of all, the data might then be more reliable, but secondly such an emphasis is reasonable because previous studies of discordant twins in general seem to indicate that the differences in childhood between the twins in a pair had been rather slight.

In this study we will also employ computer tomographic scanning. Recent findings show that cerebral ventricular size is under a high degree of genetic control, with relatively small inter-pair differences in normal MZ twins. However, among MZ pairs discordant for schizophrenia, the mean inter-pair difference is significantly greater, and schizophrenics have consistently larger cerebral ventricles than both their non-schizophrenic co-twins and the normal controls. This of course suggests that ventricular enlargement in schizophrenia reflects the presence of environmental factors (Reveley et al. 1982). Reveley et al. (1984) also observed that for schizophrenic twins without a family history of psychosis there was evidence of complications at birth and increased cerebral ventricular size. In the group of twins with a family history of major psychiatric disorder, no evidence of ventricular enlargement was observed. The most reasonable interpretation of this finding is that ventricular enlargement is just one non-specific indicator of a past or present cerebral pathology necessary to produce a psychotic illness in those with low or no genetic predisposition.

By investigating discordance in different types of functional psychosis beyond schizophrenia, it might theoretically be possible to study the specific significance of the different life conditions and external events. Research in this area is a neglected field, partly because ordinary clinical studies cannot provide reliable data due to several sources of error, such as lack of control of the genetic and the retrospective nature of the data, which in such studies are difficult to control.

Conclusions

None of the data presented in this paper support the notion that schizophrenia is due to an underlying malignant disease process. It seems that schizophrenic disorder involves the interaction of biological and environmental factors. However, neither genetically nor environmentally oriented research has yet been able to identify the etiological factors that are necessary and/or sufficient for the disorder. Evidently, the genes for schizophrenic disorder are not sufficient for the development of the illness. But are the genes necessary? Are not adverse environmental conditions in some cases sufficient? The task now ought to be to define the specific biological and psychosocial factors involved, and to establish the mechanism by which they interact in the development of various forms of schizophrenic disorder. However, this is not easy.

References

Baron M, Gruen R, Asnis L, Kane J (1982) Schizoaffective illness, schizophrenia and affective disorders: morbidity risk and genetic transmission. Acta Psychiatr Scand 65:253–262

Essen-Møller E (1941) Psychiatrische Untersuchung an einer Serie von Zwillingen. Acta Psychiatr Scand [Suppl 23]

Fischer M (1973) Genetic and environmental factors in schizophrenia. Acta Psychiatr Scand [Suppl 238]

Gershon ES, Hamovit J, Guroff JJ et al. (1982) A family study of schizoaffective, bipolar I, bipolar II, unipolar, and normal control probands. Arch Gen Psychiatry 39:1157–1167

Gottesman II, Shields J (1966) Schizophrenia in twins: sixteen years' consecutive admissions to a psychiatric clinic. Br J Psychiatry 112:809–818

Gottesman II, Shields J (1972) Schizophrenia and genetics: a twin study vantage point. Academic, New York

Grove WM (1983) Comment on Lidz and associates: critique of the Danish/American studies of the offspring of schizophrenic parents. Am J Psychiatry 140:998–1002

Heston LL (1966) Psychiatric disorders in foster home reared children of schizophrenic mothers. Br J Psychiatry 112:819–825

Inouye E (1961) Similarity and dissimilarity of schizophrenia in twins. In: Proceedings of the Third World Congress of Psychiatry, vol 1. University of Toronto Press, Montreal, pp 524–530

Kallmann FJ (1946) The genetic theory of schizophrenia: an analysis of 691 schizophrenic twin indedx families. Am J Psychiatry 103:309–322

Kallmann FJ (1950) The genetics of psychoses: an analysis of 1,232 twin index families. In: Congres International de Psychiatrie. Rapport VI: Psychiatrie Sociale. Hermann, Paris

Kendler KS, Greuenberg AM (1984) An independent analysis of the Danish adoption study of schizophrenia. Arch Gen Psychiatry 41:555–564

Kendler KS, Hays P (1982) Familial and sporadic schizophrenia: a symptomatic prognostic and EEG comparison. Am J Psychiatry 139:1557–1562

Kety SS (1983) Letter to the editor. Am J Psychiatry 140:964

Kety SS, Rosenthal D, Wender PH, Schulsinger F (1968) The types and prevalence of mental illness in the biological and adoptive families of adopted schizophrenics. In: Rosenthal D, Kety SS (eds) The transmission of schizophrenia. Pergamon, New York

Kety SS et al. (1975) Mental illness in the biological and adoptive families of adopted individuals who have become schizophrenic: a preliminary report based on psychiatric interviews. In: Fieve RR, Rosenthal D, Bill H (eds) Genetic research in psychiatry. The John Hopkins University Press, Baltimore

Kringlen E (1967) Heredity and environment in the functional psychoses: an epidemiological-clinical twin study. University Press, Oslo. Reprinted by Heinemann, London (1968)

Kringlen E (1978) Adult offspring of two psychotic parents, with special reference to schizophrenia. In: Wynne LC, Cromwell RL, Matthysse S (eds) The nature of schizophrenia: new approaches to research and treatment. Wiley, New York

Kringlen E, Cramer G (1986) Genes and eye-movement dysfunctions and schizophrenia. A study of offspring of MZ and DZ twin pairs discordant for functional psychosis. Paper at Royal Society of Medicine, London

Lidz T, Blatt S (1983 a) Critique of the Danish/American studies of the biological and adoptive relatives of adoptees who became schizophrenic. Am J Psychiatry 140:426–435

Lidz T, Blatt S (1983 b) Letter to the editor. Am J Psychiatry 140:963

Luxenburger H (1928) Vorläufiger Bericht über psychiatrische Serienuntersuchungen an Zwillingen. Z Gesamte Neurol Psychiatr 116:297–326

Mosher LR, Pollin W, Stabenau JR (1971) Families with identical twins discordant for schizophrenia: some relationships between identification, thinking styles, psychopathology and dominance-submissiveness. Br J Psychiatry 118:29–42

Pollin W, Stabenau JR, Tupin J (1965) Family studies with identical twins discordant for schizophrenia. Psychiatry 28:60–78

Pollin W, Stabenau Jr, Mosher L, Tupin J (1966) Life history differences in identical twins discordant for schizophrenia. Am J Orthopsychiatry 36:492–509

Reveley AN, Revely MA, Clifford CA, Murray RN (1982) Cerebral ventricular size in twins discordant for schizophrenia. Lancet:540–541

Reveley AM, Reveley NA, Murray RM (1984) Cerebral ventricular enlargement in non-genetic schizophrenia: a controlled twin study. Br J Psychiatry 1:10–15

Rosanoff AJ, Handy LM, Plesset IR et al. (1934) The etiology of so-called schizophrenic psychoses: with special reference to their occurrence in twins. Am J Psychiatry 91:247–286

Rosenthal D (1961) Sex distribution and the severity of illness among samples of schizophrenic twins. J Psychiatr Res 1:26–36

Rosenthal D (ed) (1963) The Genain quadruplets. Basic, New York

Rosenthal D (1966) The offspring of schizophrenic couples. J Psychiatr Res 4:169–188

Rosenthal D (1970) Genetic theory and abnormal behaviour. McGraw-Hill, New York

Rosenthal D (1971) Two adoption studies of heredity in the schizophrenic disorders. In: Bleuler M, Angst J (eds) Die Entstehung der Schizophrenie. Huber, Bern

Rosenthal D, Wender PH, Kety SS et al. (1968) Schizophrenics' offspring reared in adoptive homes. In: Rosenthal D, Kety SS (eds) The transmission of schizophrenia. Pergamon, Oxford

Rosenthal D, Wender PH, Kety SS et al. (1971) The adopted-away offspring of schizophrenics. Am J Psychiatry 128:307–311

Siever LJ, Gunderson JG (1979) Genetic determinants of borderline conditions. Schizophr Bull 5:59–86

Slater E (1953) Psychotic and neurotic illnesses in twins. Her Majesty's Stationery Office, London (Medical Research Council Special Report Series 278)

Tienari P (1963) Psychiatric illnesses in identical twins. Acta Psychiatr Scand 39 [Suppl 171]

Tienari P (1975) Schizophrenia in finish male twins. In: Lader MH (ed) Studies of schizophrenia. Br J Psychiatry Spec Publ No 10

Tienari P, Sorri A, Naarala M et al. (1981) The Finnish adoptive family study. Psychiatry Soc Sci 1:107–116

Tienari P, Sorri A, Naarala M et al. (1983) The Finnish adoptive family study: adopted-away offspring of schizophrenic mothers. In: Sterlin H et al. (eds) Psychosocial intervention in schizophrenia. Springer, Berlin, Heidelberg, New York, Tokyo

Tienari P, Sorri A, Naarala M et al. (1984) Interaction of genetic and psychosocial factors in schizophrenia. Paper presented at WPA Regional Symposium, Helsinki

Torgersen S (1984) Genetic and nosological aspects of schizotypical and borderline personality disorders. Arch Gen Psychiatry 41:546–554

Tsuang MT (1979) "Schizo-affective disorder": dead or alive? Arch Gen Psychiatry 36:633–634

Wahl OF (1976) Monozygotic twins discordant for schizophrenia: a review. Psychol Bull 83:91–106

Walker E, Shaye J (1982) Familial schizophrenia: a predictor of neuromotor and attentional abnormalities in schizophrenia. Arch Gen Psychiatry 39:1153–1156

Wender PH, Rosenthal D, Kety SS et al. (1974) Crossfostering: a research strategy for clarifying the role of genetic and experimental factors in the etiology of schizophrenia. Arch Gen Psychiatry 30:121–128

Modern Diagnostic Criteria and Genetic Studies of Schizophrenia

P. McGuffin [1], A. E. Farmer [1], and I. I. Gottesman [2]

Operational Criteria: Help or Hindrance in Genetic Research?

In 1972 Gottesman and Shields published their definitive work *Schizophrenia and Genetics*, presenting their own twin study findings and critically reviewing other twin, family and adoption evidence. So compelling was the case for an important genetic contribution to schizophrenia that Professor Paul Meehl, in a "critical afterword", expressed the view that this was "the final step in a purely behavioural study of the genetics of schizophrenia". The implication was that further advances would surely come from techniques which took the researchers past purely surface clinical phenomenon, moving a step or two closer towards the primary gene product and revealing the causal origins of schizophrenia, "the thing in itself". It is, perhaps, chastening to consider that a decade and a half later only modest progress has been achieved. Over this period two major trends have been discernible in schizophrenia research. To be sure, one has been of an increasing concern with biological aspects of the condition. However, the other has centred on definitions and classifications of schizophrenia, such that it has now become virtually mandatory to employ operational criteria in any research paper which aims at publication.

The year 1972 also saw the birth of the criteria of Feighner et al., providing the first definition of schizophrenia to be cast explicitly in an operational form. The intention of these authors was clearly to enhance reliability and hence improve the repeatability of research findings. Feighner's criteria and subsequent operational definitions (e.g. Spitzer et al. 1975) offered the potential advantages of operationalism (Hempel 1961) and came to be widely prescribed as the "remedy for diagnostic confusion" in schizophrenia (Kendell 1975). However, with adherence to operational definitions as the prevailing philosophy, some authors began to question the veracity of *any* findings which had been reported prior to the operational criteria era. Such an overall view is regrettably shortsighted and likely to lead to errors, for it fails to see that reliable definitions provide no sure guarantee of validity.

Numerous operational definitions of schizophrenia have now been produced (see e.g. Berner et al. 1983) with considerable variation in their constituent items, their combinatorial rules and the amount of emphasis each places upon longitudinal as against cross-sectional aspects of schizophrenia. It is scarcely surprising,

[1] Dept. of Psychological Medicine, University of Wales College of Medicine, Cardiff CF4 4XN, United Kingdom
[2] Department of Psychology, University of Virginia, Charlottesville, Virginia, USA

therefore, that when a variety of operational definitions is employed to classify the same sample of patients there is frequently poor concordance over which subjects are or are not diagnosed as suffering from schizophrenia (Brockington et al. 1978). Therefore the most important question must be which of these many definitions has the greatest utility or validity. In the absence of any clear understanding of the pathophysiology of schizophrenia the question has to be answered by indirect means. For example, it might be asked which definition best predicts outcome or response to treatment, or best delineates a disorder with high heritability (Robins and Guze 1970). It is the latter approach with which we are chiefly concerned in this paper. Regrettably some authors have stood the question on its head and instead of asking whether definition X is useful, have asked whether schizophrenia is truly a familial/genetic condition given that we now have definition X? Therefore, although we would prefer to start from the premise that schizophrenia is a genetic condition and use this knowledge to assess which is the most useful operational definition, we must also consider whether, once schizophrenia has been operationally defined, there is still evidence for genetic transmission.

A further consequence of the introduction of operational definitions has been a rekindling of interest in heterogeneity. The application of operational criteria for schizophrenia subtypes to twins or other pairs of related individuals provides a means of assessing whether clinical heterogeneity reflects aetiological heterogeneity. We will therefore spend the first part of this paper considering the issue of operational definitions and the genetics of schizophrenia as a whole and will then go on to discuss what recent studies have so far told us about heterogeneity.

Family and Adoption Studies

The tendency for schizophrenia to run in families is accepted by most as a long-established fact. For example, the contribution of heredity was allowed by Jaspers (1962) as one of the few reasonably firm "causal connections" in schizophrenia. The facts and figures are now well known. The most authoritative summary has been produced by Gottesman and Shields (1982) who show, in a compilation of many studies, that the average morbid risk (or lifetime expectancy) of schizophrenia is around 10% in the first-degree relatives of index cases. The rates are lower in parents than in siblings or offspring, but if allowances are made for the fact that parents are "selected for health" and suitable statistical adjustments made for the reduced period of risk, then the expectancy for parents is close to that for other first-degree relatives (Essen-Møller 1955). The morbid risk is lower in second-degree relatives, at around 3%–4%, and higher in first-degree relatives where there are multiple members affected, so that, for example, in the offspring of two schizophrenic parents the risk is well over 40%. Such figures must be compared with a population morbid risk of around 1%. Some of the studies on which such figures are based date back over a period of almost 60 years and have been criticised for such shortcomings as absence of controls, failure to make diagnoses "blind" and, of course, a lack of explicit diagnostic criteria. Furthermore, some workers (e.g. Kallmann 1938) selected probands, or index cases, with "definite" schizophrenia but widened the criteria for relatives, including "probable" cases. Nevertheless, until recently, few challenged the facts of familiality of schizophrenia and the only controversy hinged upon whether genes or family environment were mainly responsible.

Challenges to the idea that schizophrenia is familial have, however, arisen recently. These come not from partisan environmentalists, but from researchers mainly interested in classification and the application of modern explicit diagnostic criteria. Pope and colleagues (1983) reported that on applying DSM-III criteria to family history information recorded in casenotes, none of a total of 199 first-degree relatives of schizophrenics had an illness which fulfilled the definition of schizophrenia. Subsequently, Abrams and Taylor (1983) used their own criteria to diagnose a sample of 128 first-degree relatives of schizophrenics. They reported that only two were schizophrenic, providing a lifetime prevalence of 1.6%. How could such results have arisen, and do they seriously challenge the conventional belief that schizophrenia is familial? The answers are less difficult than they would at first sight seem. Pope and colleagues used only family history information, which inevitably yields a lower rate of psychopathology among relatives than do personal interviews. Abrams and Taylor apparently had more satisfactory sources of information, but even here the method fell well short of a full-blown family interview study. Neither group of workers had any independent estimate of the frequency of operationally defined schizophrenia in the general population and neither had a control sample. However, we know from other studies that the frequency of operationally defined schizophrenia among the relatives of non-schizophrenics may be as low as 0.2% (Kendler et al. 1985), and if this is so, then the sample size required to confidently *reject* the idea that schizophrenia is familial would need to be considerably higher than that obtained in either of these two "negative" studies. Thus it seems quite possible that the combination of methods of low sensitivity, insufficient sample size and restrictive criteria conspired to produce falsely negative results.

It is fortunate that there have now been a number of studies with more satisfactory methodologies and, not surprisingly, these have yielded positive results. Tsuang et al. (1980) performed personal interviews and assessments of clinical records on 375 first-degree relatives of schizophrenics and 543 relatives of controls. On using modified Feighner criteria the morbid risks of schizophrenia were 5.5% and 0.6% respectively. A subsequent reassessment using DSM-III criteria produced essentially similar results. Also using Feighner-like criteria, Guze et al. (1983) in St. Louis carried out a follow-up and family study with "blind" diagnoses based on personal interviews with relatives. Again, a significant excess of schizophrenia was found in the relatives of schizophrenics compared with the relatives of other psychiatric patients. More recently, Baron et al. (1985) have added to the evidence that schizophrenia does not cease to be a familial condition once it has been narrowly and explicitly defined.

Confirmation of familiality does not, of course, necessarily mean that the genetic contribution to schizophrenia is established. For many, the most convincing evidence for a genetic contribution to schizophrenia has come from adoption studies. Unfortunately, up until the present, no adoption studies have been "purpose-built" to examine the transmission of schizophrenia employing modern op-

Table 1. A comparison of adoptees' family study results with and without application of operational criteria

Authors	Diagnosis	Genetic relationship to a schizophrenic?			
		Yes[a]		No[b]	
		n	Affected	n	Affected
Kety et al. (1976, 1983)	Chronic schizophrenia plus "latent" or "uncertain" cases	118	20.3	224	5.8
Kendler et al. (1981)	DSM-III schizophrenia plus schizotypal personality disorder	105	13.3	224	1.6

[a] Biological relatives of adopted-away schizophrenics
[b] Adoptive relatives of schizophrenics and relatives of control adoptees

erational criteria. However, the Danish adoption material collected by Kety et al. (1976) provided sufficient clinical detail for Kendler and coworkers (1981) to carry out a reassessment of the adoptees family material applying DSM-III criteria, blind as to whether the subject was biologically related to the schizophrenic index adoptee. The earlier finding of the Danish adoption studies was that the biological relatives of schizophrenics appeared to have high rates of schizophrenia and of schizoid or paranoid traits which, although not qualifying for the diagnosis of schizophrenia, were grouped by the researchers under the term "schizophrenia spectrum disorder" (Rosenthal et al. 1971). The notion of spectrum disorder later influenced the authors of DSM-III, who produced a category of *schizotypal personality* which is operationally defined, more restrictive and (in our view) probably preferable to its forerunner. Therefore Kendler and colleagues (1981) employed the DSM-III definitions of both schizophrenia and schizotypal personality disorder in their study. The essential findings were that 13.3% of 105 biological relatives of adopted-away schizophrenics were diagnosed as having either DSM-III schizophrenia or schizotypal personality disorder, compared with only 1.3% of 224 adoptive relatives of schizophrenics and relatives of control adoptees. While it would be desirable to carry out a study designed specifically with DSM-III in mind, the results of this reassessment provide a robust defence against suggestions that earlier findings based on clinical descriptive criteria gave schizophrenia a misleadingly "genetic" appearance. Indeed, as Table 1 indicates, the introduction of more restrictive criteria *increases* the difference in rates of illness between those who are genetically related and those not genetically related to a schizophrenic index adoptee.

Twin Studies

The evidence reviewed above encourages our confidence in the important genetic contribution to schizophrenia as defined using modern criteria. Therefore, in considering twin studies we will focus less on this issue than on the question of which set of criteria provides the most useful and valid definition. The use of twins as a guide to positioning the boundaries of schizophrenia was suggested by Gottesman and Shields (1972). The basic premise of the classical twin method is of course that monozygotic (MZ) twins share all of their genes plus a common environment, whereas dizygotic (DZ) twins share only half of their genes and a common environment. Therefore any greater similarities in MZ than in DZ pairs should reflect genetic influences. Gottesman and Shields (1972) showed that employing either very broad or very narrow diagnostic criteria for schizophrenia tended to lower the MZ/DZ concordance ratio, whereas using a "middle of the road" clinical definition provided the highest MZ/DZ differences.

As with adoption studies, no twin studies as yet have been designed specifically with the application of operational criteria for schizophrenia in mind. Such a study is currently in progress at the Maudsley Hospital, London, but fortunately, because of the detailed case material collected by Gottesman and Shields (1972) on their twins, we do not have to wait for the new study's completion to obtain some notion of how operational criteria perform in this context. The Gottesman and Shields series consisted of 22 MZ pairs (26 probands) and 32 DZ pairs (34 probands) ascertained through the Maudsley Hospital twin register. The 60 probands had received a hospital diagnosis of schizophrenia with blind confirmation by a consensus of six diagnosticians. In our recent study using modern criteria (McGuffin et al. 1984), two raters reassessed the detailed clinical abstracts which were identified only by a code number so that zygosity and identity of the co-twin were unknown. A variety of operational diagnostic criteria were applied using a checklist containing all of the constituent items. Reliability was established by having both raters score 20 abstracts independently. The kappa coefficients (Cohen 1968) ranged from 0.48 to 1 (Table 2). It is noteworthy that schizophrenia as defined by presence or absence of one or more Schneiderian first-rank symptoms provided perfect inter-rater agreement. [We note that Schneider (1959) did not set out to produce criteria which were "operational"; however, it has been pointed out (Kendell 1975) that first-rank symptoms are sufficiently explicit to be cast into an operational form and used in the same way as other more recent criteria.]

Although MZ/DZ concordance ratios as used by Gottesman and Shields (1972) provide some crude indication of the size of the genetic contribution, correlations in liability and approximately heritability provide more satisfactory

Table 2. Inter-rater reliability of operational criteria for schizophrenia

Authors/criteria	Kappa coefficient
Schneider (1959)	1.0
Feighner et al. (1972)	0.80
Carpenter et al. (1973)	0.86
Spitzer et al. (1975)/RDC	0.79
Taylor et al. (1975)	0.48
American Psychiatric Association (1980)/DSM-III	0.84

statistics. We therefore assumed a multifactorial/threshold model of schizophrenia in which liability to the disorder is contributed by multiple environmental and genetic factors acting in a predominantly additive fashion, such that only those individuals whose liability is beyond a certain threshold manifest the disorder. It was also assumed that the distribution of liability within the population is normal or that it could be transformed to a normal distribution. It has been shown (Falconer 1965; Reich et al. 1972) that knowing the frequency of such a trait in the population and in a particular class of relatives, it is posssible to calculate a *correlation in liability*. It can also be simply shown that heritability, or the proportion of the variance in liability which is due to additive gene effects, can be estimated as twice the difference between the MZ and the DZ correlations (Falconer 1981). Further statistical details, including the approach to estimating population frequencies and standard errors, have been described by us elsewhere (McGuffin et al. 1984).

A summary of the more important results obtained from our reassessment of Maudsley twins (McGuffin et al. 1984; Farmer et al. 1987) is given in Table 3. It can be seen that all of the criteria lead to a reduction in the number of probands (originally 60). The most restrictive criteria prove to be Schneider's first-rank symptoms [We have omitted from the table the results based on the criteria of Carpenter et al. (1973) and Taylor et al. (1975) which were included in our original study. Both of these criteria proved to be almost as restrictive as Schneider's and both resulted in low rates of disorder and zero concordance among DZ twins, so that we were unable to provide an estimate of heritability using the conventional formula.]

High and closely similar heritabilities are provided by DSM-III and its forerunners, the criteria of Spitzer et al. (1975) and of Feighner et al. (1972). We must

Table 3. Twin concordance and heritabilities of operational criteria for schizophrenia. (Data from McGuffin et al. 1984; Farmer et al. 1987)

Criteria	MZ twins			DZ twins			h^2 ($\pm$SE)
	n	Concordance (%)	r	n	Concordance (%)	r	
Spitzer et al. (1975							
Broad	22	45.5	0.86	23	8.7	0.45	0.83±0.4
Narrow	19	52.6	0.90	21	9.5	0.48	0.84±0.4
Feighner et al. (1972)							
Probable	21	47.6	0.88	22	9.1	0.46	0.84±0.4
Definite	19	47.4	0.88	18	11.1	0.52	0.72±0.4
DSM-III (American Psychiatric Association 1980)	21	47.6	0.87	21	9.5	0.44	0.85±0.4
Schneider (1959)	9	22.2	0.74	4	50.0	0.91	0±0.49

Concordance is expressed probandwise
r, correlation in liability; h^2, approximate broad heritability

note that for all definitions the estimates of heritability have high standard errors. Furthermore the study is, in effect, a repeated reassessment of the same subjects, so that the estimates of heritability cannot be assumed to be independent. Thus there is no straightforward answer to the question of whether they differ significantly. Nevertheless, the modern North American criteria must all be regarded as satisfactory, whereas Schneider's first-rank symptoms, with a heritability effectively of zero, appear to be must less useful.

Why might Schneider's definition have performed so poorly? As clinicians educated in a "Schneider-orientated" environment, we confess that this is disappointing. Schneider's symptoms afforded outstandingly good inter-rater agreement, but it could be that this result, achieved by rating conservatively, sacrificed sensitivity. Thus only one-quarter of probands were classified as schizophrenic. A further difficulty is that we were using material which was not purpose-built to provide Schneider-orientated information. By contrast, previous studies of schizophrenics, using instruments such as the Present State Examination (Wing et al. 1974) which lay emphasis on Schneiderian symptoms, have found that the majority of patients with schizophrenia are Schneider-positive (Brockington et al. 1978). Indeed, a study of our own (McGuffin et al. 1978) was in keeping with previous British findings (Mellor 1970) that over 70% of patients with a teaching hospital diagnosis of schizophrenia exhibited first-rank symptoms. On the other hand, recent outcome studies of schizophrenia (Brockington et al. 1978; Stephens et al.1982; Bland and Orn 1979) have also cast doubt on the validity of the Schneiderian system, finding that its predictive power is low. Kendell (1982) has pointed out that "outcome validity" and "aetiological validity" are not necessarily one and the same, but it must be noted that the satisfactory results produced in our genetic study of DSM-III, Feighner's criteria and Spitzer's Research Diagnostic Criteria accord well with the results of follow-up studies (Brockington et al. 1978; Stephens et al. 1982; Helzer et al. 1981) which find such criteria to be effective in predicting outcome.

In summary, the application of operational criteria to twin data confirms that earlier findings implicating genetic factors in the aetiology of schizophrenia cannot be ascribed simply to the use of "subjective" clinical judgements as the criterion for diagnosis. More importantly, however, our results suggest that not all criteria are equally useful or valid from a genetic viewpoint. In particular, reliance on Schneider's first-rank symptoms markedly reduces the number of probands and fails to yield a heritable syndrome. Modern North American criteria, on the other hand, define a highly heritable condition. The main caveat here is that the sample (although based on one of the largest reported twin series) is small and, as we have discussed in greater detail elsewhere (McGuffin et al. 1984) allows us insufficient statistical power to reach a definitive conclusion. Such a conclusion must await enlargement of the sample size and an investigation which is specifically focused on the constituent items contained in the various sets of operational criteria.

Heterogeneity

Although Kallmann (1938) was apparently unimpressed by the homotypia for clinical subtypes in his family study of schizophrenia, a reanalysis by Slater (1947) showed a tendency for like to go with like in affected parent-offspring pairs at a level which was significantly better than chance. Other researchers have subsequently shown that in pairs of first-degree relatives where both are affected by schizophrenia there is a tendency for both to exhibit the same subtype when "traditional" categories such as paranoid or hebephrenic schizophrenia are employed (Tsuang et al. 1974; Scharfetter and Nusperli 1980). However, there is also an overall tendency for probands with a paranoid form of disorder to have a lower frequency of secondary cases among relatives than probands with nonparanoid or hebephrenic illness (Kendler and Davis 1981). We have therefore suggested (McGuffin et al. 1987) that a possible explanation for this finding, together with the finding of incomplete homotypia, is that traditional categories of disorder occupy different positions on a multifactorial continuum of liability. Thus, for example, we suggest that the patients described by Kallmann (1938) as having "nuclear" schizophrenia (hebephrenics and catatonics) lie beyond a more extreme, more severe threshold than do those patients with "peripheral" forms (i.e. simple and paranoid schizophrenics). It has previously been suggested that a multiple-threshold model provides a poor statistical fit (Baron 1982) but we find that on applying the isocorrelational version of the threshold model of Reich et al. (1972, 1979), we obtain an excellent fit providing we permit different correlations in liability for sibling and parent-offspring pairs (McGuffin et al. 1987).

Unfortunately, extensive family data are not available for modern subtyping systems which incorporate explicit operational definitions. However, we have again gone back to the Gottesman and Shields (1972) schizophrenia twin series and have applied subtyping criteria. Three different approaches to subtyping were taken. Tsuang and Winokur (1974) have devised an operational version of the traditional hebephrenic and paranoid categories, adding also a third "undifferentiated" group. More novel approaches have been put forward by Farmer et al. (1983, 1984) and by Crow (1980). Farmer's subtypes were based upon a multivariate statistical analysis. Two stable and apparently distinct groups of schizophrenics were delineated by cluster analysis (Farmer et al. 1983), and subsequently the characteristics of the subtypes were examined in further detail by analysing a separate sample using discriminant analysis (Farmer et al. 1984). Interestingly, the characteristics of the subtypes to some extent resembled traditional categories, and hence the group of patients with onset before 25 years, poor premorbid work adjustment and such clinical features as blunting of affect were named hebephrenic-like or "H type" while a group with later onset, poor premorbid *social* adjustment and well-organised delusions were named paranoid-like or "P type". By contrast, Crow's subtypes were derived more directly from aetiological hypotheses. Crow (1980) proposed that a type I schizophrenia is characterised by prominence of positive symptoms and good response to neuroleptics and is usually associated with a normal CT brain scan appearance and absence of negative features or cognitive impairment. Type II schizophrenia is associated with negative symptoms, a poor response to neuroleptics and a tendency to show

Table 4. Concordance for subtype in the Maudsley (1948–1964) twin series where both twins were diagnosed schizophrenic

Authors, typology	Concordance for subtype	
	MZ (%)	DZ (%)
Tsuang and Winokur (1974) paranoid/non-paranoid	$\frac{13}{15}$ (87)	$\frac{3}{3}$ (100)
Farmer et al. (1983, 1984) H type/P type	$\frac{11}{15}$ (73)	$\frac{4}{4}$ (100)
Crow (1980) type I/type II/mixed	$\frac{11}{15}$ (73)	$\frac{3}{4}$ (75)

Table 5. Concordance for schizophrenia in the Maudsley (1948–1964) twins as a function of the proband's subtype

Authors	Subtype	Concordance	
		MZ (%)	DZ (%)
Tsuang and Winokur (1974)	Paranoid	$\frac{2}{5}$ (40)	$\frac{1}{14}$ (7)
	Non-paranoid	$\frac{13}{21}$ (62)	$\frac{3}{20}$ (15)
Farmer et al. (1983, 1984)	P type	$\frac{4}{12}$ (33)	$\frac{1}{17}$ (6)
	H type	$\frac{11}{14}$ (79)	$\frac{3}{17}$ (18)
Crow (1980)	Type I	$\frac{8}{15}$ (53)	$\frac{4}{21}$ (19)
	Type II/mixed	$\frac{7}{11}$ (64)	$\frac{0}{13}$ (0)

enlarged lateral cerebral ventricles on a brain scan. Type I disorder, it is postulated, reflects abnormalities in brain dopaminergic systems, while type II disorder has a different pathogenesis, which may even be infective in origin. Crow allows that these categories overlap to a considerable extent and so in casting them into an operational format we incorporated a "mixed" group.

As Table 4 shows, all three subtyping systems produce a marked tendency towards homotypia but this is incomplete in the MZ twins. Since such pairs are genetically identical we cannot therefore argue in favour of a complete separation of subtypes at a genetic level for any of the three systems.

Table 5 presents the data in a slightly different form. Here we divide up the probands according to subtype but give the probandwise concordance including any form of schizophrenia in the co-twin. It appears that all three systems separate schizophrenia into "less genetic" (paranoid, P type, type 1 schizophrenia) and "more genetic" (nonparanoid, H type, type 2/mixed schizophrenia) forms.

Here we have not attempted any sort of model-fitting exercise but it is tempting to speculate that, as with out findings based upon reanalysis of Kallmann's (1938) data, these subtyping schemes are merely finding somewhat different ways of placing two thresholds on a liability continuum. Thus all three approaches, although offering subtyping schemes which are demonstrably reliable (Farmer et al. 1983; McGuffin et al. 1984; Farmer et al. 1987), enable us to detect subgroups within schizophrenia which are probably quantitatively rather than qualitatively different from each other.

The Kraepelinian Dichotomy

Most genetic studies have commenced from the premise that schizophrenia and manic-depressive psychosis are quite separate disorders. However, a number of findings prevent a complacent acceptance that this is true at a genetic level. Slater (1953) remarked on the fact that depression was more common in the parents of his schizophrenic twins than was schizophrenia. Ødegaard (1972) found that nearly one in three of the *psychotic* relatives of schizophrenics had a diagnosis of affective psychosis when the proband had the disorder with obviously affective features or one resulting in "no defect". However, where the proband was considered to have severe schizophrenia the proportion of psychotic relatives diagnosed as having affective psychosis fell to one in six. Ødegaard commented that the categories of manic-depressive illness and schizophrenia "are helpful in the same way as degrees of latitude and longitude for ocean navigation and not as unsurpassable walls erected between two parts of a population." Some evidence tending to confirm this dimensional view comes from recent studies employing operational criteria. Thus in a family study (Guze et al. 1983), when the diagnosis in schizophrenic probands was widened to include "questionable" cases of schizophrenia there was a small excess not only of schizophrenia but also of depressive illness among relatives. Elsewhere, Tsuang et al. (1980) found a less clear distinction between the family histories of schizophrenic and affective disorder probands when the affective disorder consisted of mania rather than of depression.

Against such a background, studies of genetically identical individuals might be particularly illuminating. McGuffin et al. (1982) reported a set of identical triplets where two had received hospital diagnoses of schizophrenia, while the third, treated elsewhere, was considered to have manic depressive illness. A re-evaluation of their illnesses (Table 6) using standardised methods and diagnosis by blind raters suggested that the discordance was not due simply to misdiagnosis or to a different diagnostic bias between psychiatrists. Thus the triplets perhaps illustrate some of the shortcomings of a strictly applied Kraepelinian dichotomy and warn us against an uncritical acceptance of operational criteria. Similar findings have since been reported in twins by Dalby et al. (1986). Furthermore, Farmer et al. (1987) have shown that on applying DSM-III criteria, five MZ schizophrenic probands in the Gottesman and Shields (1972) series have co-twins who could be assigned to DSM-III affective disorder categories. Four of these affectively ill co-twins could not be regarded as psychotic and so perhaps do not greatly embarrass the neo-Kraepelinian DSM-III dichotomy. However, the fifth

Table 6. Comparison of diagnoses on the "Z" triplets (McGuffin et al. 1982)

Triplet	Hospital diagnosis	Blind assessors			CATEGO[a]	RDC
		First	Second	Third		
G	Manic-depressive psychosis, manic type	Manic-depressive psychosis, manic type	Manic-depressive psychosis, manic type	Manic-depressive psychosis, manic type	NSMN/DSMN	Episodes of mania and major depressive disorder (age 14–21). One episode of schizoaffective psychosis, manic type (age 26)
R	Schizophrenia, unspecified	Schizophrenia, paranoid type	Schizophrenia, unspecified	Schizophrenia, schizoaffective type	NS+	Episodes of schizoaffective psychosis manic and depressed type (age 15–20). Schizophrenia chronic course (age 20–)
M	Schizophrenia, unspecified	Schizophrenia, paranoid type	Schizophrenia, unspecified	Manic-depressive psychosis, circular type	NS+	Episodes of schizoaffective psychosis manic and depressed type (age 15–17. Schizophrenia, chronic course (age 17–)

RCD, Research Diagnostic Criteria (Spitzer et al. 1975)
[a] CATEGO diagnosis at the X50 stage: NSMN/DSMN=nuclear syndrome plus mania/schizophrenia without first-rank symptoms plus mania; NS+ =nuclear syndrome. The diagnosis of all three triplets resolved to S+ (schizophrenic) at the X9 stage

was diagnosed as having major affective disorder with mood-incongruent delusions. Farmer and her colleagues point out that although there is no wholly satisfactory solution to such an apparent anomaly it may be more reasonable, for the present, to classify such "mood-incongruent" delusional patients as having schizophrenia. Thus DSM-III, while in some respects performing well, as we have described earlier, cannot be regarded as an entirely trouble-free diagnostic system.

Conclusions

Despite the drawbacks and limitations of operational definitions of schizophrenia, their continued use would seem to be essential given that we are dealing with a condition (or group of conditions) where the pathogenesis remains obscure. Operational definitions lack subtlety and flexibility compared with the diagnostic practice of the experienced clinician. There is little room for such notions as "praecox feeling", and, disappointingly, a straightforward "Chinese menu" set of criteria such as DSM-III appears to be more servicable than the (to us) intuitively more appealing Schneiderian system. However, we consider that the work of constructing appropriate criteria is not yet done and that there must still be a continuing process of revision and reassessment. Hence utility and validity must be scrutinised as well as reliability. Luxenburger (quoted in Jaspers 1962) expressed the view that schizophrenia, for the purposes of genetic research is no more than a "working hypothesis". It is essential that we continue to accept that operational versions of schizophrenia are also no more than useful working hypotheses based on observable phenomena, and we must beware of adopting a convention whereby DSM-III or any other definition, however useful, becomes an immutable codification which somehow is believed to embody schizophrenia, the thing in itself.

References

Abrams R, Taylor MA (1983) The genetics of schizophrenia: a reassessment using modern criteria. Am J Psychiatry 140:171–175

Baron M (1982) Genetic models of schizophrenia. Acta Psychiatr Scand 65:263–275

Baron M, Gruen R, Kane J, Asnis L (1985) Modern research criteria and the genetics of schizophrenia. Am J Psychiatry 142:697–701

Berner P, Gabriel E, Katschnig A, Kieffer W, Kohler K, Leng G, Simhandel CH (1983) Diagnostic criteria for schizophrenia and affective psychoses. World Psychiatric Association, American Psychiatric Press, Washington DC

Bland RC, Orn H (1979) Diagnostic criteria and outcome. Br J Psychiatry 143:34

Brockington IF, Kendel RE, Leff JP (1978) Definitions of schizophrenia: concordance and prediction of outcome. Psychol Med 8:387–398

Carpenter WT, Strauss JS, Bartko JJ (1973) Flexible system for the diagnosis of schizophrenia: report from the WHO pilot study of schizophrenia. Science 182:1275–1278

Cohen J (1968) Weighted kappa: nominal scale agreement with provision for scaled disagreement or partial credit. Psychol Bull 70:213–20

Crow TJ (1980) Molecular pathology of schizophrenia: more than one disease process? Br Med J 280:66–68

Dalby JT, Morgan D, Lee ML (1986) Single case study. Schizophrenia and mania in identical twins. J Nerv Ment Dios 174:304–308

Essen-Møller E (1955) The calculation of morbid risk in parents of index cases, as applied to a family sample of schizophrenics. Acta Genet (Basel), 5:334–342

Falconer DS (1965) The inheritance of liability to cotwin diseases, estimated from the incidence among relatives. Ann Hum Genet 29:51–76

Falconer DS (1981) Introduction to quantitative genetics, 2nd edn. Longman, London

Farmer AE, McGuffin P, Spitznagel E (1983) Heterogeneity in schizophrenia: a cluster analytic approach. Psychiatry Res 8:1–12

Farmer AE, McGuffin P, Gottesman II (1984) Searching for the split in schizophrenia: a twin study perspective. Psychiatry Res 13:109–118

Farmer AE, McGuffin P, Gottesman II (1987) Twin concordance for DSM-III schizophrenia: scrutinising the validity of the definition. Archives of General Psychiatry (in press)

Feighner JP, Robins E, Guze SB, Woodruffe RA, Winokur G, Munoz R (1972) Diagnostic criteria for use in psychiatric research. Arch Gen Psychiatry 26:57–63

Gottesman II, Shields J (1972) Schizophrenic and genetics: a twin study vantage point. Academic, London

Gottesman II, Shields H (1982) Schizophrenia, the epigenetic puzzle. Cambridge University Press, Cambridge

Guze SB, Cloninger CR, Martin RL, Clayton PJ (1983) A follow-up and family study of schizophrenia. Arch Gen Psychiatry 40:1273–1276

Helzer JE, Brockington IF, Kendell RE (1981) Predictive validity of DSM-III and Feighner definitions of schizophrenia: a comparison with Research Diagnostic Criteria and CATEGO. Arch Gen Psychiatry 38:791–797

Hempel CG (1961) Introduction to the problems of taxonomy. In: Zubin J (ed) Field studies in the mental disorders. Grune & Stratton, New York, pp 3–22

Jaspers K (1962) General psychopathology. Manchester University Press, Manchester

Kallmann FJ (1938) The genetics of schizophrenia. Augustin, New York

Kendell RE (1975) Schizophrenia: the remedy for diagnostic confusion. In: Silverstone T, Barraclough B (eds) Contemporary psychiatry. Headley Brothers, Ashford, Kent, pp 11–17 (Br J Psychiatry, special publication no. 9)

Kendell RE (1982) The choice of diagnostic criteria for biological research. Arch Gen Psychiatry 39:1334–1339

Kendler KS, Davis KL (1981) The genetics and biochemistry of paranoid schizophrenia and other paranoid psychoses. Schizophr Bull 7:689–709

Kendler KS, Gruenberg AM, Strauss JS (1981) An independent analysis of the Copenhagen sample of the Danish adoption study of schizophrenia. II. The relationship between schizotypal personality disorder and schizophrenia. Arch Gen Psychiatry 38:982–984

Kendler KD, Gruenberg AM, Tsuang MT (1985) Psychiatric illness in first degree relatives of schizophrenic and surgical control patients. Arch Gen Psychiatry 42:770–779

Kety SS (1983) Mental illness in the biological and adoptive relatives of schizophrenic adoptees: Findings relevant to genetic and environmental factors in etiology. Am J Psychiatr 140:720–727

Kety SS, Rosenthal D, Wender PH, Schulsinger F, Jacobsen B (1976) Mental illness in the biological and adoptive families of individuals who have become schizophrenic. Behav Genet 6:219–225

McGuffin P, Farmer AE, Rajah SM (1978) Histocompatibility antigens and schizophrenia. Br J Psychiatry 132:149–151

McGuffin P, Reveley AM, Holland A (1982) Identical triplets: non-identical psychosis? Br J Psychiatry 140:1–6

McGuffin P, Farmer AE, Gottesman II, Murray RM, Reveley A (1984) Twin concordance for operationally defined schizophrenia. Confirmation of familiality and heritability. Archives of General Psychiatry 41:541–545

McGuffin P, Farmer AE, Gottesman II (1987) Is there really a split in schizophrenia? The genetic evidence. Br J Psychiatry (in press)

Mellor CS (1970) First rank symptoms of schizophrenia. Br J Psychiatry 117:15–23

Ødegaard Ø (1972) The multifactoral theory of inheritance in predisposition to schizophrenia. In: Kaplan AR (ed) Genetic factors in schizophrenia. Thomas CC, Springfield, Illinois, pp 256–275

Pope HG, Jonas J, Cohen BA, Lipinski JF (1983) Heritability of schizophrenia. Am J Psychiatry 140:132–133

Reich T, James JW, Morris CA (1972) The use of multiple thresholds in determining the mode of transmission of semi-continuous traits. Ann Hum Genet 36:163–184

Reich T, Cloninger CR, Wette R, James J (1979) The use of multiple thresholds and segregation analysis in analysing the phenotypic heterogeneity of multifactorial traits. Ann Hum Genet 32:371

Robins E, Guze SB (1970) Establishment of diagnostic validity in psychiatric illness: its application to schizophrenia. Am J Psychiatry 126:983–987

Rosenthal D, Wender PH, Kety SS, Welner J, Schulsinger F (1971) The adopted away offspring of schizophrenics. Am J Psychiat 128:307–311

Scharfetter C, Nusperli M (1980) The group of schizophrenias, schizoaffective psychoses, and affective disorders. Schizophr Bull 6:586–591

Schneider K (1959) Clinical psychopathology. Grune & Stratton, London

Slater E (1947) Genetical causes of schizophrenic symptoms. Monatsschr Psychiatr Neurol 113:50–58

Slater E (1953) Psychotic and neurotic illness in twins. H.M. Stationery Office, London (Medical Research Council special report series No 278)

Spitzer RL, Endicott J, Robins E (1975) Research Diagnostic Criteria, instrument No 58. New York State Psychiatric Institute, New York

Stephens JH, Astrup C, Carpenter WT, Schaffer JW, Goldberg J (1982) A comparison of nine systems to diagnose schizophrenia. Psychiatry Res 6:127–143

Taylor MA, Abrams R, Gaztanga P (1975) Manic depressive illness and schizophrenia: a partial validation of research diagnostic criteria utilising neuropsychological testing. Compr Psychiatry 16:9

Tsuang MT, Winokur G (1974) Criteria for sub-typing schizophrenia. Arch Gen Psychiatry 31:43–47

Tsuang MT, Fowler RL, Cadoret RJ, Monnelly E (1974) Schizophrenia among first degree relatives of paranoid and nonparanoid schizophrenics. Compr Psychiatry 15:295–302

Tsuang M, Winokur G, Crowe R (1980) Morbidity risks of schizophrenia and affective disorders among first degree relatives of patients with schizophrenia, mania, depression, and surgical conditions. Br J Psychiatry 137:497–504

Wing JK, Cooper JE, Sartorius N (1974) The measurement and classification of psychiatric symptoms. Cambridge University Press, Cambridge

Genetic Models and the Transmission of Schizophrenia *

M. BARON

Introduction

The role of heredity in schizophrenia is generally accepted; however, the underlying genetic mechanisms remain obscure. The failure to identify and quantitate specific genetic components is partly attributable to etiologic heterogeneity, diagnostic uncertainties, simplistic genetic formulations and incomplete knowledge of the human genome. Drawing on recent advances in statistical and molecular genetics, and on diagnostic concepts of mental illness, I will attempt to address these issues as they relate to the genetic hypothesis of schizophrenia. Following discussion of diagnostic issues and methods for collecting family data, I will consider two research strategies: (a) mathematical models that examine specific patterns of familial transmission and (b) studies with biological traits and gene markers. Some of these issues have been discussed in greater detail elsewhere (Baron 1986 a, b; Baron and Rainer 1987).

Diagnosis and Case Ascertainment

Before we turn our attention to specific genetic strategies it is important to focus on phenotypic classification.

An accurate definition of the phenotype is crucial in genetic studies. However, defining the disorder in question may not be a straightforward task; that is, the question of who is ill and who is well depends on how "broad" or "narrow" our criteria are. The structured, criterion-based approach to psychiatric diagnosis has added an important dimension to modern psychiatry by greatly improving reliability and consensus among clinicians and investigators; however, questions remain about external validity and clinical heterogeneity. Additional data such as differential familial patterns, symptom picture, illness course and outcome, treatment response, and biological correlates may aid in dissecting diagnostic categories into more homogeneous subtypes; this subdivision may, in turn, reflect etiologic heterogeneity or gradation in genetic severity.

* Some of the studies reported in this presentation were supported by a Research Scientist Development Award MH00176 and by grants MH30608 and MH30906 from the National Institute of Mental Health

Department of Psychiatry, Columbia University College of Physicians and Surgeons; Division of Psychogenetics, Department of Medical Genetics, New York State Psychiatric Institute, 722 West 168th Street, New York, NY 10032, USA

Generally, the "affected" category can be defined in two ways: (1) "Narrow" versus "broad" schizophrenia. This classification stems from the incomplete concordance between different sets of diagnostic criteria; that is, the rate at which the disorder is diagnosed depends on the particular diagnostic system under consideration. Since the rate varies seven-fold (review: Endicott et al. 1982), the guiding principle should be to select a system which is neither too restrictive, so as to render the phenotype a rare event, nor too broad, a situation which may compromise phenotypic homogeneity. An example of a most restrictive definition is provided by the criteria of Taylor and Abrams (1975) as compared to the much broader New Haven Schizophrenia Index (Astrachan et al. 1972). The Research Diagnostic Criteria (RDC; Spitzer et al. 1978) and the DSM-III provide a middle-ground definition of schizophrenia. Whatever criteria are chosen, the system used to collect the data should allow a comprehensive evaluation of psychopathology such that potentially related clinical states can be identified and tagged for possible future analysis. (2) Disorders which do not fit criteria for schizophrenia but are thought to be genetically related to the "core" disorder as evidenced by familial aggregation. These clinical states reportedly include schizotypal personality disorders (Kendler et al. 1981; Baron et al. 1985a; Torgersen 1985).

Once an operational definition of the phenotype is agreed upon, further steps should be taken to ensure the adequacy of the data for genetic analysis. These include: (a) Prospective ascertainment of probands and families obtained from a single population pool (to minimize selection bias and to reduce heterogeneity). (b) Personal interviews as the chief source of information on family members (a measure deemed more sensitive and accurate than the indirect family history method). (c) Blind assessment of family members with respect to diagnosis and kinship status (to minimize bias with respect to the clinical diagnosis). (d) Although nuclear families are adequate for some types of genetic analysis, extended pedigrees, especially those with multiple affected members, contain more genetic information than smaller families and generally constitute a more suitable target for segregation and linkage analysis.

Genetic Formulations

Segregation Analysis and Related Techniques

Objective and Significance. The use of mathematical models in genetic analysis is a basic tool in human genetics. An important goal of this approach is to determine from family data the mode of inheritance of a particular phenotype. Knowledge of mode of inheritance is useful for a number of reasons. First, it points to a specific genetic mechanism. Second, it can be used in genetic counseling. Third, it can aid in the design of genetic research paradigms with a special view to elucidating the underlying genetic defect. Additionally, when complex disorders are considered, mathematical techniques can shed light on two types of heterogeneity: (1) A situation where several genetic and nongenetic mechanisms converge on a single phenotype. For example, a single major gene operating in conjunction with polygenic effects and environmental factors. (2) A scenario where different disease subtypes, or symptom clusters, diverge from a single genetic disposition. Variable phenotypic manifestations may occur when the genes involved in the disease process are pleiotropic; that is, the genes express themselves in several different traits.

As reviewed (Gottesman and Shields 1982; Baron 1986a), there have been numerous attempts to fit genetic models to empirical risk data; by and large, however, genetic modeling in schizophrenia has not fully met the aforementioned requirements; namely, a convergence of advanced methodologies for diagnosis, case ascertainment, and mathematical formulations (Baron, 1986a). In the following passages I will describe a series of analyses where some of these issues were taken into account.

Data. The sampling and diagnostic procedures have been described in detail elsewhere (Baron et al. 1985a, b, c). Briefly, using systematic ascertainment of families derived from a New York-based population, we obtained diagnostic information on the first-degree relatives of chronic schizophrenic patients, schizotypal subjects, and normal controls. Probands and relatives were evaluated using the Schedule for Affective Disorders and Schizophrenia (SADS; Endicott and Spitzer 1978) and the Schedule for Interviewing Borderlines (SIB; Baron et al. 1981). Diagnostic classification followed the RDC augmented by the DSM-III. The majority of relatives were interviewed directly; family history data and medical records supplemented the personal interviews. In most cases the diagnosis was determined blindly with respect to the clinical and kinship status of other family members.

Computational Models. Two models were applied to the data: (1) an extension of the "mixed" model, originally described by Morton and MacLean (1974); (2) an extended version of Reich et al.'s (1979) multivariate-multifactorial model. A more detailed presentation of these genetic formulations has been given elsewhere (Risch and Baron 1984; Baron and Risch 1987).

The mixed model incorporates the combined effect of a major locus, polygenic background, and environmental influences. The model is illustrated in Fig. 1. The data were analyzed allowing for several distinct phenotypes – schizophrenia, schizotypal personality disorder, and normal. Affection was defined in terms of a continuous liability scale with different thresholds corresponding to the different phenotypes. That is, only individuals with liability greater than the high threshold were susceptible to schizophrenia; individuals with liability between the high and the low thresholds were susceptible to schizotypal personality disorder; and those below the low threshold were normal. Contributions to the liability occurred through a single major locus with two alleles, polygenic variation, and two types of environmental background: environment common to sibs, and random environment. The overall population mean for liability was assumed to be 0, and total variance within each major locus genotype was 1. The parameters of the model were the frequencies of the three genotypes (the two homozygotes and the heterozygotes); the probabilities that individuals of each genotype transmit the abnormal allele; the mean liability of individuals of each of the three genotypes; the different thresholds; the proportions of within-genotype variance due to poly-

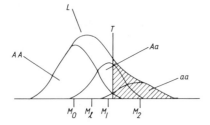

Fig. 1. The mixed model. The distribution of the overall liability to the disorder [comprising single-major-locus (SML), polygenic, and environmental components] is denoted by L. The mean of the distribution is M_l. The SML components are the three genotypes (AA, Aa, aa) and their respective means (M_0, M_1, M_2). The threshold for the disorder is T, and the *shaded area* above the threshold stands for the expression of illness. (Adapted from Morton and MacLean 1974)

genic background, common sib environment, and random environment; and the mean and standard deviation of the age-of-onset distribution, which was assumed to be the same for the different disease phenotypes. The penetrances could be calculated from the mean liabilities and the thresholds. Likelihoods of the model were calculated conditional on the parents' phenotypes and ages of onset (if affected) to account both for the reduced fertility of schizophrenics and the tendency of affected parents to have later onset. Since all families were ascertained through a single proband we assumed single ascertainment. Tests of hypotheses were performed using the likelihood-ratio criterion.

The main advantage of this model over the more commonly used single-major-locus and polygenic models is that the latter formulations are now subsumed under the same general model, rather than being considered separately; therefore, their relative contributions to the overall liability can be quantitated. Thus, the mixed model can examine three patterns of genetic transmission: a "pure" single gene inheritance; a "pure" polygenic inheritance; and concurrent contributions from both types of transmission.

The multivariate-multifactorial model invokes multiple genetic and environmental factors (each of small and additive effect) which contribute to the liability to the disorder. Under the model it is assumed that the liability in the population is distributed as a normal curve. When the liability exceeds a threshold the disorder becomes manifest. If more than one illness form is assumed to exist, each form is allowed to have a separate liability. In our version of the model we allowed three disease states, or phenotypes enumerated as 1, 2, and 3 respectively: schizophrenia as defined by Taylor and Abrams criteria (narrow definition), schizophrenia as defined by less restrictive criteria (RDC; broad definition), and schizotypal personality disorder. The components of the variance for the liability to phenotype 1 were the transmitted component common to all three phenotypes; the transmitted component common to phenotypes 1 and 2; the transmitted component common to phenotypes 1 and 3; the transmitted component unique to phenotype 1; and a random environmental component unique to phenotype 1. The components of the variance for liabilities 2 and 3 were defined similarly. The transmitted components are also the heritability parameters. The three additional

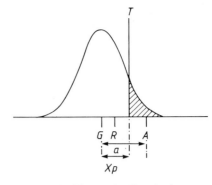

Fig. 2. The multivariate-multifactorial model. The underlying liability to the disorder is represented on the horizontal axis. The normal curve depicts the phenotypic distribution in the general population; the mean of the distribution is denoted by G. T is the threshold of the liability above which all individuals whose liability to the disorder exceeds T are affected with the disorder. Thus the *shaded area* represents the prevalence of the disorder in the general population. The liability at point T exceeds G by X_p (the distance between the two points). A is the mean liability of affected individuals, and a is the distance between A and the mean of the phenotypic distribution G. R is the mean liability of the relatives of affected persons

parameters of the model are the thresholds for the three disease states. Two submodels were examined. Submodel I determines whether the data can be explained by the transmitted component common to all three phenotypes (the other components being zero); if consistent with the data, this model would suggest that the three phenotypes represent different manifestations of the same disease process. A simplified version of submodel I is presented in Fig. 2. In submodel II we assumed that all the common transmission parameters are equal to zero but the transmission components unique to each of the three phenotypes were allowed to have values other than zero; that is, it was assumed that each phenotype has a distinct liability and the three disease states are transmitted independently. The two submodels were tested against a general model where the different transmitted components were allowed to have arbitrary values. Tests of hypotheses were done using the likelihood-ratio criterion.

Unlike the mixed model, the multivariate-multifactorial formulation does not allow more than one type of genetic mechanism; however, in the current analysis it allows greater phenotypic diversity which in turn may reflect genetic gradation.

Namely, in addition to subdividing the broad phenotypic "spectrum" to schizophrenia proper and schizotypal personality disorder, the schizophrenic category is further broken down to narrow and broad subtypes.

Results. Segregation analysis using the mixed model suggested a mixed pattern of transmission, with a single major locus making a large contribution to the genetic liability; the single locus was more likely to be recessive than dominant, with high gene frequency (61.1%) and low penetrance (1.7%). The components of liability variance for the recessive mixed model were: major locus 62.9%; polygenes

19.5%; common sib environment 6.6%; random environment 11.0%: Single-locus inheritance without polygenic background was rejected, as was a pure environmental hypothesis. A pure polygenic model also gave good agreement with
the data, although the mixed model was more parsimonious. The components of
variance for the polygenic model were: polygenes 81.9%; common sib environment 6.9%; random environment 11.2%.

The analysis using the multivariate-multifactorial model gave the following
results: When tested against the general model, submodel II (independent transmission) was rejected, whereas submodel I (common transmission) was compatible with the data. The heritability component (the transmitted component common to all three phenotypes) in submodel I was 72%, indicating that most of the
variance can be explained by transmitted factors.

Both the mixed model and the multivariate-multifactorial models provided
further evidence that schizotypal personality disorder is in the genetic spectrum
of schizophrenia. Overall, the results suggested a gradation in genetic severity
from normal to schizotypal personality disorder (mild phenotype) to schizophrenia (severe phenotype). Additionally, the multifactorial model indicated that
when schizophrenia is subclassified according to Taylor-Abrams criteria, "non-
Taylor-Abrams schizophrenia" (broad illness form) occupied an intermediate position between schizotypal personality disorder and "Taylor-Abrams schizophrenia" (narrow illness form). There was no evidence for separate liabilities for the
different disease states; that is, the different illness forms were not transmitted independently.

Similar models were applied by Carter and Chung (1980) and Tsuang et al.
(1983), although the analyses were less comprehensive than those presented
herein. Carter and Chung applied the mixed model to data on "hospitalized"
schizophrenia; they found that the model could not be rejected and that there was
little statistical power to distinguish between the single-locus and polygenic alternatives. However, their study may have been compromized by the adherence to
hospital chart diagnosis and the failure to consider the milder phenotypes as part
of the schizophrenia "spectrum." Tsuang et al., using the Iowa 500 data, examined a multifactorial model similar to our submodel I; they concluded that the
model was not compatible with their data. However, they did not consider schizophrenia subtypes, and their definition of the milder phenotypes deviated from the
conventional classification; also, their analysis did not allow for separate liabilities for the different conditions (our submodel II).

Limitations and Prospects. Although in some respect the studies I have described
represent an advance over previous familial analyses, a unique solution that discriminates between alternative genetic hypotheses was not found. The ambiguous
results can be ascribed to several potential sources of error: (a) The analysis of
illness distributions is likely to be compromised by etiologic heterogeneity. Although the models I have discussed allow for some heterogeneity – for example,
the mixed model involves a single gene, polygenic inheritance, and environmental
factors, and both the mixed model and the multivariate-multifactorial model examine phenotypic heterogeneity as a possible correlate of genetic variation – these
models are limited in that more involved types of heterogeneity, such as multiple,

independent etiologies (for example, several different loci with two or more alleles) were not taken into account. (b) The heterogeneity problem is compounded by reduced fertility and assortative mating, and by potentially inaccurate assumptions that underlie the mathematical models, including the absence of epistasis (namely, the interaction between genes in multiple gene systems), and differential effects of loci across the gene pool. (c) The sample was small and was limited to nuclear families. More extensive date on extended pedigrees might allow a more informative analysis. (d) In the absence of biological correlates or linked gene markers, the definition of the phenotype leaves much to be desired. I noted earlier the disparity among the different diagnostic systems of schizophrenia. A further diagnostic complication concerns the milder phenotypes, where considerable overlap has been noted between schizotypal and other personality disorder features (review: Baron et al. 1985a).

At our present state of knowledge, the limitations inherent in genetic modeling mandate caution in interpreting the results of segregation analysis. Nevertheless, the following observations can be made: (1) Regardless of the model examined, the analyses described suggest a substantial transmitted component in the liability to schizophrenia. As I indicated earlier, the transmitted components of the variance in the mixed-recessive model (single locus and polygenes combined) and in the pure polygenic model were 82.4% and 81.9% respectively. Similarly, 72% of the variance in the multivariate-multifactorial model was due to transmitted factors; that is, the environmental component was 28%. (2) In conjunction with morbid risk and adoption studies (reviews: Torgersen 1985; Baron et al. 1985a, b), the different genetic models suggest that schizophrenia has a polychotomous nature and that the various manifestations of the phenotype, such as schizophrenia subtypes and schizotypal personality disorder, appear to be different degrees of the same underlying process and therefore may share a common etiology. (3) Many inherited traits with uncertain mode of inheritance (as judged by segregation analysis techniques) have subsequently been shown to be controlled by a small number of major loci. Further refinement of mathematical techniques, in conjunction with clearer clinical distinctions and sizable pedigree samples, may shed light on this issue. However, as I will discuss below, information on genetic linkage or associated biological traits will be necessary for unraveling the genetic defect.

Biological Traits and Gene Markers

Objective and Significance. In the absence of a linked marker locus or an associated biological trait mathematical techniques can merely point to the consistency of family data with a particular genetic model. Moreover, as I noted earlier, these techniques may be compromised by etiologic heterogeneity and diagnostic uncertainties. The use of biological vulnerability traits and gene markers holds promise for redressing these issues.

Biological vulnerability traits are correlated with the genetic susceptibility to the disorder; presumably they are part of the pathway from genotype to phenotype with various degrees of proximity to the original gene product. These traits may include various biochemical, neurophysiological, and morphological measures, and they generally stem from etiologic or pathophysiological hypotheses of the disorder of interest. The underlying genetic mechanism of biological vulnerability traits is not always known; however, as will be explained below, knowledge of the specific genetic mechanism is not always critical for the design and implementation of experimental paradigms.

Gene markers are genetic loci with known chromosomal assignment. Studies with gene markers enrich our understanding of human genetics in several ways: (a) Since gene loci follow a simple mendelian mode of inheritance (a single locus with two or more alleles), the demonstration of linkage (the tendency of loci to segregate together) between the disorder of interest and a specific gene locus offers conclusive proof of the underlying genetic nature of the illness. (b) Linkage with separate genetic loci would suggest the presence of several genetic types of the illness; thus the gene marker strategy is an excellent tool for unraveling genetic heterogeneity. (c) Genetic marker information can increase the precision of genetic counseling and risk prediction. This is particularly true in the case of complex disorders, where simulation studies have shown that under certain assumptions concerning genetic parameters and mode of inheritance, single gene transmission may be undetectable by analysis of illness distributions unless a linked genetic marker is added to the information available (Goldin et al. 1984). The linkage approach has been successful in several heterogeneous disorders which were considered genetically intractable by statistical modeling techniques; prime examples are mental retardation and retinitis pigmentosa. Gene markers can generally be classified into the classical markers (including cellular antigens, enzymes and other serum proteins detected electrophoretically, and some observable traits such as color blindness) and the DNA or "new generation" markers (inherited variations at the DNA level which are detectable by molecular genetic techniques).

Methods. To qualify as an etiological vulnerability trait a variable must meet the following requirements: (a) genetic control, i.e., resemblance among biologically related individuals – a higher correlation in monozygotic than in dizygotic twins, and significant correlations between both siblings and parents and offspring; (b) state independence, i.e., the stability of the trait over time regardless of the individual's clinical state; (c) association with the disease both at the population level and in families, as evidenced by differences between affected and unaffected subjects with respect to the biological trait. Since schizophrenia is likely to be etiologically heterogeneous, the relevance of a particular "candidate trait" may be limited to a subset of the disorder. Several genetic strategies have been conceived in an attempt to identify biologically homogeneous subsets. Generally, a biologically "deviant" subgroup may be selected based on either observed deviations from control values or admixture analysis (a statistical method which examines the presence of multiple distributions subsumed under a single curve). Using this approach, the relatives of biologically "deviant" probands are examined for an association between deviant biological values and the occurrence of illness. Both univariate (the study of a single variable) and multivariate (the study of multiple variables) approaches have been described; the multivariate approach is more comprehensive in that it ascertains the relative contribution of several biological traits to the development of the disorder, as well as the degree of interaction between the different factors. Finally, although these strategies do not require mode of inheritance as input, statistical models that examine specific genetic hypotheses (see Computational Models above) can incorporate the biological variable and examine its relation to the transmission of the disorder. The methodologies for disease-trait associations have been described in greater detail elsewhere (Rieder and Gershon 1978; Elston and Namboodiri 1980; Cloninger et al. 1981; Baron et al. 1985d, e).

When gene markers are considered, the primary method of interest is pedigree linkage analysis. Linkage occurs when two loci on the same chromosome are sufficiently near each other so that recombination (rearrangement of the alleles due to an exchange of chromosomal material during the meiosis phase of cell division) is not likely to occur. The distance between loci can be inferred from the number of recombinations; the closer the loci, the less likely is recombination to occur. The most commonly used method in determining linkage is based on the odds ratio, i.e., the ratio between the probability of there being linkage at a given recombination frequency, or fraction (θ) ranging from 0.0–0.5, and that of there being no measurable linkage ($\theta = 0.5$):

$$\text{odds ratio} = \frac{\text{probability of observing the pedigree when } \theta = 0.0\text{–}0.5}{\text{probability of observing the pedigree when } \theta = 0.5}.$$

The odds ratio is usually expressed as its logarithm, also known as the lod score. The larger the lod score, the stronger the evidence for linkage (the conventional cutoff is a lod score of 3.0). The lod score method requires specification of mode of transmission and the associated genetic parameters such as gene frequency and geneotypic penetrances. Variable expressivity of the phenotype can be taken into account. A less commonly used method for measuring linkage is sib-pair analysis; using this method, linkage is likely to exist if pairs of affected siblings are more likely to have the same gene marker than expected by change. The sib-pair approach is useful in the study of disorders with unknown mode of inheritance because it does not require specification of the genetic mechanism; however, it is limited to the study of siblings and relative to the lod score method is lacking in genetic informativeness. Finally, when a gene marker is associated with an increased likelihood of the illness in the general population, the gene locus is said to be associated with the disease. The statistical measure for disease-marker associations, also known as the relative incidence (RI) of the marker, is equal to the ratio hk/HK, where h and H correspond to the number of patients and controls who have the marker, and k and K denote the number of subjects (patients vs controls) where the marker is absent. More involved methods which test the significance of disease-marker associations across different populations are also available. Further details on statistical methodologies for gene marker studies can be found elsewhere (Ott 1985).

Applications. Studies of biological vulnerability traits and gene markers have been reviewed in detail elsewhere (Baron 1986b). The hallmarks of these studies are furnished below.

The search for biological vulnerability traits in schizophrenia has encompassed biogenic amine enzymes and metabolites, neuromuscular abnormalities, immune response mechanisms, psychophysiological and attentional measures, electrophysiological variables, and variations in brain morphology. For the most part, these studies were incomplete, mainly for want of comprehensive family data. Of the few biological measures studied systematically as potential vulnerability traits, three seem in some data sets to have satisfied the necessary requirements, i.e., genetic control, state independence, and association with the illness both at the population level and in families. These three proposed traits are reduced platelet monoamine oxidase (MAO) and plasma amine oxidase activities (Baron et al. 1985 d, e) and increased brain ventricular size (DeLisi et al. 1986). As discussed, however (Baron, 1986 b), these findings have not been observed uniformly and their interpretation is subject to methodological uncertainties such as the possible impact of extraneous factors and the extent to which they qualify as major risk factors in the liability to schizophrenia.

As for gene markers, genetic linkage studies are scarce and the results are inconsistent. As reviewed (Baron 1986 b), some studies have reported possible linkage with the immunoglobulin Gm locus, the group-specific antigen Gc, and the HLA complex. However, other investigators did not replicate these findings, and questions concerning inadequate statistical and diagnostic measures have been raised. Studies of disease-marker associations seem to have met a similar fate. Some authors have reported associations between schizophrenia, or schizophrenic subtypes, and HLA antigens, ABO blood groups, or the group-specific antigen Gc, while other investigators have failed to replicate these results. Moreover, some of the studies may have been compromised by methodological uncertainties including diagnostic and statistical methods and issues relating to population stratification (Baron 1986 b).

Limitations and Prospects. The prospects of future research in this area hinge upon several methodological issues.

Heterogeneity. Heterogeneity can be reduced by refinement of diagnostic criteria or by biological or genetic "dissection" of the schizophrenic phenotype. These two strategies can complement each other; for example, classifying schizophrenia into clinical subtypes may facilitate the detection of biological or genetic linkages which may otherwise be obscured by clinical heterogeneity. Conversely, the presence of genetic linkage in one group of pedigrees may pave the way to identifying the clinical and biological correlates that characterize genetically linked vs unlinked cases; thus, genetics and classification may be intertwined. However, should multiple etiologies exist with each etiology accounting for a very small proportion of cases, the task of identifying all the genetic factors that contribute to the etiology of schizophrenia may be hopelessly complex.

Mode of Inheritance. The experimental paradigms proposed for biological vulnerability traits are robust; that is, they do not require knowledge of the underlying mode of transmission. However, since studies with gene markers are predicated on single-gene transmission, the efficiency of such studies in genetically heterogeneous disorders may be reduced. In addition, some of the underlying assumptions, particularly those related to the specification of genetic parameters in linkage analysis, may not be accurate. Nevertheless, the linkage strategy has been fruitful in other heterogeneous disorders (see p. 64); therefore it is my opinion that a priori knowledge of mode of inheritance should not be a prerequisite for conducting similar studies in schizophrenia.

Specificity. Should linkage or association with gene markers or biological traits be established, it will be important to determine whether these genetic factors are specific to schizophrenia, or nonspecific determinants of the predisposition to psychopathology, with other genetic or nongenetic constituents being required for the development of specific clinical syndromes. Indeed, this already seems to be the case with some of the proposed biological vulnerability traits such as altered activity levels of platelet MAO and increased brain ventricular volume.

Extraneous Factors. The proposed biological traits may be sensitive to a variety of extraneous factors such as psychiatric medications, diet, hospitalization, and diurnal and seasonal variation. These variables require careful consideration both in the research design and in the interpretation of the empirical data. In contrast, the study of gene markers is not susceptible to these limitations.

Environment. Genetic strategies may provide an incisive look into the question of gene-environment interaction. For example, subjects at genetic risk, as determined by a closely linked gene marker or an associated biological trait, can be studied prospectively with the aim of identifying environmental events that could bring about, or protect against, genotypic expression. Conversely, affected and unaffected biologically related individuals (assuming the latter have completed their risk period) who are identical with respect to the genetic factor can be compared for the presence of specific environmental events; if these events interact with the genetic make-up to produce the phenotype, they should be more likely to be present in the affected than in the normal relatives.

Future Advances. As I noted earlier, the search for biological vulnerability traits is contingent upon the prevailing biological hypotheses. New or revised formulations will be required to enable the researcher to cast a wider net. In contrast, gene markers are not subject to this particular restriction because they can be studied independently of the biochemistry or physiology of the disease. Until recently, however, the study of gene markers in human disease has been hindered by the paucity of known marker loci. Specifically, the classical markers scan a small portion (approximately 20%) of the human genome; this has resulted in low probability of assigning genes for the disorder in question to their respective chromosomal locations through linkage to a known marker. New developments in genetics – specifically, recombinant DNA techniques – have revolutionized genetic research by greatly expanding the number of available gene markers. Since these methods have made it possible to detect all inherited variations at the DNA level (regardless of whether the marker locus gives rise to a biochemical phenotype or other visible characteristics, a requirement which limited the utility of the conventional genetic methodologies involving classical gene markers), they can lead to a construction of a complete linkage map of the human genome. As reviewed (Botstein et al. 1980; White et al. 1985), some of the advantages of the new technology over the "old genetics" are as follows: (a) The DNA markers that can be generated by these techniques are numerous and can, in principle, map each region of the human genome. This set of new markers should enable the chromosomal localization of the genes responsible for many types of inherited disorders. (b) Many of these markers have high polymorphism frequency, which makes them particularly suitable for linkage studies. (c) Once linkage is established the new methods can lead to the identification and characterization of the gene itself. Eventually, the gene products can be identified and shed light on the biochemistry and physiology of the disease. Thus, clinically important genes can be mapped, localized, and characterized and their biological function (or dysfunction) can be subjected to direct scrutiny. The new vistas opened for human genetics by the DNA methods have led several research groups to urge the use of these methods in psychiatric genetics (Gershon 1984; Baron 1985); studies applying these techniques to schizophrenia have already begun (Feder et al. 1985; Detera-Wadleigh et al. 1986).

Conclusions

Genetic modeling techniques suggest a substantial heritable component in the liability to schizophrenia. However, despite the advances in mathematical and clinical tools the underlying genetic mechanisms remain unclear. This is partly attributable to etiologic heterogeneity and diagnostic uncertainties.

While further refinement of statistical methodology and diagnostic categories might shed more light on these issues, it may be unrealistic to expect a breakthrough in this area unless specific biological correlates or linkage markers are added to the information available.

With the advent of the new DNA technology the prospects for such a breakthrough seem increasingly brighter. Since these techniques can scan the entire human genome, all major genes operating in diesease transmission are likely to be uncovered; subsequently, the gene products could be identified, thus elucidating pathophysiological processes and paving the way to specific preventive and treatment measures.

Optimism over the new opportunities must be tempered with caution. First, barring a fortuitous finding, the task at hand may be lengthy, tedious, and costly. However, the use of "candidate" probes, i.e., DNA clones of genes coding for proteins implicated in the biology of schizophrenia (neurotransmitters, enzymes, hormones, etc.) is a potential shortcut. Second, diagnostic uncertainties constitute an impediment to genetic studies. However, genetics and classification may have to go hand in hand, for genetic tools can contribute to nosological distinctions. Third, while the gene marker strategy is a powerful method for sorting out etiologic homogeneity and unraveling mode of inheritance in some pedigrees, multiple etiologies each accounting for a small fraction of cases may render the search for a linked marker locus impractical. There are, to be sure, other methodological issues to contend with, including pleiotropic effects, crude estimates of genetic parameters, environmental influences, reduced fertility, and overall low morbidity risk, which, with the exception of genetic isolates, reduce the likelihood of identifying suitable pedigrees for linkage analysis. On balance, however, it is my opinion that the "new genetics" deserves special attention in schizophrenia research.

Acknowledgements. Thanks are due to Neil Risch, Ph.D., Morton Levitt, Ph.D., John Kane, M.D., John D. Rainer, M.D., Rhoda Gruen, M.A., Lauren Asnis, M.S., and Sally Lord, M.S.W. for participation in these studies.

References

Astrachan BM, Harrow M, Adler D et al. (1972) A checklist for the diagnosis of schizophrenia. Br J Psychiatry 121:529–539

Baron M (1985) Molecular genetics and psychiatry: a new frontier. Paper presented at the World Psychiatric Association Regional Symposium, Athens

Baron M (1986a) Genetics of schizophrenia: I. Familial patterns and mode of inheritance. Biol Psychiatry 21:1051–1066

Baron M (1986b) Genetics of schizophrenia: II. vulnerability traits and gene markers. Biol Psychiatry 21:1189–1211

Baron M, Rainer JD (1987) Molecular genetics and human disease: implications for modern psychiatric research and practice. (submitted)

Baron M, Risch N (1987) The spectrum concept fo schizophrenia: evidence for a genetic-environmental continuum. J Psychiatr Res (in press)

Baron M, Asnis L, Gruen R (1981) The Schedule for Schizotypal Personalities: a diagnostic interview for schizotypal features. Psychiatr Res 4:213–228

Baron M, Gruen R, Rainer JD, Kane J, Asnis L, Lord S (1985a) A family study of schizophrenic and normal control probands: implications for the spectrum concept of schizophrenia. Am J Psychiatry 142:447–454

Baron M, Gruen R, Kane J, Asnis L (1985b) Modern research criteria and the genetics of schizophrenia. Am J Psychiatry 142:697–701

Baron M, Gruen R, Asnis L, Lord S (1985c) Familial transmission of schizotypal and borderline personality disorders. Am J Psychiatry 142:927–934

Baron M, Risch N, Levitt M et al. (1985d) Genetic analysis of platelet monoamine oxidase activity in families of schizophrenic patients. J Psychiatr Res 19:9–21

Baron M, Risch M, levitt M et al. (1985e) Genetic analysis of plasma amine oxidase activity in schizophrenia. Psychiatr Res 15:121–132

Botstein D, White RL, Skolnick M et al. (1980) Construction of genetic linkage map in man using restriction fragment length polymorphisms. Am J Hum Genet 32:314–331

Carter CL, Chung (1980) Segregation analysis of schizophrenia under a mixed genetic model. Hum Heredity 30:350–356

Cloninger CR, Lewis C, Rice J et al. (1981) Strategies for resolution of biological and cultural inheritance. In: Gershon ES, Matthysse S, Breakefield RD, Ciaranello RD (eds) Genetic research strategies in psychobiology and psychiatry. Boxwood Press, Pacific Grove

DeLisi LE, Goldin LR, Hamovit JR, Maxwell ME, Kurtz D, Gershon ES (1986) A family study of the association of increased ventricular size with schizophrenia. Arch Gen Psychiatry 43:148–153

Detera-Wadleigh SD, DeLisi L, Berrettini WH et al. (1986) DNA polymorphisms in schizophrenia and affective disorders. In: Shagass C, Josiassen RC, Bridger WH et al. (eds) Biological psychiatry 1985. Elsevier, New York, pp 66–69

Elston RC, Namboodiri KK (1980) Types of disease and models for their genetic analysis. Schizophr Bull 6:368–374

Endicott J, Spitzer RL (1978) A diagnostic interview: the Schedule for Affective Disorders and Schizophrenia. Arch Gen Psychiatry 35:837–844

Endicott J, Nee J, Fleiss J et al. (1982) Diagnostic criteria for schizophrenia: reliabilities and agreement between systems. Arch Gen Psychiatry 39:884–889

Feder J, Gurling HMD, Darby J et al. (1985) DNA restriction fragment analysis of the proopiomelanocortin gene in schizophrenia and bipolar disorders. Am J Hum Genet 37:286–294

Gershon ES (1984) Biological approaches to neuropsychiatric genetics. Paper presented at the CINP congress, Florence

Goldin LR, Cox NJ, Pauls DL et al. (1984) The detection of major loci by segregation and linkage analysis: a simulation study. Genet Epidemiol 1:285–296

Gottesman II, Shields J (1982) Schizophrenia: the epigenetic puzzle. Cambridge University Press, New York

Kendler KS, Gruenberg AM, Strauss JS (1981) An independent analysis of the Danish adoption study of schizophrenia. II: The relationship between schizotypal personality disorder and schizophrenia. Arch Gen Psychiatry 38:982–984

Morton NE, MacLean CJ (1974) Analysis of family resemblance. III. Complex segregation analysis of quantitative traits. Am J Hum Genet 26:489–503

Ott J (1985) Analysis of human genetic linkage. The John Hopkins University Press, Baltimore

Reich T, Rice J, Cloninger CR et al. (1979) The use of multiple thresholds and segregation analysis in analyzing the phenotypic heterogeneity of multifactorial traits. Ann Hum Genet 42:371–390

Rieder RO, Gershon ES (1978) Genetic research strategies in biological psychiatry. Arch Gen Psychiatry 35:866–873

Risch N, Baron M (1984) Segregation analysis of schizophrenia and related disorders. Am J Hum Genet 36:1039–1059

Spitzer RL, Endicott J, Robins E (1978) Research Diagnostic Criteria: rationale and reliability. Arch Gen Psychiatry 35:773–782

Taylor MA, Abrams R (1975) A critique of the St. Louis psychiatric research criteria for schizophrenia. Am J Psychiatry 132:1276–1280

Torgersen S (1985) Relationship of schizotypal personality disorder to schizophrenia: genetics. Schizophr Bull 11:554–563

Tsuang MT, Bucher KD, Fleming JA (1983) A search for "schizophrenia spectrum disorder": an application of a multiple threshold model to blind family data. Br J Psychiatry 143:572–577

White RL, Leppert M, Bishop DT et al. (1985) Construction of linkage maps with DNA markers for human chromosomes. Nature 313:101–105

The Genetics of Schizophrenia: Discussion

E. Strömgren

Drs. Kringlen, McGuffin and Baron have given excellent reviews of their respective areas of the genetics of schizophrenia. I do not intend to review the reviews. Rather, I shall discuss a few points in more detail.

Dr. Kringlen concerned himself with the problem of to what extent the schizophrenic syndrome can be supposed to be especially influenced by genetic factors, Dr. McGuffin discussed the problems connected with providing diagnostic criteria which can serve as a sufficiently solid basis for exact calculations of modes of inheritance, whereas Dr. Baron outlined different possibilities for modes of transmission and the degrees to which empirical data fit the different modes. Together, the three readers have really given us a view of the status of genetic research in schizophrenia today. It might be interesting to see how this present-day status compares with that, say, 50 years ago. One of the best describers of the status during the 1930s was Hans Luxenburger in Munich (Luxenburger 1936). At that time the first really solid, methodologically sound family and twin studies on schizophrenia had been completed, so it was a good time to formulate theories. Luxenburger's formulations were very simple. He distinguished between the specific genes for schizophrenia, the internal environment and the external environment, the internal environment consisting of all those genes which could influence the penetrance of the specific genes. Luxenburger was inclined to think of the specific genes as recessive major genes. If that were true, some simple calculations could be made: If the concordance rate in twin pairs in which one twin was a schizophrenic proband was called a, the force of the external environment would be $1-a$. Next, if among the children of two schizophrenic parents the expectation for schizophrenia was b, the force of external + internal environment would be $1-b$ and the force of the internal environment would then be $a-b$. If, as was assumed at that time, concordance in monozygotic twins was 75%, this would leave 25% for the external environment; and if the expectation for the children of schizophrenic dual matings was 50%, this would leave 25% for the internal environment and 50% for the specific genes. It can be debated whether we have in principle got much further today. We would, of course, have to change the figures a little, but not radically. We may doubt whether any of the underlying genes are more specific than others, and whether any of them are major genes, but the practical consequences of this would not be conspicuous.

Dr. Kringlen discussed especially twin studies and adoption studies. With regard to twin studies there is now probably general agreement that the concor-

Aarhus Psychiatric Hospital, 8240 Risskov, Denmark

dance in monozygotic twins is somewhere between 30% and 50%, which deviates radically from Kallmann's figures of about 85% that dominated the literature during the 1940s and 1950s. I agree with Dr. Kringlen that the difference may be ascribed partly to differences in diagnostication. On the other hand, I am not so sure that there were serious errors with regard to the sampling of Kallmann's material. We have enough knowledge about the incidence of schizophrenia in the New York State area which was studied by Kallmann, and also about the incidence of twins. If these two incidences are combined, it seems evident that Kallmann really did find a great majority of schizophrenic twins in the area. In that respect his material should therefore be relatively representative. So I still think the problem mainly lies in diagnostic procedures.

Dr. Kringlen drew attention to the highly interesting observation that in most twin materials there seems to be a higher concordance of schizophrenia in females than in males. The difference may be even larger than what is generally assumed; when age correction is applied in the calculation of concordance, it should be taken into consideration that the age of onset of schizophrenia is higher in females than in males. This again means that if age correction were performed correctly, the difference between female and male pairs would be even greater. Attempts have been made to explain the difference as a consequence of greater proximity of female twins and less opportunity for social contacts outside the home, but there are other possible explanations. I have had access to Luxenburger's original twin material and was struck that in the male co-twins it had often been rather difficult to reach a certain diagnosis, they were more difficult to trace, and their whole situation was often complicated by alcoholism which might conceal mild schizophrenia. In any case, it seems very difficult to find a plausible genetic explanation for the differences found between the sexes.

Dr. Kringlen mentioned the very important question of incidence of schizophrenia in the offspring of twin pairs discordant for schizophrenia. In his own large material Dr. Kringlen found that the incidence of schizophrenia was lower in the offspring of the non-schizophrenic twin than in that of the schizophrenic twin. This would point to environmental rather than genetic causation. The dif-

Table 1. Schizophrenia and schizophrenia-like psychoses in offspring of schizophrenic twins. (Personal communication from A. Bertelsen and I. Gottesman)

	No.		S+S-like	
	Total	At risk	n	MR (%)
MZ Schizophrenic twins	47	38.8	6	15.5
Normal co-twins	24	23.0	4	17.4
DZ Schizophrenic twins	27	22.2	4	18.0
Normal co-twins	52	37.6	1	2.7

Age correction according to the method of Strömgren
MZ, monozygotic; DZ, dizygotic; S, Schizophrenia; S-like, schizophrenia-like psychosis; MR, morbid risk

ferences were, however, not significant. In this connection it is relevant to mention Fischer's study (1971) on the same topic; she found the expectation for schizophrenia to be the same among the offspring of schizophrenic and non-schizophrenic twin partners. These figures can be supplemented by the results of a follow-up study performed by Dr. Aksel Bertelsen and Dr. Irving Gottesman on Fischer's material (Table 1, Fig. 1). Sixteen years have now elapsed since Fischer published her results, and what has happened in the meantime strongly confirms her conclusions: the expectation for schizophrenia seems to be the same in both groups of offspring. It is also the same in the offspring of schizophrenic members of dizygotic twin pairs, but much lower in the offspring of non-schizophrenic dizygotic twins. So this rather large material tends to support the idea of a strong genetic factor in the causation of schizophrenia.

With regard to adoption studies I agree with Dr. Kringlen that the results indeed indicate some genetic contribution to the causation of schizophrenia, but that the studies can be criticised in different respects. It is to be regretted that in general in these studies true morbid risks have not been calculated. On the other hand, it is clear that a correct age correction procedure would be very laborious,

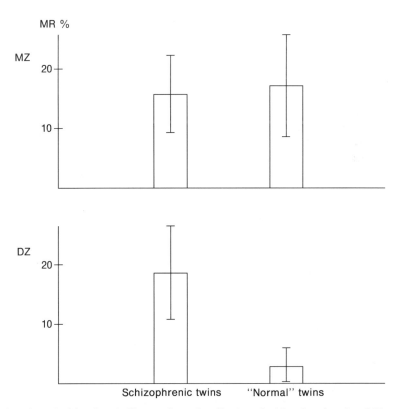

Fig. 1. Schizophrenia and schizophrenia-like psychoses in offspring of schizophrenic twins. *MZ*, monozygotic; *DZ*, dizygotic; *MR*, morbid risk (Personal communication from A. Bertelsen and I. Gottesman)

especially because these studies usually operate with the concept of "schizophrenia spectrum" which comprises a number of different syndromes with very different ages of onset. This implies that age corrections would have to be calculated separately for each of the syndromes. Special difficulties arise because for some spectrum disorders no standard materials exist which give sufficient information about age of onset.

With special regard to the Danish/American adoption studies, it is important that in recent years the size of the sample has been very much enlarged and that the material must now be supposed to be fully representative of the Danish population. If, in addition, adequate methods for determination of disease expectancies are now applied to the material, still more interesting results may be obtained.

A special remark with regard to the concept of schizophrenia spectrum: It was an excellent idea to introduce this concept when the adoption studies started. All disorders were included within this spectrum which *might* have a genetic relationship to schizophrenia. It was never claimed that they all did have such a relationship. Unfortunately, there is obviously the danger that those who are not too familiar with the nature of these studies get the impression that everything which can be labelled as belonging to the schizophrenia spectrum necessarily has a genetic relationship to schizophrenia. Many misunderstandings have arisen in this way.

Dr. McGuffin has given an excellent description of the advantages and risks implied in the use of standardised diagnostic criteria. For many purposes it seems necessary to apply such criteria, but unfortunately the different systems do not coincide, and who shall determine which of them comes closest to any nosological entity which may be suspected to exist behind the diagnosis schizophrenia? It is of course necessary that the diagnostic systems have a high reliability. But it should never be forgotten that reliability is not enough. As long as we have no markers whatsoever for any nosological entity within the field of schizophrenia, validity is a quite arbitrary concept. Most diagnostic criteria systems also have the drawback that they only give a point diagnosis, disregarding clinical changes over time.

As things stand, the so-called polydiagnostic approach is the most realistic, as described so usefully in the monograph edited by Berner et al. (1983). It should never be forgotten, however, that the diagnostic criteria are tools, just tools – they should never seize power.

Dr. Baron has given us an admirably clear and comprehensive view of the genetic models which can be applied for the understanding of the transmission of schizophrenia. Dr. Baron apparently feels that today the most likely model, the one which is most compatible with existing data, is the so-called mixed model implying a major gene, probably of a recessive nature, a polygenic background and environmental influences. This is exactly the model which Luxenburger had in mind 50 years ago.

Dr. Baron has demonstrated that by now we are in possession of statistical methodologies which can handle the very heterogeneous factors operant in the causation of schizophrenia. The weak point that remains is that the data to which these methods should be applied are as soft as they are in the case of schizophrenia. I think everybody will agree with Dr. Baron in his conclusion that "it may be unrealistic to expect a breakthrough ... unless specific biological correlates or linkage markers are added to the information available." Unfortunately, the existence of biological or genetic markers has not yet been demonstrated with any degree of certainty. If, in the future, some markers are identified, it is most probable that they are only of relevance for some part of the whole field of schizophrenic disorders.

In any case, it seems that the highly qualified research performed during the last half-century has not brought us much closer to solving the riddle of schizophrenia. An enormous amount of useful observations have been made, and we must of course continue to collect facts, and to refine our methodology so that what we find really are facts. It is like in court: we should provide the truth, the whole truth, and nothing but the truth. With regard to the causes of schizophrenia, we seem by now to have found nearly everything – except the truth.

References

Berner P, Gabriel E, Katschnig H, Kieffer W, Koehler K, Lenz G, Simhandl Ch (1983) Diagnostic criteria for schizophrenic and affective psychoses. World Psychiatric Association: distributed by American Psychiatric Press, Washington DC

Fischer M (1971) Psychoses in the offspring of schizophrenic twins and their normal co-twins. Br J Psychiatry 118:43–52

Luxenburger H (1936) Untersuchungen an schizophrenen Zwillingen und ihren Geschwistern zur Prüfung der Realität von Manifestationsschwankungen. Z Neurol Psychiatr 154:351–394

Part IV
Psychological and Psychophysiological Models of Schizophrenia

An Experimental Psychological Model for Schizophrenia

D. R. HEMSLEY

Introduction

The disorder which we refer to as schizophrenia is characterized by a wide range of disturbances of behaviour and experience. It we accept the utility of the concept of schizophrenia, how might we link such diverse phenomena as auditory hallucinations, poverty of speech and delusions? The present paper will consider the relevance of abnormalities of perception and cognition for our understanding of schizophrenic symptoms.

A major difficulty for any such formulation is that many of the key symptoms of schizophrenia, such as hallucinations, thought withdrawal and thought insertion, clearly represent alterations in conscious experience. Psychological constructs which have been generated to explain performance on cognitive tasks are not easily mapped onto experiential phenomena, although attempts have been made to do this. For example, Erdelyi (1979) speculates that "the processing region at which conscious identification (experience, phenomenal awareness, focal attention) of the input is finally achieved is proposed to be in or near the short-term storage system" (p. 13). It is worth recalling James' (1891) view that certain forms of psychopathology correspond to a disruption in the stream of conscious experience. Two of the characteristics of normal thought proposed by James are the following: "within each personal consciousness, thought is sensibly continuous" and "it is interested in some parts of objects to the exclusion of others" (p. 225). Both of these are disturbed in schizophrenia. I shall argue that the processes underlying cognitive abnormalities may be understood with reference to recent models of normal information processing, and, more importantly, that these may be relevant to the abnormal intrusions into conscious experience characteristic of schizophrenia.

Cognitive Abnormalities in Schizophrenia

A disturbance of cognition has long been viewed as one of the most distinguishing features of schizophrenia. Thus Kraepelin (1919) wrote "the patients lose in a most striking way the faculty of logical ordering of their trains of thought" (p. 19). On attention he observed "It is quite common for them to lose both inclination

Institute of Psychiatry, Department of Psychology, University of London, De Crespigny Park, London SE58AF, United Kingdom

and ability on their own initiative to keep their attention fixed for any length of time ... there is occasionally noticed a kind of irresistible attraction of the attention to casual external impressions" (pp. 6–7). More generally, he noted "Mental efficiency is always diminished to a considerable extent" (p. 23).

The most ambitious aim of current psychological research in this area is to specify a single cognitive dysfunction, or pattern of dysfunction, from which the various abnormalities resulting in a diagnosis of schizophrenia might be derived. This is clearly in the tradition of Bleuler (1911/1950), who attempted to account for the symptoms of the disorder in terms of a single underlying psychological defect. In his view the symptoms resulted from a disruption of the associative processes, these being the connections between ideas which enable normals to organize and interrelate many single thoughts and exclude irrelevant thoughts. It will be seen below that this has intriguing similarities to many recent formulations as to the nature of schizophrenic disorganization.

Also influential have been reports by the patients themselves. McGhie and Chapman (1961) carried out an extended interview study of newly admitted schizophrenics, concentrating on changes in the patients' experiences and presenting the findings in the form of selected quotations. Typical were the following: "My thoughts get all jumbled up. I start thinking or talking about something but I never get there"; "Things are coming in too fast. I lose my grip of it and get lost. I am attending to everything at once and as a result I do not attend to anything." McGhie and Chapman argued that such reports indicated that the primary disorder in schizophrenia is a decrease in the selective and inhibitory functions of attention. They went on to suggest that many other cognitive, perceptual, affective and behavioural abnormalities could be seen as resulting from this primary attentional deficit.

Current psychological research aims to specify cognitive abnormalities specific to schizophrenia. The results of such research are often theoretically elaborated in two ways. Oltmanns and Neale (1978) write "First, the single empirical measure which has been assessed is assumed to index a more general construct. Second, it is then postulated that the construct which is implicated in the deficit is causally related to schizophrenia and can account for a variety of schizophrenic behaviours. In other words it is held to be a primary symptom of schizophrenia" (p. 198).

The first stage is dependent on an agreed model of normal functioning, and the use of tasks which tap a particular function. The information processing approach is dominant in research into adult cognitive processes and forms the basis for most current work on schizophrenics' cognitive abnormalities. It is not, however, without its difficulties. Although current models of human cognition share many important features, it cannot be claimed that there is an agreed model. They are constantly changing, and there are frequently opposing models to explain the same phenomena. A further problem is that schizophrenics tend to perform poorly on most cognitive tasks.

Before attempting to formulate a model of schizophrenia I shall indicate briefly the kind of experimentation upon which such models are based. Much of my own work derives from Broadbent's (1971, 1977) model of selective attention. This makes the important distinction between stimulus set (filtering) and response set (pigeon-holing). The latter mechanism acts as a bias towards certain categories of response at the expense of others by allocating larger or smaller numbers of "states of evidence" to each category state. An example may make this clearer. Consider a subject who is required to shadow a lengthy series of numbers against a white noise background – 9, 4, 1, 7, etc. If then the sound "ee" is presented this "evidence" may be sufficient to produce the response "3". The subject is biased towards perception of digits rather than letters. Thus when the actual stimulus is unexpected, normal biases may act to impair performance. The mechanism may be seen as a way of making use of the redundancy and patterning of sensory input to reduce information processing demands, redundancy being defined by Garner (1962) as "the amount of correlation between events" (p. 143). I have argued that a disturbance at this level may be basic to the schizophrenic condition, and that the poor performance of schizophrenics on certain cognitive tasks is interpretable in terms of such an abnormality (e.g. Hemsley and Richardson 1980). However, as was noted previously, schizophrenics tend to perform more poorly on most tasks, and their abnormal performance may be attributable simply to the difficulty level of this task.

This formulation suggesting that schizophrenics are less able to make use of the redundancy and patterning of sensory input, does, however, raise the possibility that we may be able to construct tasks where schizophrenics would be predicted to perform better than normals due to the latter forming inappropriate expectancies. However, the endeavour to demonstrate such an effect is unlikely to be straightforward since its magnitude must be great enough to counteract the generally lowered performance of schizophrenics resulting from such factors as poor motivation. A recent study did indicate superior performance by non-paranoid schizophrenics (Brennan and Hemsley 1984). This made use of the phenomenon of "illusory correlation" (Chapman 1969). This refers to the report by observers of correlation between two events which in reality are not correlated. It can be demonstrated by repeatedly presenting pairs of words in a random order, some of these pairs having strong associative connections. Each pairing is presented an equal number of times. When normal subjects are required to report how frequently the paris were presented they overestimate the co-occurrence of pairs having a strong associative connection. It may be viewed as a demonstration of the way in which prior expectations influence, and in this case mislead subjects. It was therefore predicted that non-paranoid schizophrenics would produce weaker illusory correlations (i.e. more accurate performance) than normals. This was found to be the case.

An Integration of Models of Cognitive Abnormality in Schizophrenia

Research on schizophrenia has drawn upon several models of information processing, employed a wide range of experimental tasks, and resulted in hundreds of publications. What conclusions may be drawn from this research effort? Let us consider seven current views as to the nature of schizophrenics' cognitive impairment (Table 1).

Table 1. Current views on the nature of schizophrenics' cognitive impairment

1. "The basic cognitive defect ... is an awareness of automatic processes which are normally carried out below the level of consciousness" (Frith 1979, p. 233)
2. "There is some suggestion that there is a failure of automatic processing in schizophrenia so that activity must at proceed the level of consciously controlled sequential processing" (Venables 1984, p. 75)
3. Schizophrenics "concentrate on detail, at the expense of theme" (Cutting 1985, p. 300)
4. Schizophrenics show "some deficiency in perceptual schema formation, in automaticity, or in the holistic stage of processing" (Knight 1984, p. 120)
5. Schizophrenics show a "failure of attentional focusing to respond to stimulus redundancy" (Maher 1983, p. 19)
6. "Schizophrenics are less able to make use of the redundancy and patterning of sensory input to reduce information processing demands" (Hemsley 1987)
7. Schizophrenics "do not maintain a strong conceptual organization or a serial processing strategy ... nor do they organize stimuli extensively relative to others" (Magaro 1984, p. 202)

How might these be brought together and related to the abnormal experiences characteristic of schizophrenia? Several models of normal cognition suggest that the awareness of redundant information is inhibited to reduce information processing demands on a limited capacity system. Thus the change from controlled to automatic processing on a task as a result of prolonged practice may be seen as including a gradual inhibition of awareness of redundant information (Schneider and Shiffrin 1977; Shiffrin and Schneider 1977). A related position is that developed by Posner and his colleagues. They distinguish automatic processes and conscious attention, the former not giving rise to awareness, the latter involving awareness and closely associated with "a general inhibitory process" (Posner 1982, p. 173). The cognitive abnormalities in schizophrenia would therefore be viewed as related to a weakening of inhibitory processes which are seen as crucial to conscious attention. This would be seen as mediating the intrusions into awareness of aspects of the environment not normally perceived, as reported by the patients in McGhie and Chapman's (1961) study.

In a very general sense the models of Broadbent, Shiffrin and Schneider, and Posner and his colleagues may be seen as illustrating the way in which the spatial and temporal regularities of past experience influence the processing and, more speculatively, awareness of current sensory input. *It is a weakening of the influences of stored memories of regularities of previous input on current perception which is postulated as basic to the schizophrenic condition.*

Let us therefore return to Table 1. Two quotes (1 and 3) clearly indicate that cognitive performance is disrupted by the intrusion of material normally below awareness. The remainder may be viewed as related to a weakening of the influence of spatial and temporal regularities on perception. The present formulation has attempted to link these views.

Cognitive Abnormalities and the Symptoms of Schizophrenia

Spohn (1984) writes "I consider it of some importance that information processing deficits such as Knight's 'perceptual organization deficit' be shown to be related to more complex forms of psychopathology in schizophrenia, as a means of validating the deficit and demonstrating that it is not trivial" (p. 347). Although the possible link between disordered thinking and an information-processing disturbance is easily understood – indeed Maher's (1983) formulation derives largely from research on language – this is not the case for other important schizophrenic phenomena such as hallucinations and delusions. The present model is illustrated in Fig. 1.

Many authors have argued that delusions represent attempts to explain and understand hallucinatory experiences. Frith's (1979) model goes further in attempting to account for delusions in the absence of hallucinations. The basic defect is seen as involving the mechanism that controls and limits the contents of consciousness, as described above. Thus, on occasions, a correct perception of an aspect of a situation may reach awareness; the abnormality lies in the fact that it would not normally do so. Its registration leads to a search for the reasons for its occurrence. Maher and Ross (1984) argue that the process whereby delusions are formed is the same as that used by normals to explain their experiences. This is seen as a five-stage process, beginning with the observation of something unusual, followed by a feeling of puzzlement. This may lead to a search for further information, and at some point subsequently there follows an explanatory insight

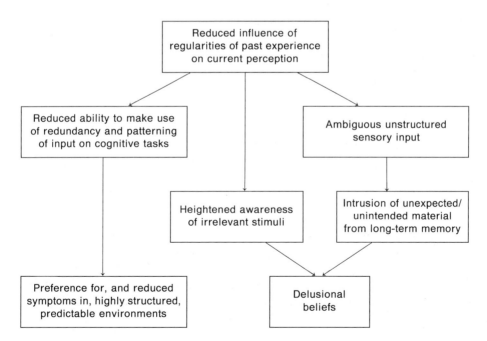

Fig. 1. Model of cognitive abnormalities and symptoms of schizophrenia

where all becomes clear. Once this explanation has emerged, any further exploration is of a confirmatory nature rather than a search for defects in the explanation in an impartial way.

In a general sense, hallucinations may be seen as the intrusion into conscious experience of material from long-term memory (LTM), this then being attributed to an external source. George and Neufeld (1985) have rephrased this in information-processing terms by referring to an interaction between the "spontaneous retrieval of information stored in long term memory and sensory processing, the latter having an inhibitory effect on the former" (p. 268). This view has been influenced by the extensive research on perceptual deprivation on the perceptual experiences of normal subjects (e.g. Jakes and Hemsley 1986). It appears to be the lack of structured input which is of importance in producing the abnormal perceptual experiences which Leff (1968) suggested "overlap considerably with those of mentally ill patients" (p. 1507).

It has also proved possible to demonstrate the short-term manipulation of auditory hallucinations in a group of schizophrenic patients by means of variations in auditory input (Margo et al. 1981). The greatest reduction in hallucinatory experiences occurred when a response was required of the subject; for the passive conditions, the experiences were inversely related to the structure and attention-commanding properties of the input. This is consistent with Frith's (1979) suggestion that hallucinations are dependent on the meaningfulness of sensory input. Such findings offer no direct explanation of the occurrence of schizophrenic hallucinations, only of the extent to which they may vary under short-term manipulations of sensory input. However it is tempting to speculate, following Hartmann (1975, p. 73), that "possibly something in the realm of ability to pattern sensory input or interact with it may be involved in the inhibitory factor" (for hallucinatory experience). It was suggested above that schizophrenics may be less able to make use of the structure in presented material – one might therefore argue that hallucinations are related to a cognitive impairment which, even under normal conditions of sensory input, results in ambiguous messages reaching awareness and therefore fails to inhibit the emergence of material from LTM.

The emphasis of the above is clearly on what have come to be referred to as positive symptoms – delusions, hallucinations and thought disorder. In contrast are the negative symptoms – the absence of a behaviour that would ordinarily exist in a person who is functioning and coping well. They include such abnormalities as poverty of speech, social withdrawal and affective flattening. However, it is unclear whether the distinction represents (a) two underlying disorders, (b) differing severity of the same disorder, (c) individual differences in reaction to the same disorder, (d) different stages of the same disorder, or a combination of (b), (c), and (d).

In 1977, I argued that the pattern of cognitive deficits shown by schizophrenics might usefully be seen as resulting in a stage of "information overload" and that the strategies of processing employed by normal subjects in situations of experimenter-induced overload could be relevant to an understanding of schizophrenic behaviour. In particular, it was suggested that certain of the negative symptoms of schizophrenia, such as poverty of speech, social withdrawal and retardation, might for certain individuals represent adaptive strategies, learnt over time, to minimize the effects of the cognitive impairment. Factors which might be expected to determine preferred strategies, and hence the form of behavioural abnormality, would include severity of impairment, personality factors independent of the psychosis, and environmental influences. It is possible that the most acceptable methods of adaptation within some institutions involve withdrawal and lowered responsiveness.

Implications for Treatment

1. It is necessary to consider the possibility that certain of the behavioural abnormalities shown by schizophrenics represent "adaptive strategies" to cope with the disorganization resulting from the cognitive abnormality. A similar point was made by Wing (1975) who suggested that "it could be argued that social withdrawal and flatness of affect are in fact a means of coping with severe thought disorder" (p. 241). Thus it might be expected that for those in whom cognitive impairment remains prominent, and who have reacted by withdrawing from situations requiring complex decision-making, any attempt to increase social interaction may result solely in an increase in florid symptomatology. In contrast, for those patients in whom the cognitive disturbance has largely remitted or been successfully treated, certain abnormalities of behaviour resulting from previously adaptive strategies may no longer be serving a useful function. This brings us to the second point.

2. There is a need to take into account the level of residual cognitive impairment when planning rehabilitation programmes; the assessment should be carried out once optimal levels of medication have been achieved. Recently, Wykes (1985) has demonstrated a significantly greater level of cognitive impairment in chronic schizophrenics requiring continuous hospital care in a long-stay ward than in those able to function more independently.

3. It is of interest to consider the predictability of the environment in which the schizophrenic is expected to function. This is difficult to quantify, but it is clear that a long-stay ward is more regular and predictable than life outside hospital. It is also apparent, and expected on the basis of the present formulation, that those in whom cognitive abnormalities remain prominent will function best in a highly predictable setting.

Recently we have attempted to assess the predictability of relatives' behaviour towards schizophrenic patients who are discharged from hospital to live at home (MacCarthy et al. 1986). It is clear that the family environment has an important effect on the prognosis of such patients. The expressed emotion (EE) rating technique is a reliable method of assessing certain aspects of the family atmosphere (Vaughn and Leff 1976). If relatives are highly critical or too emotionally involved, the patient is more likely to relapse within 9 months. However, it is not clear how the EE measure relates to actual communication patterns within the home, nor do we understand the mechanism by which the behaviour of relatives precipitates relapse. The main hypothesis of the study was that high-EE relatives provide a more complex home environment by responding to problem behaviours in a more unpredictable way. As a result they provide more ambiguous information about their own feelings and the kind of behaviour they expect from the patient. We found that highly critical relatives tended to deal with problems in a variable or unpredictable fashion.

Possible Links with Biological Models of Schizophrenia

This section will attempt to indicate the way in which links might be forged between biological and psychological models of schizophrenia. To do so it will focus on one biochemical theory, that which emphasizes a disturbance in the dopamine system. This is not to imply acceptance of the theory, which is not without its critics. Rather, it will serve as an illustration of how different levels of explanation for schizophrenic phenomena might be related. Recently there has been a growth of interest in the effects of amphetamine on attention and the possible implications for models of schizophrenia. Lubow et al. (1982) have argued that the latent inhibition (LI) paradigm is an effective way of manipulating attention in animals and that this may provide a link with the attentional disturbance prominent in schizophrenia. In the first stage of the LI paradigm a stimulus is repeatedly presented to the organism. In the second stage, the pre-exposed stimulus is paired with reinforcement in any of the standard learning procedures, classical or instrumental. When the amount of learning is measured relative to a group that did not receive the first stage of stimulus pre-exposure, it is found that the stimulus pre-exposed group learn the new association much more slowly. This is interpreted as indicating a reduction in the deployment of attention to a predictable redundant stimulus. Lubow et al. (1982) have shown in animals that LI is disrupted if amphetamine is administered in both the pre-exposure and the test phase. They write "output is controlled, not like in the intact animal, by the integration of previous stored inputs and the prevailing situational conditions, but only by the latter" (p. 103). Recall the discussion above of the way in which optimal performance is dependent on an interaction between the stimulus presented and stored memories of regularities in previous inputs which result in expectancies or response biases. Lubow et al. (1982) suggest that animals under the influence of amphetamine may be viewed as unable to utilize acquired knowledge in a newly encountered situation. They write, "Not having the capacity to 'use' old stimuli, all stimuli are novel. Therefore such an organism will find itself endlessly bombarded with novel stimulation, resulting perhaps in the perceptual inundation phenomena described in schizophrenia" (p. 104). There are intriguing similarities to the suggestion that schizophrenics fail to make use of the redundancy and patterning of sensory input to reduce information-processing demands.

Conclusions

Clearly in schizophrenia there are dysfunctions at a number of levels – social, cognitive, psychophysiological and biochemical. A major task is to demonstrate how these are interrelated. While there is no agreed psychological model for the abnormalities of behaviour and experience characteristic of the disorder, there is some

Table 2. Summary of evidence relevant to the model. (From Hemsley 1987)

Direct

1. Schizophrenics' performance deficits (e.g. Hemsley and Richardson 1980)
2. Lack of "illusory correlations" in non-paranoid schizophrenics (Brennan and Hemsley 1984)

Indirect

Unstructured (i.e. low redundancy) sensory input leads to (a) increased hallucinatory experiences in chronically hallucinating schizophrenics (Margo et al. 1981) and (b) "hallu-cinatory" experiences in normal subjects, the extent of which is related to the dimension of psychoticism (Jakes and Hemsley 1986)

Very indirect

1. A known correlate of relapse (critical comments) is related to unpredictable key relatives' behaviour (MacCarthy et al. 1986)
2. Animals under amphetamine behave as if "all stimuli are novel" (Lubow et al. 1982)

---

convergence of views as to the form of perceptual/cognitive abnormalities. I have attempted to link them to the major schizophrenic symptoms.

The evidence upon which such a formulation is based is diverse and, it must be acknowledged, often indirect. It may be classified somewhat arbitrarily as direct, indirect and very indirect, and is summarized in Table 2.

However, it is clear that an approach based on the study of abnormalities of information processing may be extended to a consideration of environmental factors leading to relapse and of possible biological bases of the disorder.

References

Bleuler E (1911/1950) Dementia praecox or the group of schizophrenias. International Universities Press, New York

Brennan JH, Hemsley DR (1984) Illusory correlations in paranoid and non-paranoid schizophrenia. Br J Clin Psychol 23:225–226

Broadbent DE (1971) Decision and stress. Academic, London

Broadbent DE (1977) The hidden preattentive processes. Am Psychol 32:109–118

Chapman LJ (1969) Illusory correlation in observational report. J Verb Learn Verb Behav 6:151–155

Cutting J (1985) The psychology of schizophrenia. Churchill Livingstone, London

Erdelyi MH (1979) A new look at the new look: perceptual defense and vigilance. Psychol Rev 81:1–25

Frith CD (1979) Consciousness, information processing and schizophrenia. Br J Psychiatry 134:225–235

Garner WR (1962) Uncertainty and structure as psychological concepts. Wiley, New York

George L, Neufeld RWJ (1985) Cognition and symptomatology in schizophrenia. Schizophr Bull 11:264–285

Hartmann E (1975) Dreams and other hallucinations: an approach to the underlying mechanism. In: Siegel RK, West LJ (eds) Hallucinations: behavior, experience and theory. Wiley, New York

Hemsley DR (1977) What have cognitive deficits to do with schizophrenic symptoms? Br J Psychiatry 130:167–173

Hemsley DR (1982) Cognitive impairment in schizophrenia. In: Burton A (ed) The pathology and psychology of cognition. Methuen, London
Hemsley DR (1987) Information processing and schizophrenia. Paper presented at EABT conference, Munich 1985. In: Straube E, Hahlweg K (eds) Schizophrenia, models and intervention. Springer, Heidelberg (in press)
Hemsley DR, Richardson PH (1980) Shadowing by context in schizophrenia. J Nerv Ment Dis 168:141–145
Jakes S, Hemsley DR (1986) Individual differences in reaction to brief exposure to unpatterned visual stimulation. Pers Individ Diff 7:121–123
James W (1891) The principles of psychology, vol I. MacMillan, London
Knight RA (1984) Converging of models of cognitive deficit in schizophrenia. In: Spaulding WE, Cole JK (eds) Theories of schizophrenia and psychosis. University of Nebraska Press, London, pp 93–156
Kraepelin E (1919) Dementia praecox and paraphrenia. Livingstone, Edinburgh
Leff JP (1968) Perceptual phenomena and personality in sensory deprivation. Br J Psychiatry 114:1499–1508
Lubow RW, Weiner J, Feldon J (1982) An animal model of attention. In: Speigelstein MY, Levy A (eds) Behavioural models and the analysis of drug action. Elsevier, Amsterdam pp 89–107
MacCarthy B, Hemsley DR, Schrank-Fernandez G, Kuipers E, Katz R (1986) Unpredictability as a correlate of expressed emotion in the relatives of schizophrenics. Br J Psychiatry 148:727–731
Magaro PA (1984) Psychosis and schizophrenia. In: Spaulding WD, Cole JK (eds) Theories of schizophrenia and psychosis. University of Nebraska Press, London, pp 157–230
Maher BA (1983) A tentative theory of schizophrenic utterance. In: Maher BA, Maher WB (eds) Progress in Experimental Personality Research, vol 12. Academic, New York, pp 1–52
Maher B, Ross JS (1984) Delusions. In: Adams HE, Sutker P (eds) Comprehensive handbook of psychopathology. Plenum, New York, pp 383–409
Margo A, Hemsley DR, Slade PD (1981) The effects of varying auditory input on schizophrenic hallucinations. Br J Psychiatry 139:122–127
McGhie A, Chapman J (1961) Disorders of attention and perception in early schizophrenia. Br J Med Psychol 34:103–116
Oltmanns TF, Neale JM (1978) Abstraction and schizophrenia: problems in psychological deficit research. In: Maher BA (ed) Progress in Experimental Personality Research, vol 8. Academic, New York, pp 197–243
Posner MI (1982) Cumulative development of attentional theory. Am Psychol 37:168–179
Schneider W, Shiffrin RM (1977) Controlled and automatic human information processing: I. Detection, search, and attention. Psychol Rev 84:1–66
Shiffrin RM, Schneider W (1977) Controlled and automatic human information processing: II. Perceptual learning, automatic attending and a general theory. Psychol Rev 84:127–190
Spohn HE (1984) Discussion. In: Spaulding ND, Cole JK (eds) Theories of schizophrenia and psychosis. University of Nebraska Press, London, pp 345–359
Vaughn CE, Leff JP (1976) The influence of family and social factors on the course of psychiatric illness: a comparison of schizophrenic and depressed neurotic patients. Br J Psychiatry 129:125–137
Venables PH (1984) Cerebral mechanisms, autonomic responsiveness and attention in schizophrenia. In: Spaulding WD, Cole JK (eds) Theories of schizophrenia and psychosis. University of Nebraska Press, London, pp 47–91
Wing JK (1975) Impairments in schizophrenia: a rational basis for social treatment. In: Wirt RD, Winokur G, Roff M (eds) Life history research in psychopathology, vol 4. University of Minnesota Press, Minneapolis, pp 237–268
Wykes T (1985) Cognitive impairment in a psychiatric population – its relationship to chronic disabilities and some implications for rehabilitation. M. Phil. thesis, University of London

Psychological Models of Schizophrenic Impairments

R. COHEN and U. BORST

This paper will not deal with psychological models which focus on the etiology and the course of schizophrenic disorders. Instead, it will concentrate on models that try to elucidate impairments considered characteristic of schizophrenic patients. By leaving out models of etiology and course, we exclude some outstanding accomplishments, such as Meehl's (1962) conception of schizotaxia, schizotypy, and schizophrenia, or Zubin and Spring's (1977) vulnerability model, which succeeded in integrating vast amounts of accumulated knowledge into coherent stories, into narratives covering the most diverse areas of research. We shall also exclude the many theories that discuss family dynamics as the basis for the development of schizophrenia (see Hirsch and Leff 1975) or attitudes of the relatives as critical for evoking schizophrenic episodes. The most notable example of the latter is the booming research which embarked from Brown's concept of expressed emotion (Leff and Vaughn 1985), and has surpassed most other approaches in the prediction of relapse, no matter how nebulous the mechanisms that link these familial attitudes to relapse. Most recently, this research has even been linked to the earlier work about communication deviance in the parents as a causative factor in the development of schizophrenia (Miklowitz et al. 1986).

The models we shall discuss all have in common the attempt to specify psychological determinants of schizophrenic impairments by relating the concepts and objects of clinical observation to the concepts and experimental data from general psychology. Usually this is done by looking for differences between groups of schizophrenics and controls in test variables that are selected as being both central to the cultivation of certain models in the garden of psychological research, and as having interpretive connections to concepts of the model which in turn seem to bear a close semantic resemblance to the concepts used by clinicians in explaining symptomatic behavior. If differences are found in such key variables, the psychological model is taken to "explain" not only the specific behavior measured, but also more general characteristics of schizophrenic functioning, possibly even particular symptoms. In most cases there is no information available that would allow one to decide whether a difference is better conceived of as an expression of the psychotic episode, as a sequel of the response to the breakdown and its treatment, or as an indication of more enduring characteristics that might reflect basic deficiencies (Huber 1983) and even qualify as markers of vulnerability (Zubin et al. 1985).

Sozialwissenschaftliche Fakultät, Fachgruppe Psychologie, Universität Konstanz, Postfach 5560, 7750 Konstanz, Federal Republic of Germany

Trends and Limitations of Psychological Models in Schizophrenia Research

Most contemporary research in this area relates the performance of schizophrenics to highly developed models of cognitive functioning in normals and tries to specify which of the stages and processes defined within these models might be crucial for the impairments. This research has largely replaced the earlier attempts to explain schizophrenic behavior by imaginatively elaborating on the concepts of clinical psychiatry with reference to research in general psychology. When Buss and Lang reviewed the psychological research on schizophrenia in 1965, they arrived at basically five models advanced to explain the disorder: (1) social censure, (2) sensitivity to affective stimuli, (3) insufficient motivation, (4) repression, and (5) interference theory. They felt that the most promising of the five was interference theory, which stresses the well-documented fact that when a schizophrenic is faced with a task, he often cannot attend properly or in a sustained fashion, nor can he maintain a set or change the set quickly when necessary. This is the only model among the older ones to which the present models, with their parochial exclusion of social and emotional elements, can still be easily related. In the more recent models emotions find a place at best as autonomic or central arousal, usually assuming schizophrenics, and especially chronic nonparanoid schizophrenics, to be overaroused (e.g., Gjerde 1983; Mirsky 1969). This assumption is based on reasonably good evidence from cardiovascular, electroencephalographic, and some pupillometric data, although the results with electrodermal measures are highly inconclusive (see Zahn 1986), and although it is extremely difficult to maintain a concept of unitary arousal.

Most of these earlier models have largely disappeared from the literature. They did not fare better than seems typical for theories in "soft psychology" (Meehl 1978): after a period of enthusiasm there is a period of growing bafflement about inconsistent results that lead to an increasing number of plausible ad hoc interpretations with hardly any risk that the model be liquidated, until people just lose interest in the model and turn to something else. The half-life seems to be longest for those models which have only a rather limited scope (see Chapman and Chapman 1973) and which usually focus on the performance in highly specific tasks with superior discriminative power. Typical examples are the segmental set theory of Shakow (1962; see Nuechterlein 1977), which discusses primarily certain differences in reaction times dependent on the length and the regularity of the intervals between warning and imperative stimuli, Cohen's perseverative-chaining model for self-editing deficits in referent communication (Cohen et al. 1974), Zubin's (1975) neural trace theory, focusing on the increase in reaction times following a modality shift even if that shift is expected, and the seminal work of Holzman about smooth pursuit eye movement (see Lipton et al. 1983). All of these models still provoke quite a few experimental attempts to test some of their specific assumptions. Usually, such studies are still firmly attached to the experimental conditions of the original work and rather devoid of unseemly philandering with possible generalizations. We shall not discuss these models in any detail, since it is impossible to do them justice within the framework of this paper. The emphasis of this paper will be on the dominant trend of today's psychological research on schizophrenic impairments, and that is the attempt to take advantage of the rapid and fascinating development of theories about information processing in normals.

Two implications should be stressed whenever research about schizophrenics is firmly lodged within models about normal functioning – as is true for the mainstream of contemporary research: (1) Collecting information not about symptomatic behavior but about behavior considered relevant primarily within the framework of a model about normal functioning implies that the aim of the research is not to develop diagnostic devices, but rather to interpret the performance of the schizophrenics according to rules found useful to describe the behavior of normals. To this end, negligible differences between schizophrenics and other groups, as found for instance in most recognition as compared to recall tasks (see Koh 1978), can be just as informative as large differences, provided reliability and variance of the measures allow the detection of differences where differences really exist. (2) Whatever is specific to the psychological functioning of psychiatric patients is likely to be overlooked. Accordingly, none of these models takes account of the obvious fact that schizophrenics typically behave normally most of the time, and that sporadic intrusions of deviant (though usually still associated) responses, as well as the more persistent omissions of normal responses, rarely extend over long periods of time.

Strangely enough, none of the models has allotted much attention to the specific determinants and regularities of those symptoms that are considered essential for the diagnosis, e.g., according to the criteria for schizophrenic disorders as listed in the *Diagnostic and Statistical Manual* (DSM-III; American Psychiatric Association 1980). Usually, the relationship between the concepts of the model and symptomatic behavior is simply assumed; only very rarely it is also tested. It was only for hallucinations that we found at least a few studies which either compared the telemetered EEG from periods with and without the symptom – defined by experienced observers or the patients themselves – (e.g., Serafetinides et al. 1986; Stevens and Livermore 1982), or which manipulated the environment of the patients and asked them about their experiences (e.g., Alpert 1985; Margo et al. 1981). According to these reports the likelihood of hallucinations is decreased when the patient is engaged in goal-directed activity and if the situation is highly structured. This explanation might also hold for reports of behavior therapists who applied operant conditioning techniques to reduce the frequency of disturbing behavior apparently related to hallucinations (see Redd et al. 1979).

The paucity of research on the immediate determinants and regularities of symptomatic behavior might partly be due to the fact that it is usually sufficient for clinical purposes to know only about the occurrence and severity of symptoms over prolonged periods of time. This can now be done with considerable reliability by the use of standardized interviews and a variety of rating scales. Another reason for the paucity of research is that not many patients are cooperative enough for time-consuming within-subject comparisons, and that only a few are able to indicate the onset or offset of symptomatic experiences. Even about hallucinations, for example, our patients could only report in the past tense. Finally, this neglect of symptomatic behavior in psychological research may reflect the state of the development of scientific psychology. The best measures are available for formal thought disorder (e.g., Andreasen et al. 1985; Bannister and Fransella

1966; Rochester and Martin 1979), and there is also some recent progress with regard to motor abnormalities (see Manschreck 1986) and even to affective deficits (see Knight and Roff 1985). By and large it appears that the greatest deficiencies in psychological research are found exactly in those areas which are considered to be of primary importance for the impairments characteristic of schizophrenic patients: affect, volition, sense of self, and the relationship to the external world (American Psychiatric Association 1980).

Coping with Interindividual Heterogeneity in a Jungle of Confounding Variables

A perpetual hindrance in schizophrenia research is the clinical, and probably also the etiological, heterogeneity of the patients. Certainly, this heterogeneity has been considerably reduced by the introduction of more stringent diagnostic criteria, albeit at the expense of a decreased comparability with earlier work. But even within the narrower concept of schizophrenia, heterogeneity is still so overwhelming that most researchers seek help in subclassifications. While the classical subtypes of hebephrenic, paranoid, catatonic and simple schizophrenia have not fared very well with respect to reliability or prognostic validity, many researchers have followed Silverman (1964) and Venables (1964) in differentiating between acute and chronic patients, between paranoids and nonparanoids, and/or between good and poor premorbids. The latter classification is closely related to the reactive/process dichotomy and is defined primarily by the quantity and quality of work and social relations prior to hospitalization (Kokes et al. 1977). Unfortunately, life does not keep these categories decently apart, and all of them are intractably confounded by sex, age, marital status, and other nuisance variables such as social status and education, severity and length of illness, and neuroleptic medication. These conflations are particularly troublesome, since we quite often cannot even guess the direction of a causal path. Matching subjects according to one of these confounding variables will lead inevitably to biased samples and easily to statistical artifacts.

There is no psychological or statistical model which allows one to approach these naturally occurring confoundations in a systematic and comprehensive way. To give just a few examples: The more stringent the diagnostic criteria, the more we find a preponderance of men (Lewine et al. 1984). Men are hospitalized earlier while women are more often married, and marital status turns out to be about the most powerful item in premorbid adjustment scales for predicting good outcome. Finally, while good premorbids may be either paranoid or nonparanoid, poor premorbids almost always tend to be nonparanoid (Goldstein et al. 1968) and are most frequently found among those with long periods of hospitalization (Strauss 1973). These latter confoundations make it nearly impossible to test the validity of the widespread and plausible supposition that the differences between paranoid and nonparanoid patients can be understood as the result of an intraindividual development from acute to chronic stages with a "reduction in cue utilization and scanning" (Broen 1968) and an increased tendency toward "sensory input processing – ideational gating" (Silverman 1967). It has even been suggested that the whole range of "intra- and intersubject variability in symptomatology ... may represent differing adaptations to similar cognitive disturbances" (Hemsley 1977) or protective strategies against the "information overload" in the acute phases of the illness. Positive evidence for such a development can only come from longitudinal studies. Thus far research has not been conclusive.

In more recent years this entanglement of premorbid adjustment with paranoid vs. nonparanoid symptomatology is frequently discussed in the context of Crow's (1980) distinction between type I patients with predominantly positive and reversible symptoms such as delusions and hallucinations and type II patients with intellectual impairment and a predominance of negative symptoms such as affective flattening, loss of drive, and poverty of speech. Type I patients are considered to have reversible, dopamine-related functional dysregulations, while the symptoms of type II patients are considered to be largely irreversible or even progressive and to reflect structural brain abnormalities, which Crow (1985) recently assumed to be localized in the temporal lobe. For a long time the differentiation between positive and negative symptoms did not attract much interest, except for the seminal paper by Strauss et al. (1974) and the outstanding work by Wing and Brown (1970). The most recent surge of interest in this field is probably due primarily to the wealth of etiological and therapeutic implications of Crow's typology but also to Andreasen's (1982) development of highly reliable scales to assess a more broadly defined array of negative symptoms.

It was largely the research instigated by Crow himself which revealed a number of conceptual ambiguities in this typology: (1) Most studies found positive and negative symptoms not as opposite poles of a common dimension, but as largely uncorrelated clusters (e.g., Owens and Johnstone 1980; Pogue-Geile and Harrow 1984; Rosen et al. 1984) which may coexist in the same patient but follow different time courses. (2) The cluster of negative symptoms itself seems to comprise at least two independent factors, apathy and psychomotor retardation, both of which are independent of thought disorder and loss of goal orientation (Gibbons et al. 1985). (3) Virtually the same list of symptoms that defines negative symptoms in schizophrenia also characterizes poor premorbid adjustment, nonspecific depressive syndromes, defect states following an acute psychotic episode, some side effects of neuroleptic medication, and most likely also those of prolonged institutionalization (Carpenter et al. 1985; Sommers 1985).

This conceptual ambiguity of negative symptoms allows for all possible correlations to be found between negative symptomatology and any other variable such as response to neuroleptic treatment. It might also explain why an enlargement of the lateral ventricles correlates not with negative symptoms but rather with the absence of positive symptoms and with behavioral deterioration (Owens et al. 1985). Such ventricular enlargement is frequently found among chronic poor premorbid schizophrenics (see Goetz and van Kammen 1986). Apparently, it does not reflect some kind of progressive atrophy, and is unrelated to duration of illness (Andreasen et al. 1986; Weinberger 1985). Negative symptoms are correlated not only with poor pre- as well as postmorbid adjustment, but also with long-term outcome and the performance in quite a variety of neuropsychological tests (e.g., Andreasen and Olsen 1982; Opler et al. 1984; Pogue-Geile and Harrow 1984). This long-term consistency of general adjustment and of features that may also qualify as negative symptoms in schizophrenia is certainly impressive, but up to now there is no way to decide whether they have anything to do with the psychotic episode and whether and when they might even indicate something like a schizophrenic defect (Zubin et al. 1985).

From a clinical as well as from a scientific point of view there can hardly be a more timely task for psychological models than to unravel the interplay of both positive and negative symptoms with the highly confounded variables of premorbid adjustment, sex, social status, age, the response to treatment, and, finally, the response to the psychotic episode itself. The challenge has been recognized since the early work of Kraepelin, but progress has been very, very slow.

Models of Information Processing as a Frame of Reference to Elucidate Schizophrenic Impairments

Most clinicians and experimental researchers will agree that it is not unreasonable to discuss schizophrenic impairments under the heading of information processing, a concept that holds modern psychology under its spell. They might also agree that the impairments of schizophrenics are most conspicious in tasks that could be described as "effortful" and "attention-demanding," or as requiring "controlled processes" or "attentional capacity," to use the terms from some highly favored and elaborate models of modern cognitive psychology (Kahneman 1973; Posner 1978; Shiffrin and Schneider 1977). All these terms refer primarily to later stages of information processing on the way from sensory input to some response system or just to long-term memory. Deficiencies of schizophrenics in tasks requiring these more demanding modes of later processing are so ubiquitous that they are often considered to reveal nothing but a rather unspecific, "general deficit" of the patients (Chapman and Chapman 1973).

Controversies and conjectures prevail only with respect to the question of whether there are also impairments in earlier stages of processing, given that pure sensory deficits have been excluded by definition. The earlier processes are assumed to function largely unconsciously, automatically, and effortless, although Frith (1979) drew attention to the fact that schizophrenics might have a pathological awareness of automatic processes which are normally carried out below the level of consciousness. Quite a few of the controversies probably stem primarily from the bedeviling diversity of methods used to investigate early stages of processing and from the fact that so far only event-related potential research has allowed a comparison of relatively early and late stages of the responses to the same stimuli.

Nearly all studies applying event-related potential methodology concur that there is a substantial attenuation of amplitudes only in the late and slow components (see Roth 1977; Zahn 1986), which are often considered to reveal some of the late "controlled processes" (Callaway and Naghdi 1982). Also with respect to the middle components, the weight of the evidence points to smaller amplitudes in schizophrenics than in normals (see Buchsbaum 1977). But contrary to the late components, these middle components sometimes still show a differential response to selective attention demands, at least when stimulation rate is relatively fast (Baribeau-Braun et al. 1983). The early components, finally, are usually within normal range. Sometimes, but only rarely, they have been found to be even augmented, as stressed by Shagass (1976) and reported for early components of somatosensory potentials. Taken together, these findings argue against primary deficiencies in the earliest stages of information processing or in the basic mechanisms of selective attention, and suggest that there are mainly severe difficulties in organizing and maintaining an effective strategy for processing the information.

There is not much support in the literature for the notion, so popular in the last decades, that schizophrenics have defective mechanisms of filtering or gating sensory input. Only two sets of data might be taken as indicating a reduction of such early inhibitory mechanisms: Freedman et al. (1983) reported less reduction of an early auditory component in the responses to the second of the clicks in repeatedly presented pairs, and Braff et al. (1978) found less reduction of blink amplitude and latency if a warning stimulus preceded the blink-reflex-inducing noise.

While the earliest iconic stages of visual information processing seem to be normal according to the results of two stimulus integration studies (Knight et al. 1978; Spaulding et al. 1980), a number of backward masking studies (e.g., Saccuzzo and Braff 1981) indicate a prolonged vulnerability of the icon to interfering effects from a subsequent pattern mask. This has been found most pronounced in poor premorbid schizophrenics and in those with negative symptoms (Green and Walker 1986). It is interpreted as a pathological slowness of information processing from the iconic store to a more permanent memory system. A similar interpretation is usually offered for the particularly poor performance of both acutely ill and remitted schizophrenics in a variety of span of apprehension tests (e.g., Asarnow and MacCrimmon 1981). These tests usually require the patient to identify a target letter in tachistoscopically presented letter arrays, although the deficiency is not restricted to the visual modality (Harris et al. 1985).

Both the backward masking and the span of apprehension data are usually taken as support for Yates' (1966) notion of a reduced rate of information transfer in the earliest stages of information processing. Whatever its cause, such a reduction in the rate of information transfer can certainly have similar deleterious effects on later stages of processing as defective filtering. For many years the concept of defective filtering was highly in vogue in schizophrenia research to account for impairments in all kinds of attention-demanding tasks. It had been borrowed from Broadbent's original model and inflated with the many diverse meanings of "overinclusion" (see Payne 1971) to denote a deficiency in focusing attention on task-relevant stimuli. As Hemsley (1975) has shown, many of the data purportedly indicating such a filtering defect are better accounted for by difficulties in response set or "pigeon-holing" according to Broadbent's (1971) later model.

Despite the high degree of consistency in the self-reports of acutely ill patients, and despite the strong corroboration from various attention-demanding laboratory tasks, we found surprisingly little direct psychophysiological evidence for Venables' (1984, p. 49) conjecture that the patient early in the disease process "is characterized by an inability to restrict the range of his attention so that he is

flooded by sensory impressions." Again and again there has also been the notion
and even some indication of a paradoxical attenuation of responses with an increase in the intensity of the stimuli among the more acute and good premorbid
patients (e.g., Schooler et al. 1976; Gray 1975). The paucity of immediate psychophysiological support for Venables' conjecture may well be due to the scarcity of
studies that have examined patients in the earliest phases of illness. Often these
patients are not prepared to volunteer for experiments. No doubt, it is easier to
test chronic nonparanoid patients, and in these patients the picture is quite different.

A high proportion of chronic nonparanoid patients have been found to be
strikingly unresponsive or hyporesponsive to moderate-intensity stimuli, especially with respect to electrodermal activity, at least when these stimuli are task-
irrelevant (Bernstein et al. 1982; Gruzelier and Venables 1972; see Zahn 1986).
This electrodermal nonresponding appears related to symptoms of emotional
withdrawal and conceptual confusion as well as to a relatively low level of skin
conductance and low rate of spontaneous fluctuations (see Öhman 1981). One
might wonder whether it is based on the same limbic and/or attentional dysfunctions as the strikingly poor responses of chronic schizophrenics to autonomic
conditioning procedures with aversive stimuli (e.g., Ax 1975; Rist et al. 1981).
Certainly, it is not unreasonable to assume with Öhman (1981) that nonresponding might be secondary to withdrawal and confusion. But whatever is primary,
it is still difficult to understand how unexpected events can be treated in a way
not eliciting an orienting response, which, in Öhman's interpretation, indicates an
involuntary shift from the automatic to the controlled mode of processing in
order to evaluate the unexpected event.

A recent report by Knight et al. (1985) should warn us not to conclude that
chronic schizophrenics merely do not care any longer about external events. The
performance of poor premorbid schizophrenics in a picture recognition task was
compared with that of various control groups when random noise, meaningful
pictures, or patterned but meaningless masks quickly followed the tachistoscopic
presentation of the target pictures. Poor premorbid schizophrenics were the only
group that responded to the pattern mask as if it were a meaningful mask, showing poorer recognition performance than with the random mask. All the other
groups were apparently able to immediately distinguish between what was meaningful and what was just a meaningless pattern. Knight et al. (1985) take this finding to indicate a rather early perceptual organization deficit, which can render all
later controlled processes excessively vulnerable to information overload.

Searching for Neurophysiological Correlates of Schizophrenic Symptoms and Deficits

In an attempt to strengthen and stabilize the nomological network of a model it
has become increasingly popular to postulate and investigate certain relationships
between the psychological concepts and some set of neurophysiological or neuropsychological findings. In this way, Magaro (1984) summarizes the vast literature
on differences between paranoid and nonparanoid schizophrenics by suggesting

that nonparanoid schizophrenics tend to rely primarily on the automatic mode of information processing, which he relates to a preference for right hemisphere functioning, while paranoids tend to favor the controlled mode of processing, which Magaro sees as a special emphasis on left hemisphere functions.

This attempt to blend psychopathological evidence with neuropsychological knowledge or speculations about hemispheric functioning fits in well with the prevailing trend of the time. At least since Flor-Henry (1976) proposed that schizophrenia might be related to left hemisphere dysfunctions, the whole armamentarium of clinical and neuropsychological methods has been pressed into service to provide evidence for this proposition. By and large the results appear more confusing than enlightening (see Kovelman and Scheibel 1986; Seidman 1983; Walker and McGuire 1982). Nevertheless, Venables (1984) has managed to integrate them, in an amazing tour de force, by postulating an overactivation of the left hemisphere in response to a primary right hemisphere dysfunction. Another attempt to reconcile the conflicting facts and fictions was made by Gruzelier (1983), who suggested that left hemisphere overactivation is characteristic for paranoid schizophrenics while right hemisphere overactivation is typical for patients with negative symptoms such as blunted affect, withdrawal, and motor retardation. This latter group was found to have larger electrodermal responses on the right hand, apparently quite a common finding among schizophrenics (see Öhman 1981; Zahn 1986). The patients with more florid and hypomanic features had larger responses on the left side, provided the stimuli were intense enough to keep the number of nonresponders down.

Neither have the most recent technical developments been particularly successful in demonstrating a characteristic left hemisphere dysfunction in schizophrenia. Positron emission tomography has only rarely evinced any systematic group differences in hemispheric activation (see Wolkin and Brodie 1986), and the studies with regional cerebral blood flow have only rarely provided consistent results that could be interpreted without a number of ad hoc assumptions. A typical example is the series of studies by Gur (1985), who found increased left hemisphere metabolic activity of schizophrenic patients during the resting state only in unmedicated patients. During cognitive activity her schizophrenics showed some signs of left hemisphere overactivation not for the verbal but rather for a spatial task.

Following the suggestions of Magaro (1984) and the evidence of Reynolds (1983) for increased dopaminergic innervation especially of the left amygdala, it might be worthwhile to turn from global comparisons of schizophrenics and normals to studies of the specific relationship between positive symptoms and indications of left hemisphere overactivation and/or dysfunction. Negative symptoms may be related not so much to dysfunctions of the right hemisphere as to dysfunctions of the prefrontal cortex. This appears as quite a relief from the never-ending game of trying to find some match between all kinds of dubious dichotomies like positive/negative symptoms, automatic/controlled modes, or early/late stages of processing and finally the functions of the two cerebral hemispheres. The trend to relate negative symptoms to frontal lobe dysfunction has been strongly reinforced by the pioneering work of Ingvar and Franzen (1974), who found evidence for reduced frontal blood flow in the most withdrawn, mute, and indifferent of their schizophrenic patients. Intriguing results have recently been published by Weinberger et al. (1986), comparing chronic, medication-free schizophrenics with normals. For the resting state there was only weak and inconclusive evidence for the postulated "hypofrontality" of the schizophrenics. For activated states there was a drastic difference between conditions: no differences between groups were found when the subjects were engaged in either an easy matching task or in one of two versions of the Continuous Performance Test, but highly significant differences emerged when they were working on a modified Wisconsin Card Sorting test. The increase of relative blood flow at dorsolateral prefrontal areas, typical for normals working on the test, was practically absent in chronic schizophrenics, and the relative reduction of prefrontal flow in this group correlated with poor performance on the test.

These latter studies demonstrate how important it is to compare the groups not just in an ill-defined resting state but under conditions of well-defined activation. Beyond that, they inevitably lead to the question of how these results about frontal dysfunctions are related to those aspects of human performance that are usually discussed under labels like motivation, arousal, attention, and effort. It may be time to untie from the safe harbor of solidly built and prestigious models of cognitive aspects of information processing in normals and risk anew some expeditions into poorly charted seas without safe passages and full of mysteries. These are the mysteries many of the old models had tried to explore under the flags of social censure, lack of motivation, regression, interference, or just attention deficit. The questions have remained the same, and they are as urgent today as they have ever been. Only the old models have faded away or were left behind when it became obvious that they were insufficient to deal with the many inconsistencies of experimental results or that they had become so heavily loaded with ad hoc explanations that they were more of a burden than an aid in moving on to a better understanding of the intricacies of schizophrenic impairments. The models and research that have been discussed in this paper do not give us immediate directions, but do provide us with a solid basis and stable points of reference for such an endeavor.

References

Alpert M (1985) The signs and symptoms of schizophrenia. In: Alpert M (ed) Controversies in schizophrenia. Changes and constancies. Guilford Press, New York, pp 255–266
American Psychiatric Association (1980) Diagnostic and statistical manual of mental disorders, 3rd edn. American Psychiatric Association, Washington DC
Andreasen NC (1982) Negative symptoms in schizophrenia. Arch Gen Psychiatry 39:784–788
Andreasen NC, Olsen S (1982) Negative v positive schizophrenia. Definition and validation. Arch Gen Psychiatry 39:789–794
Andreasen NC, Hoffman RE, Grove WM (1985) Mapping abnormalities in language and cognition. In: Alpert M (ed) Controversies in schizophrenia. Changes and constancies. Guilford Press, New York, pp 199–227
Andreasen NC, Nasrallah HA, Dunn V, Olson SC, Grove WM, Erhardt JC, Coffman JA, Crossett JHW (1986) Structural abnormalities in the frontal system in schizophrenia. A magnetic resonance imaging study. Arch Gen Psychiatry 43:136–144
Asarnow RF, MacCrimmon DJ (1981) Span of apprehension deficits during the postpsychotic stages of schizophrenia. Arch Gen Psychiatry 38:1006–1011

Ax AF (1975) Emotional learning deficiency in schizophrenia. In: Kietzman ML, Sutton S, Zubin J (eds) Experimental approaches to psychopathology. Academic, New York, pp 255–268

Bannister D, Fransella F (1966) A grid test of schizophrenic thought disorder. Br J Soc Clin Psychol 5:95–102

Baribeau-Braun J, Picton TW, Gosselin J-Y (1983) Schizophrenia: a neurophysiological evaluation of abnormal information processing. Science 219:874–876

Bernstein A, Frith C, Gruzelier J, Patterson T, Straube E, Venables P, Zahn T (1982) An analysis of the skin conductance orienting response in samples of American, British, and German schizophrenics. Biol Psychol 14:155–211

Braff D, Stone C, Callaway E, Geyer M, Glick I, Bali L (1978) Prestimulus effects on human startle reflex in normals and schizophrenics. Psychophysiology 15:339–343

Broadbent DE (1971) Decision and stress. Academic, London

Broen WE (1968) Schizophrenia: research and theory. Academic, New York

Buchsbaum MS (1977) The middle evoked response components and schizophrenia. Schizophr Bull 3:93–104

Buss AH, Lang PJ (1965) Psychological deficit in schizophrenia: I. Affect, reinforcement and concept attainment. J Abnorm Psychol 70:2–24

Callaway E, Naghdi S (1982) An information processing model for schizophrenia. Arch Gen Psychiatry 39:339–347

Carpenter WT, Heinrichs DW, Alphs LD (1985) Treatment of negative symptoms. Schizophr Bull 11:440–452

Chapman LJ, Chapman JP (1973) Disordered thought in schizophrenia. Appleton-Century-Crofts, New York

Cohen BD, Nachmani G, Rosenberg S (1974) Referent communication disturbances in acute schizophrenia. J Abnorm Psychol 83:1–13

Crow TJ (1980) Molecular pathology of schizophrenia: more than one disease process. Br Med J 280:66–68

Crow TJ (1985) The two-syndrome concept: origins and current status. Schizophr Bull 11:471–486

Flor-Henry P (1976) Lateralized temporal-limbic dysfunction and psychopathology. Ann NY Acad Sci 280:777–797

Freedman R, Adler LE, Waldo MC, Pachtman E, Franks RD (1983) Neurophysiological evidence for a defect in inhibitory pathways in schizophrenia: comparison of medicated and drug-free patients. Biol Psychiatry 18:537–551

Frith CD (1979) Consciousness, information processing and schizophrenia. Br J Psychiatry 134:225–235

Gibbons RD, Lewine RRJ, Davis JM, Schooler NR, Cole JO (1985) An empirical test of a Kraepelinian vs. a Bleulerian view of negative symptoms. Schizophr Bull 11:390–396

Gjerde PF (1983) Attentional capacity dysfunction and arousal in schizophrenia. Psychol Bull 93:57–72

Goetz KL, van Kammen DP (1986) Computerized axial tomography scans and subtypes of schizophrenia. A review of the literature. J Nerv Ment Dis 174:31–41

Goldstein MJ, Held JM, Cromwell RL (1968) Premorbid adjustment and paranoid-nonparanoid status in schizophrenia. Psychol Bull 70:382–386

Gray AL (1975) Autonomic correlates of chronic schizophrenia: a reaction time paradigm. J Abnorm Psychol 84:189–196

Green M, Walker E (1986) Symptom correlates of vulnerability to backward masking in schizophrenia. Am J Psychiatry 143:181–186

Gruzelier JH (1983) A critical assessment and integration of lateral asymmetries in schizophrenia. In: Myslobodsky MS (ed) Hemisyndromes. Psychobiology, neurology, psychiatry. Academic, New York, pp 265–326

Gruzelier JH, Venables PH (1972) Skin conductance orienting activity in a heterogeneous sample of schizophrenics. J Nerv Ment Dis 155:277–287

Gur RE (1985) Regional cerebral blood flow in schizophrenia. In: Alpert M (ed) Controversies in schizophrenia. Changes and constancies. Guilford Press, New York, pp 79–89

Harris A, Ayers T, Leek MR (1985) Auditory span of apprehension deficits in schizophrenia. J Nerv Ment Dis 173:650–657

Hemsley DR (1975) A two-stage model of attention in schizophrenia research. Br J Soc Clin Psychol 14:81–89

Hemsley DR (1977) What have cognitive deficits to do with schizophrenic symptoms? Br J Psychiatry 130:167–173

Hirsch SR, Leff JP (1975) Abnormalities in parents of schizophrenics. Oxford University Press, London

Huber G (1983) Das Konzept substratnaher Basissymptome und seine Bedeutung für Theorie und Therapie schizophrener Erkrankungen. Nervenarzt 54:23–32

Ingvar DH, Franzen G (1974) Abnormalities of cerebral blood flow distribution in patients with chronic schizophrenia. Acta Psychiatr Scand 50:425–462

Kahneman D (1973) Attention and effort. Prentice-Hall, Englewood Cliffs NJ

Knight RA, Roff JD (1985) Affectivity in schizophrenia. In: Alpert M (ed) Controversies in schizophrenia. Changes and constancies. Guilford Press, New York, pp 280–316

Knight RA, Sherer M, Putchat C, Carter G (1978) A picture integration task for measuring iconic memory in schizophrenics. J Abnorm Psychol 87:314–321

Knight RA, Elliott DS, Freedman EG (1985) Short-term visual memory in schizophrenics. J Abnorm Psychol 94:427–442

Koh SD (1978) Remembering of verbal materials by schizophrenic young adults. In: Schwartz S (ed) Language and cognition in schizophrenia. Erlbaum, Hillsdale NJ, pp 55–99

Kokes R, Strauss J, Klorman R (1977) Premorbid adjustment in schizophrenia: II. Measuring premorbid adjustment: the instruments and their development. Schizophr Bull 3:186–213

Kovelman JA, Scheibel AB (1986) Biological substrates of schizophrenia. Acta Neurol Scand 73:1–32

Leff J, Vaughn C (1985) Expressed emotion in families. Its significance for mental illness. Guilford Press, New York

Lewine RL, Burbach D, Meltzer HY (1984) Effect of diagnostic criteria on the ratio of male to female schizophrenic patients. Am J Psychiatry 141:84–87

Lipton RB, Levy DL, Holzman PS, Levin S (1983) Eye movement dysfunction in psychiatric patients. A review. Schizophr Bull 9:13–72

Magaro PA (1984) Psychosis and schizophrenia. In: Spaulding WD, Cole JK (eds) Nebraska Symposium on Motivation 1983. Theories of schizophrenia and psychosis. University of Nebraska Press, Lincoln, pp 157–229

Manschreck TC (1986) Motor abnormalities in schizophrenia. In: Nasrallah HA, Weinberger DR (eds) The neurology of schizophrenia. Elsevier, New York, pp 65–96 (Handbook of schizophrenia, vol 1)

Margo A, Hemsley DR, Slade PD (1981) The effects of varying auditory input on schizophrenic hallucinations. Br J Psychiatry 139:122–127

Meehl PE (1962) Schizotaxia, schizotypy, schizophrenia. Am Psychol 17:827–838

Meehl PE (1978) Theoretical risks and tabular asterisks: Sir Karl, Sir Ronald, and the slow progress of soft psychology. J Consult Clin Psychol 46:806–834

Miklowitz DJ, Strachan AM, Goldstein MJ, Doane JA, Snyder KS, Hogarty GE, Falloon IRH (1986) Expressed emotion and communication deviance in the families of schizophrenics. J Abnorm Psychol 95:60–66

Mirsky A (1969) Neuropsychological bases of schizophrenia. Ann Rev Psychol 20:321–348

Nuechterlein KH (1977) Reaction time and attention in schizophrenia: a critical evaluation of the data and theories. Schizophr Bull 3:373–428

Öhman A (1981) Electrodermal activity and vulnerability to schizophrenia: a review. Biol Psychol 12:87–145

Opler LA, Kay SR, Rosado V, Lindenmayer JP (1984) Positive and negative syndromes in chronic schizophrenic patients. J Nerv Ment Dis 172:317–325

Owens DGC, Johnstone EC (1980) The disabilities of chronic schizophrenia – their nature and factors contributing to their development. Br J Psychiatry 136:384–395

Owens DGC, Johnstone EC, Crow TJ, Frith CD, Jagoe JR, Kreel L (1985) Lateral ventricular size in schizophrenia: relationship to the disease process and its clinical manifestations. Psychol Med 15:27–41

Payne RW (1971) Cognitive defects in schizophrenia: overinclusive thinking. In: Hellmuth J (ed) Deficits in cognition. Brunner/Mazel, New York, pp 53–89 (Cognitive studies, vol 2)

Pogue-Geile MF, Harrow M (1984) Negative and positive symptoms in schizophrenia and depression: a follow-up. Schizophr Bull 10:371–387

Posner MI (1978) Chronometric explorations of mind. Erlbaum, Hillsdale NJ

Redd WH, Porterfield AL, Andersen BL (1979) Behavior modification. Behavioral approaches to human problems. Random House, New York

Reynolds GP (1983) Increased concentrations and lateral asymmetry of amygdala dopamine in schizophrenia. Nature 305:527–529

Rist F, Baumann W, Cohen R (1981) Effects of awareness and motor involvement on autonomic conditioning in chronic schizophrenics. Pavlov J Biol Sci 16:8–17

Rochester SR, Martin JR (1979) Crazy talk: a study of the discourse of schizophrenic speakers. Plenum, New York

Rosen WG, Mohs RC, Johns CA, Small NS, Kendler KS, Horvath TB, Davis KL (1984) Positve and negative symptoms in schizophrenia. Psychiatry Res 13:277–284

Roth WT (1977) Late event-related potentials and psychopathology. Schizophr Bull 3:105–120

Saccuzzo DP, Braff DL (1981) Early information processing deficit in schizophrenia: new findings using schizophrenic sub-groups and manic control subjects. Arch Gen Psychiatry 38:175–179

Schooler C, Buchsbaum MS, Carpenter WT (1976) Evoked response and kinesthetic measures of augmenting/reducing in schizophrenics: replications and extensions. J Nerv Ment Dis 163:221–232

Seidman LJ (1983) Schizophrenia and brain dysfunction: an integration of recent neurodiagnostic findings. Psychol Bull 94:195–238

Serafetinides EA, Coger RW, Martin J (1986) Letter to the editor: different methods of observation affect EEG measures associated with auditory hallucinations. Psychiatry Res 17:73–74

Shagass C (1976) An electrophysiological view of schizophrenia. Biol Psychiatry 11:3–30

Shakow D (1962) Segmental set: a theory of the formal psychological deficit in schizophrenia. Arch Gen Psychiatry 6:17–33

Shiffrin RM, Schneider W (1977) Controlled and automatic human information processing. II. Perceptual learning, automatic attending, and a general theory. Psychol Rev 84:127–190

Silverman J (1964) The problem of attention in research and theory in schizophrenia. Psychol Rev 71:352–379

Silverman J (1967) Variations in cognitive control and psychophysiological defense in the schizophrenias. Psychosom Med 29:225–251

Sommers AA (1985) "Negative symptoms": conceptual and methodological problems. Schizophr Bull 11:364–379

Spaulding W, Rosenzweig L, Huntzinger R, Cromwell RL, Briggs D, Hayes T (1980) Visual pattern integration in psychiatric patients. J Abnorm Psychol 89:635–643

Stevens JR, Livermore A (1982) Telemetered EEG in schizophrenia: spectral analysis during abnormal behaviour episodes. J Neurol Neurosurg Psychiatry 45:385–395

Strauss JS (1973) Diagnostic models and the nature of psychiatric disorder. Arch Gen Psychiatry 29:445–449

Strauss JS, Carpenter WT, Bartko JJ (1974) Speculations on the processes that underlie schizophrenic symptoms and signs. Schizophr Bull 11:61–69

Venables PH (1964) Input dysfunction in schizophrenia. In: Maher BA (ed) Progress in experimental personality research, vol 1. Academic, New York, pp 1–47

Venables PH (1984) Cerebral mechanisms, autonomic responsiveness, and attention in schizophrenia. In: Spaulding WD, Cole JK (eds) Nebraska Symposium on Motivation 1983. Theories of schizophrenia and psychosis. University of Nebraska Press, Lincoln, pp 47–91

Walker E, McGuire M (1982) Intra- and inter-hemispheric information processing in schizophrenia. Psychol Bull 92:701–725

Weinberger DR (1985) Clinical-neuropathological correlations in schizophrenia: theoretical implications. In: Alpert M (ed) Controversies in schizophrenia. Changes and constancies. Guilford Press, New York, pp 92–106

Weinberger DR, Berman KF, Zec RF (1986) Physiologic dysfunction of dorsolateral prefrontal cortex in schizophrenia. I. Regional cerebral blood flow evidence. Arch Gen Psychiatry 43:114–124

Wing JK, Brown G (1970) Institutionalism and schizophrenia. Cambridge University Press, London

Wolkin A, Brodie JD (1986) Positron emission tomography in the study of schizophrenia. In: Burrows GD, Norman TR and Rubinstein G (eds) Handbook of studies on schizophrenia, part 2. Elsevier, New York, pp 163–173

Yates AJ (1966) Data-processing levels and thought disorder in schizophrenia. Austr J Psychol 18:103–117

Zahn TP (1986) Psychophysiological approaches to psychopathology. In: Coles MGH, Donchin E, Porges SW (eds) Psychophysiology. Systems, processes, and applications. Guilford Press, New York, pp 508–610

Zubin J (1975) Problem of attention in schizophrenia. In: Kietzman ML, Sutton S, Zubin J (eds) Experimental approaches to psychopathology. Academic, New York, pp 139–166

Zubin J, Spring R (1977) Vulnerability: a new view of schizophrenia. J Abnorm Psychol 86:103–126

Zubin J, Steinhauer SR, Day R, van Kammen DP (1985) Paul Hoch Award address. Schizophrenia at the crossroads: a blueprint for the 1980s. In: Alpert M (ed) Controversies in schizophrenia. Changes and constancies. Guilford Press, New York, pp 48–76

Cognitive and Attentional Disorders in the Development of Schizophrenia

P. H. VENABLES

Introduction

As suggested by its title, this chapter will consider data and theories concerned with cognitive and attentional processes in the *development* of schizophrenia. With this in mind, the role of these factors as precursors of the disorder will be the major emphasis. However, premorbid data cannot be treated in isolation, and other material discussed will be that obtained from those who are currently patients; those in a state of remission; and additionally those who are not patients but who have "schizotypal" characteristics.

An acceptable definition of cognition is that provided by Neisser (1967) in his book *Cognitive Psychology*, in which he stated "the term cognition referes to all the processes by which the sensory input is transformed, reduced, elaborated, stored, recovered and used" (p. 4).

Kraepelin (1913), in enunciating the fundamental characteristics of dementia praecox, included in his definition "The weakening of judgement, of mental activity and of creative ability ...."

Thus, the deficit in a cognitive element was included in this early description of the disorder.

Kraepelin's dementia praecox is synonymous with some but perhaps not all present definitions of schizophrenia. In an attempt to suggest a conservative view of the position, Kety (1980), in his Maudsley lecture, said:

We would define syndromes more homogeneous in symptomatology, and more useful predictors of outcome and response to therapy for clinical practice and research, were we to restrict schizophrenia to its original concept of a chronic disorder of thought and feeling in which insidious onset, the premorbid personality qualities and the fundamental features described by Kraepelin and Bleuler were the defining characteristics.

This description of schizophrenia is one that in the current climate we might probably denote as "negative symptom" schizophrenia (Andreasen 1982; Andreasen and Olsen 1982) or "type II" schizophrenia (Crow 1980).

Venables (1984), in reviewing material on attentional deficits in negative-symptom schizophrenics, concluded that such deficits could be considered as a fundamental characteristic of these patients. While many workers would consider that attention might be considered as an aspect of cognitive psychology, it is undoubtedly difficult to define simply (Mostovsky 1970), and it would be appropri-

Department of Psychology, University of York, Heslington, York, Y01 5DD, United Kongdom

ate to think that cognitive deficits do not necessarily include attentional disorders. One aspect of cognitive deficit which will be considered later in this chapter is that of intellectual deficit or low IQ as a characteristic of schizophrenia. As an exercise it is therefore appropriate at this point to consider how attentional processes and intelligence might interact in the production of disorder.

Lehmann (1966) suggested a model based on the notion that (non-paranoid) schizophrenics may be constitutionally prone to be more "open" to the environment than normal persons. For instance, Venables (1964), using reports from McGhie and Chapman's (1961) description of the experiences of early schizophrenic patients, suggested that "the patient is characterised by an inability to restrict the range of his attention so that he is flooded by sensory impressions from all quarters." Lehmann's suggestion was that both the creative person and the schizophrenic may be "subject to the impact of a higher number of discrete sensory stimuli per time unit." He proposed that if a person can cope with this supernormal influx of stimuli, because he has an adequate central processing apparatus (which we might possibly translate as intelligence), then he will have exceptional ability. On the other hand, if this central processing apparatus is unable to cope with the influx of sensory stimuli "then the person's integration breaks down and he may become psychotic."

This brief introduction provides the basis for the remainder of the chapter. What will now be discussed is material suggesting that lower than normal IQ is a precursor of schizophrenia, and that an attentional deficit is characteristic of the schizophrenic condition, both in the morbid and the premorbid states. Finally data on the interaction of intellectual level and aspects of attention will be presented.

Intellectual Impairment in Schizophrenia

The publications in this area have recently been extensively reviewed by Aylward et al. (1984). This was the first major review in this area for some 20 years and presents data from a much more convincing set of studies than had been available to previous reviewers.

The early work had tended to concentrate of findings of lower levels of intelligence in those who were patients at the time of testing and to contrast their IQs to population norms. This procedure, of course, confounded what might be an actually lower IQ with a lowered measure of IQ which might be thought realistically to be due to the patient's currently disordered state.

Data reviewed by Aylward et al. (1984) showed that "premorbid scores of schizophrenic patients obtained during childhood, adolescence and early adulthood are lower than the scores of their siblings and peers with similar social class origins." The other outcome of Aylward et al.'s analysis of the available material is to indicate that "premorbid IQ deficit may be an exclusive, or more pronounced characteristic of schizophrenic males."

Of particular interest at this point are studies carried out in the context of longitudinal investigations. One such study, not reviewed by Aylward et al., is that of Gruzelier et al. (1979), which compared the verbal and performance IQs of children of schizophrenic parents with those of children of parents with other psychiatric diagnoses and children of normal controls. All children were between the ages of 10 and 13. It was found that the verbal, but not the performance IQ was significantly lower among the children of schizophrenic parents than in the other two groups. This finding of a low verbal IQ in the children of schizophrenic parents is replicated in the report of Winters et al. (1981), who showed that among children in the age range 6–16, the verbal IQ of children of schizophrenic parents (and also those of unipolar but not bipolar depressives) was lower than that of controls. The performance IQ of the children of unipolar depressive patients was also significantly lower than that of normal controls. Other data of relevance to this issue are provided by material from the earliest of the high-risk studies, that by Mednick and Schulsinger (1968). This material is available in a paper by Griffith et al. (1980), who find, in comparing the total WISC IQs of a high- and a low-risk group, that the high-risk group has a significantly lower mean IQ than the low-risk group. The high-risk group consisted of 207 subjects, while the low-risk group numbered 104 when originally tested in 1962. However, it is to be noted that by 1972, 17 of the high-risk group had developed schizophrenia, so that it was possible to compare the premorbid IQ of the high-risk subjects who had broken down with that of a control group, which in this instance consisted of their siblings who remained normal. In this instance there was no difference between the IQ of the patients and that of the controls after age was taken into account. It would, perhaps, have been more interesting to have compared the IQs of the sick group of high-risk subjects with a matched subgroup from the same at-risk population who had not become psychotic. Another major study of children at risk for schizophrenia which provides relevant data is that by Erlenmeyer-Kimling and colleagues (1984a) in New York. Using the data from this study, Watt et al. (1982) reported that the mean IQ of the high-risk group of children was significantly lower than that of normal controls. More interestingly, however, Erlenmeyer-Kimling et al. (1984b) report on the IQs of those of the high-risk sample who have become clinically deviant. They show that the full-scale IQ of the deviant subjects is 11 points below that of the entire high-risk group, and that the biggest difference between sick and well subjects is in verbal IQ, thus replicating the findings reviewed above. One recent report that does not replicate the findings of other investigations is that from the Israeli high-risk study (Sohlberg 1985; Sohlberg and Yaniv 1985), which showed no difference between high- and low-risk groups on overall WISC and verbal scores of intelligence. There was a nonsignificant tendency for poorer performance on Raven's matrices in the index group, but the noteworthy result was on the arithmetic subtest of the WISC, where the high-risk subjects had lower scores than controls.

In these studies we are looking at data from groups at high risk for schizophrenia because the children in the groups have a parent who is schizophrenic. In comparison to the general population, where the morbid risk is 0.85%, among these groups the risk of developing schizophrenia is around 15%; however, because only a small number of subjects in the high-risk groups are likely to develop the disorder, the differences which have been obtained are striking. It is of course likely that a considerably greater proportion than 15% are likely to be classed as borderline schizophrenic (or schizotypal personality disorder in DSM-III parlance), and if these persons also have impaired intelligence this could explain the strength of the difference between high- and low-risk groups which has been reported. No work appears to have been carried out on the intellectual level of subjects classified as having schizotypal personality disorder. Indeed, bearing in mind the hypothesis of Lehmann (1966), introduced above, and the findings (Jones 1973; Jones and Offord 1974) of the independent inheritance of IQ and schizophrenia, it is not unlikely that those having schizotypic characteristics but not being schizophrenics might in certain instances be expected to have higher than normal IQs, as a high IQ can be seen to be protective. Claridge (1972) made the same point in suggesting that "the very creative person, though highly disposed to schizophrenia does not become clinically psychotic because high general intelligence confers some immunity in the form of adequate intellectual and personality reserves."

There are data which enable the position to be examined in a slightly different way. This involves some speculation, but the exercise may be worthwhile from an heuristic viewpoint. In particular it involves the extrapolation of data on obstetric or perinatal factors from one study to another, a procedure not without some danger (McNeil and Kaij 1978).

Reider et al. (1977) in a study of children of schizophrenic parents, showed that at the age of 7 these children had lower IQ scores than those of controls and that this finding could be attributed entirely to male offspring. These lower IQs were correlated with the incidence of adverse perinatal events. This relationship was found where the parents were "continuous" (chronic and borderline) but not when they were diagnosed as being acute schizophrenics. The IQ of these high-risk children was not related to socioeconomic status, as is the case in general population samples. Thus in this study the data suggest that the low IQ, which has previously been suggested to be a factor in the development of schizophrenia, may, at least in part, be determined by perinatal rather than genetic factors.

One further link in the chain is provided by a recent analysis of data from the Copenhagen high-risk study, (Schulsinger et al. 1984). This study examines the ventricle/brain ratio (VBR) assessed by the use of computed tomographic (CT) scanning techniques on subjects from the original high-risk group (children of schizophrenic mothers) who had been diagnosed as schizophrenic, borderline schizophrenic or with no mental disorder. In accord with other studies (e.g. review by Seidman 1983), those with a schizophrenic diagnosis had higher VBR than those with no mental illness; on the other hand, those with a diagnosis of borderline schizophrenia had a lower than normal VBR. The authors also show that VBR is significantly correlated with certain perinatal complications, particularly low birth weight. The suggestion that enlarged cerebral ventricles are a result of some environmental insult and not genetically determined is in accord with the earlier work by Reveley et al. (1982), who showed that in monozygotic twins discordant for schizophrenia, the sick twin exhibited larger cerebral ventricles. Schulsinger et al. (1984) interpret their findings within a diathesis-stress model (e.g. Meehl 1962) and suggest that what is perhaps inherited is a predisposition to schizophrenia, and that when this occurs in conjunction with a stressor such as a perinatal complication then it results in schizophrenia, whereas when the same possible stressor is at a level which is below normal then the result is borderline schizophrenia. In the present context, the interpretation should perhaps be that the birth complications suffered by those who became schizophrenic mediated their effect by the production of low IQ, particularly as we know (see the study by Griffith et al. 1980, reviewed above) that a low IQ is reported in the high-risk group in this study. This suggestion should be viewed with care, however, as in reviewing the literature to date, Goetz and van Kammen (1986) state that attempts to demonstrate an association between structural abnormalities on the CT scan and a deterioration of intellectual function have been mixed, and hence it would be premature to infer a direct relationship between the two. One possibility, bearing in mind that as reviewed above, in some studies it is verbal IQ that shows the deficit in function in comparison to performance IQ, is that what is involved is a left hemisphere abnormality; indeed, this is the interpretation given by Gruzelier et al. (1979) to their findings of lower verbal than performance IQ in high-risk children. Luchins et al. (1982) provide relevant data. They assessed occipital cerebral asymmetry using CT scans on a large group of schizophrenic or schizoaffective patients and, as controls, neurological or medical patients. In normal subjects there is an asymmetry of the cerebral hemispheres, with the left lobe being larger than the right. This asymmetry tends to be reversed in schizophrenic patients. However, the complication raised by the Luchins et al. data is that the reversed asymmetry occurs in those patients *without* CT evidence of brain atrophy. The study also showed that the schizophrenics with reversed asymmetry had lower verbal than performance IQs.

This is clearly a finding that makes for difficulty in interpretation, for it suggests that schizophrenics with a lower verbal than performance IQ should be those without cerebral atrophy and hence should not be those with negative symptoms. This should be taken in the context of the data reviewed by Goetz and van Kammen (1986) which leads them to make the statement: "studies seem to indicate that the subgroup of patients with brain atrophy are distinguishable both by their lack of positive symptoms and by a particular predominance of negative symptoms."

Finally, in this section it is important to take note of the contribution made by one of the first studies in psychiatry to make use of the nuclear magnetic resonance imaging technique to provide measures of brain structure. The study by Andreasen et al. (1986) showed that schizophrenic patients in comparison with normal controls, had significantly smaller frontal lobes as well as smaller cerebrums and craniums. The authors were surprised to find that there was no association between decreased frontal size and negative symptoms. However, their data did suggest "an association between a relative decrease in brain and skull size, whatever the cause, and two major indexes of schizophrenia, negative symptoms and cognitive impairment." There was a suggestion in their data that the phenomena were relatively sex-specific and that smaller brain size might only occur in males; however, when height and weight were controlled by regression techniques, then it appeared that female schizophrenics might also have smaller cranial, cerebral and frontal sizes.

In the present context, therefore, the data do appear to suggest impaired intellectual status in negative-symptom schizophrenia and that this may be related to cerebral atrophy, possibly as a result of prenatal or perinatal factors. However, it is possible that the findings which suggest a lower verbal than performance IQ in schizophrenics do not apply to the negative-symptom group.

Attention, Selective, and Sustained

Bleuler (1924), in his *Textbook of Psychiatry*, distinguished two aspects of attention in the same way that they are now distinguished, although his terminology differed from present usage. What we now term selective attention, he wrote of as "vigility". He said "if we are performing an important experiment we observe what is relevant to it, everything else is entirely lost to our sense." Bleuler distinguishes this aspect of attention from "tenacity", or what we might now call sustained attention, which he defined as "the ability to keep one's attention fixed on a certain subject continuously."

In both aspects of attention schizophrenics are deficient. The area of disorders in selective attention have been extensively reviewed recently, e.g. by Nuechterlein and Dawson (1984) and Venables (1984, 1986), and consequently in this chapter the emphasis of the discussion will be on some aspects of sustained attention, and as in the earlier part of the chapter it will be those studies which involve the development of the disorder which will receive greatest attention. By far the greatest amount of work in this area has been conducted on smooth-pursuit eye movement (SPEM). The first work was carried out by Diefendorff and Dodge (1908), who reported that schizophrenics displayed deficient eye tracking and that they made steplike movements of the eyes as they attempted to maintain target fixation. Kraepelin (1913) cited this study, saying:

> In psychological experiments these patients cannot stick to the appointed exercise ... perhaps the experience related by Diefendorff and Dodge that patients do not usually follow a moving target continuously as normal persons do, but intermittently and hesitatingly may be explained by a similar disorder of attention.

The technique appeared to be forgotten until resurrected by Holzman et al. (1973), since when it has developed into an area of major study.

The essentials of the technique involve the patient following a target, either a pendulum or a spot on an oscilloscope, moving at a speed of less than 40 degrees/second. In the majority of studies the movement is sinusoidal, but in some it takes a triangular form. Recording of eye movement is most commonly undertaken by electro-oculographic (EOG) techniques, although some workers employ infra-red reflectometry (IR). Three methods of scoring the data are in common use; (1) subjective rating of tracking performance on a 4- or 5-point scale with standard exemplars of tracking at each rating point; (2) measurement of the numbers of "velocity arrests," i.e. the numbers of points at which the eye ceases to move before having to make a saccade to catch up with the target; (3) measurement of signal/noise ratio, where the recording of eye movement is subject to spectral analysis, frequencies immediately around the target movement frequency being taken to be "signal" while the extent of other movement frequencies is taken to be a measure of "noise". The natural logarithm of the ratio of signal to noise is the value of the measure commonly used. Again, work in this area has recently been extensively reviewed, by Lipton et al. (1983), and the present coverage can therefore be brief and selective.

Both Iacono (1985) and Siever and Coursey (1985) have suggested that the impaired SPEM may be said to have characteristics which make it a candidate as a biological marker for schizophrenia. It is evident in up to 86% of schizophrenics, and although present to some extent in patients with other psychotic diagnoses appears to be found in schizophrenic and not other patients in remission. It is found in a high proportion of first-degree relatives of schizophrenics and has been shown in twin studies to have a high heritable component. It has a high test-retest reliability over periods of up to 2 years.

What will now be considered is the extent to which SPEM is capable of being used in studies on the development of schizophrenia. The techniques has not been used in the major, well-known high-risk studies such as those in Copenhagen and New York, but data are available which use approaches other than familial definitions of high risk.

One pair of studies is those by Siever et al. (1982, 1984). In the first of these studies, normal subjects were selected, either on the basis of extreme values on platelet monoamine oxidase activity (which has been considered as a possible marker for psychiatric disorder – see review by Wyatt et al. 1979) or on the basis of a poor performance on the Continuous Performance Test (CPT; see Nuechterlein and Dawson 1984), also considered to be a characteristic of schizophrenics. Although poor eye tracking did not appear to be related to either of these other markers, subjects with impaired eye tracking were characterised by social introversion, perhaps akin to "social aversiveness", considered by Meehl (1962) to be a cardinal characteristic of schizophrenia. In the second study a large normal student population was screened for eye-tracking accuracy. Groups of low- and high-accuracy trackers were selected from the extremes of the distribution of tracking scores. The members of these groups were then rated by an interviewer and completed a questionnaire to determine their status for meeting the criteria for DSM-III schizotypal personality disorder (SPD). Those classified as poor eye trackers were significantly more often identified as satisfying the criteria for SPD than high-accuracy trackers.

Another approach is that of Simons and Katkin (1985), who examined the relationship between eye-tracking accuracy and the Physical Anhedonia Scale (Chapman et al. 1980). Anhedonia is considered by Meehl (1962) to be one of the four prime characteristics of schizophrenia and schizotypy, and has been shown by Chapman et al. (1980) to predict proneness to psychotic breakdown. While the results of this study were somewhat equivocal, three subjects who scored particularly highly on the anhedonia scale, all had poor eye-tracking scores. Another measure of schizotypic tendency and proneness to psychosis is the perceptual aberration scale (Chapman et al. 1980). This was used in a second study by Simons and Katkin (1985), and again the most deviant eye-movement records were found among a subgroup of schizotypic subjects.

Overall, the data suggest that where risk for the development of schizophrenia is defined by the subject having a schizotypic personality, there is a tendency for that risk to be associated with poor smooth-pursuit eye tracking.

A paper which helps to tie together the material on eye tracking with that on CT scans reviewed earlier is that of Bartfai et al. (1985), which appears to be the first study in which SPEM and CT data are available on the same patients. Clinically it was shown that positive symptoms tended to be correlated negatively with poor eye-tracking scores. These data therefore suggest that poor eye tracking may be a measure of negative-symptom tendency in schizophrenia. There was a weak tendency for poor eye tracking to be related directly to an index akin to the VBR used in other studies, and thus as a large value of this index is related to negative symptomatology, the direction of the SPEM/VBR relationship is appropriate. However, because the brain morphology indices in this study were all within normal range, not too much emphasis can be placed on these findings. Further work is required.

Eye Tracking and IQ in a High-Risk Study

As an illustration of the relationship between intellectual status and sustained attention, measured by eye tracking, the results of as yet unpublished material (Venables et al. 1987, in preparation) from an ongoing high-risk study (Venables 1978) will be described.

In 1972 a high-risk study was started on the island of Mauritius. In contrast to the Copenhagen and New York studies, which employed familial factors to identify the risk population, this study used patterns of electrodermal activity as risk identifiers.

The basis of the investigation was the finding in the Copenhagen study, (Mednick and Schulsinger 1968; Mednick et al. 1978) that electrodermal hyper-responsivity was observed in the premorbid state in those subjects who subsequently suffered psychiatric breakdown. This hyper-responsivity is also shown in a proportion of adult schizophrenics (e.g. Gruzelier and Venables 1972; Frith et al. 1979).

Data were collected from 1800 3-year-old children in 1972, and a selected group of 200 children, including 99 showing electrodermal hyper-responsivity, were studied regularly in the succeeding years. Control subjects in this group were made up from those with median electrodermal responsivity. The selection procedure is described by Venables (1978).

At the age of 11, the children were again studied psychophysiologically and measures of eye tracking obtained. If the original selection procedure at age 3 had been successful (and it should be admitted that the study was controversial; see Garmezy 1974), then it would be expected that those children who exhibited electrodermal hyper-responsivity would also show poor eye tracking.

One potential difficulty was an informal report from Holzman that eye-tracking performance did not reach a stable level until after the age of 11. However, work by one of the author's graduate students, Jaafar Behbehani, showed no effect of age on eye tracking in a population of children between 4 and 18 years of age.

Eye tracking was scored by the three methods described in the previous section. Taking the data as a whole, there was no relationship between age 3 electrodermal activity and age 11 eye tracking. However, bearing in mind the material

Table 1. Mean values of velocity arrests (VA), log signal/noise ratios (logS/N) and qualitative ratings (QR) of smooth pursuit eye movements of groups divided by "risk" (HR vs C) and intelligence (LI vs HI)

	HR–LI	HR–HI	C–LI	C–HI
VA	50.6 (31.6)	26.6 (14.9)	30.4 (19.1)	26.6 (7.5)
logS/N	3.0 (1.1)	3.7 (0.7)	3.7 (0.6)	3.7 (0.4)
QR	2.8 (1.1)	2.0 (1.7)	2.6 (0.7)	2.3 (0.9)
N	15	17	13	10

Values in parentheses are SD
HR, hyper-responders; C, controls;   LI, low intelligence; HI, high intelligence

reviewed in the first part of this paper on the relationship between premorbid IQ and later schizophrenic breakdown, and also a study by Kimmel and Deboskey (1978) which showed that gifted children, in comparison to average children, showed electrodermal hyper-responsivity, it seemed not unlikely that the group of electrodermal hyper-responders might include two subgroups: one of pre-schizophrenics with low IQs, and the other of gifted children with high IQs. It would be the former group which would be expected to exhibit poor eye tracking. The IQ data were used to divide the groups of hyper-responders and controls into three equal subgroups each and the eye tracking scores of the high and low IQ subgroups were compared. No hypothesis was put forward about the status of the average IQ groups.

It was found that the low-IQ-hyper-responsivity group, as hypothesised, exhibited poor eye tracking on all three indices (Table 1), while there was no difference between the eye tracking scores of the other three groups. That IQ itself did not relate to eye tracking was shown by the lack of difference between the eye-tracking scores in the low and high IQ control subgroups. There was no interaction between sex of subject, risk, and IQ on eye-tracking scores; thus the suggestion reviewed earlier, that the IQ-schizophrenia relationship was only to be found in male patients, was not supported by these data.

Thus, in a study which has as yet to reach a point where breakdowns occur in sufficient numbers to make analysis possible, an autonomic index of schizophrenia, moderated on the basis of IQ, has been shown to be related to an index, namely smooth-pursuit eye movement, a measure considered by Kraepelin to be an index of sustained attention and now thought to be a marker for schizophrenia. This provides some tentative support for the model suggested by Lehmann (1966) and put forword in the Introduction.

References

Andreasen NC (1982) Negative symptoms in schizophrenia. Arch Gen Psychiatry 39:784–788
Andreasen NC, Olsen S (1982) Negative v positive schizophrenia. Arch Gen Psychiatry 39:789–794

Andreasen NC, Nasrallah HA, Dunn V, Olson SC, Grove WM, Ehrhardt JC, Coffman JA, Crossett JHW (1986) Structural abnormalities in the frontal system in schizophrenia. A magnetic resonance imaging study. Arch Gen Psychiatry 43:136–144

Aylward E, Walker E, Bettes B (1984) Intelligence in schizophrenia: meta-analysis of the research. Schizophr Bull 10:430–459

Bartfai A, Levander SE, Nyback H, Berggen B-M, Schalling D (1985) Smooth pursuit eye tracking, neuropsychological test performance, and computed tomography in schizophrenia. Psychiatry Res 15:49–62

Bleuler E (1924) Textbook of psychiatry. Macmillan, New York

Chapman LJ, Edell WS, Chapman JP (1980). Physical anhedonia, perceptual aberration and psychosis proneness. Schizophr Bull 6:639–653

Claridge G (1972) The schizophrenias as nervous types. Br J Psychol 121:1–17

Crow TJ (1980) Molecular pathology of schizophrenia: more than one disease process? Br Med J 280:66–68

Diefendorff AR, Dodge R (1908) An experimental study of the ocular reactions of the insane from photographic records. Brain 31:451–489

Erlenmeyer-Kimling L, Marcuse Y, Cornblatt B, Friedman D, Rainer JD, Rutschmann J (1984a) The New York high-risk project. In: Watt NF, Anthony EJ (eds) Children at risk for schizophrenia. Cambridge University Press, Cambridge, pp 169–189

Erlenmeyer-Kimling L, Kestenbaum C, Bird H, Hilldoff U (1984b). Assessment of the New York high-risk project subjects in sample A who are now clinically deviant. In: Watt NF, Anthony EJ (eds) Children at risk for schizophrenia. Cambridge University Press, Cambridge, pp 227–239

Frith CD, Stevens M, Johnstone EC, Crow TJ (1979). Skin conductance responsivity during acute episodes of schizophrenia as a predictor of symptomatic improvement. Psychol Med 9:101–106

Garmezy N (1974) Children at risk: the search for the antecedents of schizophrenia. Part I. Conceptual models and research methods. Schizophr Bull 8:14–90

Goetz KL, van Kammen DP (1986) Computerized axial tomography scans and sub-types of schizophrenia. J Nerv Ment Dis 174:31–41

Griffith JJ, Mednick SA, Schulsinger F, Diderichsen B (1980) Verbal associative disturbances in children at high risk for schizophrenia. J Abnorm Psychol 89:125–131

Gruzelier JH, Venables PH (1972) Skin conductance orienting activity in a heterogeneous sample of schizophrenics. J Nerv Ment Dis 155:277–287

Gruzelier JH, Mednick SA, Schulsinger F (1979) Lateralised impairments in the WISC profiles of children at genetic risk for psychopathology. In: Gruzelier J, Flor-Henry P (eds) Hemisphere asymmetries of function in psychopathology. Elsevier/North Holland, Amsterdam, pp 105–110

Holzman PS, Proctor LR, Hughes DW (1973). Eye tracking patterns in schizophrenia. Science 181:179–181

Iacono WG (1985) Psychophysiological markers of psychopathology: a review. Can Psychol 26:96–112

Jones M (1973) IQ and fertility in schizophrenia. Br J Psychiatry 122:689–696

Jones M, Offord D (1975) Independent transmission of IQ and schizophrenia. Br J Psychiatry 126:185–190

Kety SS (1980) The syndrome of schizophrenia: unresolved questions and opportunities for research. Br J Psychiatry 136:421–436

Kimmel HD, Deboskey D (1978) Habituation and conditioning of the orienting reflex in intellectually gifted and average children. Physiol Psychol 6:377–380

Kraepelin E (1913) Dementia praecox and paraphrenia. Livingstone, Edinburgh

Lehmann H (1966) Pharmacotherapy of schizophrenia. In: Hoch P, Zubin J (eds) Psychopathology of schizophrenia. Grune and Stratton, New York, pp 120–133

Lipton RB, Levy DL, Holzman PS, Levin S (1983) Eye movement dysfunction in psychiatric patients. Schizophr Bull 9:13–32

Luchins DJ, Weinberger DR, Wyatt RJ (1982) Schizophrenia and cerebral asymmetry detected by computed tomography. Am J Psychiatry 139:753–757

McGhie A, Chapman J (1961) Disorders of attention and perception in early schizophrenia. Br J Med Psychol 34:103–110

McNeil TF, Kaij L (1978) Obstetric factors in the development of schizophrenia: complications in the births of preschizophrenics and in reproduction by schizophrenic parents. In: Wynne LC, Cromwell RL, Matthysse S (eds) The nature of schizophrenia. Wiley, New York, pp 401–429

Mednick SA, Schulsinger F (1968) Some pre-morbid characteristics related to breakdown in children with schizophrenic mothers. In: Rosenthal D, Kety SS (eds) The transmission of schizophrenia. Pergamon, New York

Mednick SA, Schulsinger F, Teasdale TW, Schulsinger H, Venables PH, Rock D (1978) Schizophrenia in high-risk children: Sex differences in pre-disposing factors. In: Serban G (ed) Cognitive defects in the development of mental illness. Brunner/Mazel, New York

Meehl PE (1962) Schizotaxia, schizotypy and schizophrenia. Am Psychol 17:827–838

Mostovsky DI (1970). The semantics of attention. In: Mostovsky DI (ed) Attention: contemporary theory and analysis. Appleton-Century-Crofts, New York, pp 9–24

Neisser U (1967) Cognitive psychology. Appleton-Century-Crofts, New York

Nuechterlein KH, Dawson ME (1984) Information processing and attentional functioning in the developmental course of schizophrenic disorders. Schizophr Bull 10:160–203

Reider RO, Broman SH, Rosenthal D (1977) The offspring of schizophrenics. II. Perinatal factors and IQ. Arch Gen Psychiatry 34:789–799

Reveley AM, Reveley MA, Clifford CA, Murray RM (1982) Cerebral ventricular size in twins discordant for schizophrenia. Lancet 1:540–541

Schulsinger F, Parnas J, Petersen ET, Schulsinger H, Teasdale T, Mednick SA, Moller L, Silverton L (1984) Cerebral ventricular size in the offspring of schizophrenic mothers. Arch Gen Psychiatry 41:602–606

Seidman LJ (1983) Schizophrenia and brain dysfunction: an integration of recent neurodiagnostic findings. Psychol Bull 94:195–238

Siever LJ, Coursey RD (1985) Biological markers for schizophrenia and the biological high risk approach. J Nerv Ment Dis 173:4–16

Siever LJ, Haier RJ, Coursey RD, Sostek AJ, Murphy DL, Holzman PS, Buchsbaum MS (1982) Smooth pursuit eye tracking impairment. Relation to other "markers" of schizophrenia and psychologic correlates. Arch Gen Psychiatry 39:1001–1005

Siever LJ, Coursey RD, Alterman IS, Buchsbaum MS, Murphy DL (1984) Impaired smooth pursuit eye movement: vulnerability marker for schizotypal personality disorder in a normal volunteer population. Am J Psychiatry 141:1560–1566

Simons RF, Katkin W (1985) Smooth pursuit eye movements in subjects reporting physical anhedonia and perceptual aberrations. Psychiatry Res 14:275–289

Sohlberg SC (1985) Personality and neuropsychological performance of high-risk children. Schizophr Bull 11:48–60

Sohlberg SS, Yaniv S (1985) Social adjustment and cognitive performance of high-risk children. Schizophr Bull 11:61–65

Venables PH (1964) Input dysfunction in schizophrenia. In: Maher B (ed) Progress in experimental personality research. Academic, New York, pp 1–41

Venables PH (1978) Psychophysiology and psychometrics. Psychophysiology 15:302–315

Venables PH (1984) Cerebral mechanisms, autonomic responsiveness and attention in schizophrenia. In: Spaulding WD, Cole JK (eds) Theories of schizophrenia and psychosis. University of Nebraska Press, Lincoln, pp 47–91

Venables PH (1986) Psychophysiology and psychiatry. In: Rosenberg, Schulsinger F, Strömgren E (eds) Psychiatry and its related disciplines – the next 25 years. World Psychiatric Copenhagen, Association, pp 79–96

Venables PH, Mitchell DA, Dalais JC (1987) Smooth pursuit eye movements in children psychophysiologically identified as at risk for schizophrenia. (in preparation)

Watt NF, Grubb TW, Erlenmeyer-Kimling L (1982) Social, emotional, and intellectual behaviour ot school among children at high risk for schizophrenia. J Consult Clin Psychol 50:171–181

Winters KC, Stone AA, Weintraub S, Neale JM (1981) Cognitive and attentional deficits in children vulnerable to psychopathology. J Abnorm Child Psychol 9:435–453

Wyatt RJ, Potkin SG, Murphy DL (1979) Platelet monoamine oxidase activity in schizophrenia: a review of the data. Am J Psychiatry 136:377–385

Psychological and Psychophysiological Models of Schizophrenia: Discussion

W. T. Carpenter, Jr.

The University of Heidelberg can be justly proud of its seminal contributions to psychiatry. No other center can match the fundamental contributions to concept and methodology relevant to the study of psychoses. This work has influenced nearly every aspect of my own work as a clinician investigator – work which I have been fortunate to share with so many of the International Pilot Study of Schizophrenia (IPSS) colleagues who have gathered in Heidelberg to celebrate your history. During the years that John Strauss and I worked so closely together (with the help of John Bartko and Lyman Wynne), it seemed that with every problem we addressed in schizophrenia, the essential questions, methods, and initial contributions emanated from Heidelberg. In personal terms, I can say that in Emil Kraepelin I experienced the raw power of descriptive psychopathology and classification. The fundamental distinction of two types of psychoses permitted the application of the disease construct and the power of explanatory analysis of form [1] to be applied in schizophrenia – an approach which still typifies the most promising efforts of today. Special reference to Kraepelin's description of the enduring personal attributes, such as weakening of the will, diminution of the drive for society and occupation, and destruction of the imaginative world, as the core clinical features of schizophrenia is merited. Today we find ourselves returning to these aspects of the schizophrenic process as the most suitable focus in the application of new technologies and methods. Progress in the classification of schizophrenia has been essentially the achievement of public and reliable criteria for case ascertainment. However, these are all too often based on superficial markers of the illness rather than on observation of the psychopathologic process that Kraepelin described in depth. I believe that John Strauss and Timothy Crow will agree that our present efforts to define the deficit, or type II, syndrome with negative symptom criteria is simply an appreciation of the power of Kraepelin's original description. Psychiatric methodology needs to recapture this core psychopathology if classification is to prove an adequate guide to the study of etiology, pathogenesis, and treatment.

Kurt Schneider demonstrated to the world the value of the practical, atheoretical, and public approach to defining disease classes – approaches that could be challenged and refined. Were this not the case, it would not have been possible for us to empirically evaluate the major tenets of Schneider's approach. We were able to suggest two major modifications. First, that first-rank symptoms, although discriminating of schizophrenia, were not sufficient to signify the presence

Maryland Psychiatric Research Center, P.O. Box 3235, Baltimore, MD 21228, USA of that disease in the absence of an organic psychosyndrome. First-rank symptoms are observed with substantial frequency in other psychotic conditions [2, 3]. Second, and more importantly, we were not able to confirm that a first-rank symptom definition of nuclear schizophrenia was associated with the deteriorating course and poor outcome anticipated if nuclear schizophrenia was comparable to Kraepelin's dementia praecox [4–6]. These findings, challenged by Wing and others [7, 8], but subsequently confirmed in a number of centers [9–18], have facilitated a modification in diagnostic criteria and prompted renewed interest in prognostic variables. This illustrates the progress for which the scientific method is intended. Schneider must have been proud that he had created a system which merited empirical evaluation and was subject to modification. The flexible system we derived from IPSS data was modeled on Schneider's approach [19–20].

Karl Japsers established psychopathology as a scientific discipline and articulated the scientific basis for the psychology of meaning. He stressed the distinction between causal explanation and meaningful connections. We would be far more generously informed about the "subjective world" and reactions of the schizophrenic patient if the tradition of intensive interpersonal treatment and study of these patients had been guided by phenomenology rather than by explanatory theory and therapeutic presentiments. Jaspers drew from the philosphic tradition of phenomenology and made it applicable in the proactive world of clinical medicine. He emphasized that a comprehensive appreciation of the inner experience of psychopathology would result in the description of psychopathologic manifestations, an understanding of its appearance in the context of the person's life story, and an appreciation of the reactions of the personality to the psychopathology. Modern workers transmuted Jaspers clinical phenomenology into a descriptive psychiatry content with the mere description of psychopathologic manifestations, emphasizing only those of some essential importance to differential diagnosis. Our field is presently correcting for the loss of Kraepelin's descriptive depth associated with definitions of schizophrenia so extensively based on expediency of assessment and reliability. I predict that we will soon find it necessary to reembrace comprehensive phenomenology as we appreciate the limited power of simple descriptive techniques. The everyday life of patient and clinician requires a phenomenologic approach. It is regretful that "modern" clinical research methods often prove inadequate to the complexities of this human disorder [21–23].

How do the above considerations relate to the three presentations which I have the privilege to discuss? First, Dr. Hemsley and Drs. Cohen and Borst are descriptive and phenomenologic in the finest sense. They describe the core features of chronic schizophrenia at the level of pschological processes. Psychological models are not offered to explain the origins of schizophrenia in an etiologic sense. Rather, they are used to define basic operations which, at the psychological level, may account for disease manifestations, especially deficit functioning as defined by Kraepelin. By elaborating these processes, psychological models developed and validated apart from schizophrenia can be introduced to generate specific hypotheses about schizophrenia. Dr. Hemsley and Drs. Cohen and Borst introduce theoretically modest, but clinically important, causal hypotheses. Modest, because they presently deal with proximal causation – the "how" of pathogenesis rather than the "why" of etiology. Clinically important, because Drs. Cohen and Borst can envision the role of psychological models in unraveling the interplay between positive and negative symptoms. They also propose that these models can address the meaning of confounding variables, such as premorbid adjustment and response to treatment. The clinical importance of Dr. Hemsley's model is made evident and reaches a high plane of description. He seeks to ascertain a cognitive dysfunction distinguishing of schizophrenia and, at the same time, capable of explaining the development of generalized dysfunction in schizophrenia. His approach is phenomenologic in that he attempts to ascertain the personal reaction to, and socioenvironmental ambience for, progression from fundamental dysfunction to the multiplicity of deficits observed in chronic schizophrenia. His reasoning follows that of Eugen Bleuler, but introduces models from social psychology of direct relevance to the study of development and course of illness. These models seem particularly relevant to psychosocially based therapeutics and rehabilitation. Dr. Hemsley's model also provides an inviting alternative to viewing schizophrenia as a clinical syndrome comprising several discrete disease entities. Distal etiology and initial perturbation could be homogeneous, with heterogeneity derived from the various pathogenic and adaptive processes which mark the individual's reaction to the presence of schizophrenia. While I favor the view of schizophrenia as a heterogeneous clinical syndrome rather than a disease entity with variable manifestations [24], I believe that Dr. Hemsley's position is heuristic and that his hypothesis merits full exploration.

Dr. Venables' contribution is quite different. His work depends more on psychological methods than on models, and he seeks to address etiology or distal causation. If smooth-pursuit eye movement is a latent trait of the genotype for schizophrenia, and low IQ combined with hyperresponsive electrodermal activity at age 3 marks risk for schizophrenia, then a major step forward in the reduction of heterogeneity of the clinical syndrome can be taken. The investigator can define a subset of interest for perinatal, genetic, season of birth, or other early risk factor studies. Dr. Venables' approach utilizes a disease construct and analysis of form that has proven so powerful in the natural sciences and in medicine [1]. It is a two-stage approach: first, identifying a group distinguishable from other groups (in this case a subset of high-risk children with low IQ) and then finding a significant correlation with important validating measures. The use of smooth-pursuit eye movement is an intriguing and well-defended putative marker of genetic risk for vulnerability to schizophrenia. If the electrodermal hyperresponsivity and low IQ correlate with other markers of manifestations of schizophrenia, the confluence of evidence may point in some rather discrete directions. Dr. Venables is taking the initial steps that would eventually lead to questions such as where in embryonic development could an insult give the observed array of dysfunction, or where the genes are that control aspects of development which might underlie the observed dysfunctions.

Dr. Venables' work illustrates one method of working from the general level clinical syndrome to identification of an interesting subgroup and the confirmation of the importance of that subgroup with a predictive relationship to a performance measure which may mark the latent structure for genetic vulnerability to schizophrenia. If confirmed, working at ever increasingly lower levels of abstraction, one would hope eventually to be guided to gene products and molecular genetics associated with vulnerability. Drs. Cohen and Borst raise another example which has the potential of moving investigative questions from the general level of symptom manifestation to the discrete level of molecular genetics. They refer briefly to what is my current favorite as an illustration of the interplay between phenomenology and disease construct, and the potential for obtaining data relevant to biologic contributions to etiology by carefully descending through the levels of functional abstraction of the human organism [25]. I refer to the dorsolateral prefrontal cortex (DLPFC) story [26]. Animal and human data support the view that functional impairments of this neuronal system cause behaviours strikingly similar to the observed deficits in chronic schizophrenic patients. Psychological challenge for performance in this system on a modified Wisconsin Card Sort can distinguish a group of schizophrenic patients from controls based on a differential pattern of regional blood flow in the area where functional anatomic correlation is hypothesized [27, 28]. A clinical observation is related to behavioral observations where anatomic location of impairment is known and neuronal networks subserving dysfunction can be hypothesized. Psychological models are essential for expressing the concept, organizing the methodology, testing hypotheses, analyzing data, and attributing meaning. This work, essentially at the level of phenomenology and psychological models, can be translated to the level of neuroanatomy [29–33]. Such functional anatomic hypotheses can guide the biochemical and histologic evaluation of postmortem brain tissue, as illustrated in the work of Dr. Beckmann and Dr. Reynolds. Biochemical and histopathologic findings, if shown to be involved in pathogenesis rather than a consequence of illness or artifact, can lead to more discrete hypotheses concerning the nature and timing of etiologic insult. If there are deviant patterns of cell migration – and Goldman Rakic has postulated that cells in layer 3 of the DLPFC are good candidates for histopathologic investigation [34] – developmental biology could provide a basis for postulating timing of insult or genetic basis for the observed histopathology. In this example, we see the multiple steps of scientific inquiry. Phenomenology defines what is wrong in schizophrenia. Models drawn from psychology may best operationalize a description of what is wrong and facilitate investigation. Observations and concepts from developmental neurobiology may provide a basis for understanding the "how" of symptom manifestation and disturbed function, and lead to hypotheses as to the "why". In the illustrations discussed, the "why" question is embedded at a low level of abstraction (i.e., molecular genetics and embryonic development), but the reasoning is similar in attempting to address "why" questions at higher levels of abstraction. Altered subjective experience can modify neuronal function and structure. Alterations in human subjective experience may be initiated at the biologic, psychological, or social level, and hypotheses from each level are legitimately put forward in an etiologic framework within the context of the biopsychosocial medical model [25, 35].

It has been my privilege to discuss three papers which document the role of psychological models and techniques in the study of schizophrenia, and to consider their position in the methodologic framework in which etiologic hypotheses can be articulated and tested. In the course of this colloquium, we will hear presentations dealing with other levels of abstraction. The richness of data, the complexity and subtlety of concepts, and the vigor of scientific work on schizophrenia is exciting. To hear examples of this work and discuss schizophrenia with colleagues in Heidelberg is a unique and inspiring experience.

References

1. McHugh PR, Slavney PR (1983) The perspectives of psychiatry. Johns Hopkins University Press, Baltimore
2. Carpenter WT, Strauss JS, Muleh S (1973) Are there pathognomonic symptoms in schizophrenia? An empiric investigation of Kurt Schneider's first rank symptoms. Arch Gen Psychiatry 28:847–852
3. Carpenter WT, Strauss JS (1974) Cross-cultural evaluation of Schneider's first rank symptoms of schizophrenia: a report from the International Pilot Study of Schizophrenia. Am J Psychiatry 131:682–687
4. Strauss JS, Carpenter WT (1974) Characteristic symptoms and outcome in schizophrenia. Arch Gen Psychiatry 30:429–434
5. Hawk AB, Carpenter WT, Strauss JS (1975) Diagnostic criteria and 5-year outcome in schizophrenia: a report from the International Pilot Study of Schizophrenia. Arch Gen Psychiatry 32:343–356
6. Carpenter WT, Bartko JJ, Strauss JS, Hawk AB (1978) Signs and symptoms as predictors of outcome: a report from the International Pilot Study of Schizophrenia. Am J Psychiatry 135:940–945
7. Wing JK, Nixon J (1975) Discriminating symptoms in schizophrenia: a report from the International Pilot Study of Schizophrenia. Arch Gen Psychiatry 30:853–859
8. Chandrasena R, Rodriso A (1979) Schneider's first rank symptoms: their prevalence and diagnostic implications in an Asian population. Br J Psychiatry 135:348–351
9. McCabe MS, Stromgren E (1975) Reactive psychoses: a family study. Arch Gen Psychiatry 32:447–454
10. Newmark CS, Falk R, Johns N, Boren R, Forehand R (1976) Comparing traditional clinical procedures with four systems to diagnose schizophrenia. J Abnorm Psychology 85:66–72
11. Baron J (1977) Linkage between an X-chromosome marker (Deutan color blindness) and bipolar affective illness. Arch Gen Psychiatry 34:721–725
12. Silverstein ML, Harrow M (1978) First-rank symptoms in the postacute schizophrenic: a follow-up study. Am J Psychiatry 135:1481–1486
13. Koehler K, Seminario I (1979) Research diagnosable schizo-affective disorder in Schneiderian first rank schizophrenia. Acta Psychiatr Scand 60:347–354
14. Silverstein ML, Harrow M (1981) Schneiderian first-rank symptoms in schizophrenia. Arch Gen Psychiatry 38:288–293
15. Andreasen NC, Akiskal HS (1983) The specificity of Bleulerian and Schneiderian symptoms: a critical reevaluation. Psychiatr Clin North Am 6:41–54
16. Armbruster B, Gross G, Huber G (1983) Long-term prognosis and course of schizo-affective, schizophreniform, and cycloid psychoses. Psychiatr Clin (Basel) 156–168
17. Ndetei DM, Sinsh A (1983) Schneider's first rank symptoms of schizophrenia in Kenyan patients. Acta Psychiatr Scand 67:148–153
18. Marneros A, Deister A, Diederich N, Rohde A (1984) Schizophrenia suspecta. Eur Arch Psychiatry Neurol Sci 234:207–211
19. Carpenter WT, Strauss JS, Bartko JJ (1973) A flexible system for the identification of schizophrenia: a report from the International Pilot Study of Schizophrenia. Science 1275–1278
20. Carpenter WT, Bartko JJ, Strauss JS (1980) A postscript on the 12-point flexible system for the diagnosis of schizophrenia: a report from the International Pilot Study of Schizophrenia. Psychiatry Res 3:357–364
21. Carpenter WT, Heinrichs DW, Hanlon TE (1981) Methodologic standards for treatment outcome research in schizophrenia. Am J Psychiatry 138:465–471

22. Carpenter WT, Strauss JS; Bartko JJ (1981) Beyond diagnosis: the phenomenology of schizophrenia. Am J Psychiatry 138:948–953
23. Strauss JS; Hafez H (1981) Clinical questions and "real" research. Am J Psychiatry 138:1592–1597
24. Carpenter WT, Heinrichs DW, Wagman AMI (1985) on the heterogeneity of schizophrenia. In: Alpert M (ed) Controversies in schizophrenia. Guilford Press, New York, pp 25–37
25. Engel GL (1977) The need for a new medical model: a challenge for biomedicine. Science 196:129–136
26. Weinberger DR (1985) Clinical-neuropathological correlations in schizophrenia: theoretical implications. In: Controversies in schizophrenia. Alpert, M (ed), New York: Guilford Press, pp 92–106
27. Berman KF, Zec RF, Weinberger DR (1986) Physiologic dysfunction of dorsolateral prefrontal cortex in schizophrenia. II. Role of neuroleptic treatment, attention, and mental effort. Arch Gen Psychiatry 43:125–135
28. Weinberger DR, Berman KF, Zec RF (1986) Physiological dysfunction of dorsolateral prefrontal cortex in schizophrenia. I. Regional cerebral blood flow evidence. Arch Gen Psychiatry 43:114–124
29. Nauta WJH (1971) The problem of the frontal lobe: a reinterpretation. J Psychiatr Res 8:167–187
30. Fuster J (1980) The prefrontal cortex. Raven, New York
31. Luria AR (1980) Higher cortical functions in man. Basic, New York
32. Goldman-Rakic PS, Isseroff A, Schwartz ML, Bugbee NM (1983) The neurobiology of cognitive development. In: Mussen P (ed) Handbook of child psychology: biology and infancy development. Wiley, New York, pp 281–344
33. Goldman-Rakic PS; Selemon LKD, Schwartz MD (1984) Dual pathways connecting the dorsolateral prefrontal cortex with the hippocampal formation and parahippocampal cortex in the rhesus monkey. Neuroscience 12:719–743
34. Goldman-Rakic PS (1987) Anatomy of the primate prefrontal cortex and the regulation of behavior by representational knowledge. In: Handbook of Physiology, Blum F, Mountcastle V (eds), Am Physiological Society, NY, Vol 5, 373–417
35. Strauss JS, Carpenter WT (1981) Schizophrenia. Plenum, New York

Part V
Biological Hypotheses on Schizophrenia

The Dopamine Hypothesis of Schizophrenia 20 Years Later

A. CARLSSON

Introduction

The view that dopamine is involved in the pathogenesis of psychosis, and thus perhaps also of schizophrenia, is supported by indirect, pharmacological evidence. Excessive release of dopamine, induced by e.g. amphetamine or L-DOPA, may lead to or worsen psychotic conditions of various types, e.g. delirious states, mania and paranoid, schizophrenia-like disturbances. Conversely, psychotic conditions can be dramatically alleviated by drugs counteracting dopaminergic neurotransmission in various ways, e.g. by blocking dopamine receptors by means of phenothiazines, thiaxanthenes, butyrophenones etc., by blocking the mechanism for neurotransmitter storage by means of reserpine, or – in combination with subthreshold doses of, for example, phenothiazines – by inhibiting the synthesis of dopamine by means of alpha-methyltyrosine (for review see Carlsson 1978, 1983 a).

When discussing the "dopamine hypothesis of schizophrenia", one should remember, however, that the drugs referred to in this context do not act specifically on schizophrenia but on other psychotic conditions as well. Thus it would perhaps be more appropriate to speak of a dopamine hypothesis of psychosis. Moreover, not all cases of schizophrenia respond to drug therapy; especially patients lacking "positive" psychotic symptomatology (i.e. delusions, hallucinations, formal thought disorder and bizarre behaviour) tend to be poor responders (see Wyatt 1985).

Finally, none of the drugs referred to are entirely specific dopaminergic agents. Especially, their actions on noradrenaline and adrenaline are often similar to those on dopamine. Besides the catecholamines, a number of other neurotransmitters are also influenced by several antipsychotic agents, and this may contribute to the therapeutic response (for review see Carlsson 1980). In general, however, the antipsychotic action tends to be best correlated to the action on dopamine.

During the past 20 years basic brain research and clinical neuropsychiatric research, have undergone dramatic development. In fact, the discovery of the modern psychotropic drugs in the 1950s and the subsequent elucidation of their mode of action provided a strong impetus to this development, which among other things led to the introduction of the concept of chemical transmission into CNS research (see Carlsson 1987).

Department of Pharmacology, University of Göteborg, P.O. Box 33031, 400 33 Göteborg, Sweden

A detailed review of the evidence for a disturbance of neurotransmitter function in schizophrenia is beyond the scope of the present chapter. Suffice it to say that so far no neurotransmitter changes have been shown beyond doubt to be primarily involved in schizophrenia (for review see Wyatt 1985). It should be realized, however, that the assessment of complex neutrotransmitter functions is very difficult, especially in the clinic or in postmortem studies. Thus, a primary disturbance in dopamine neurotransmission in schizophrenia cannot be excluded at the present time. Supersensitivity of dopamine receptors has been proposed to be responsible for schizophrenic symptomatology. In postmortem studies an increased density of dopamine receptors has been recorded in certain brain areas in cases of schizophrenia and taken as evidence for receptor supersensitivity; however, opinions differ as to whether this change is primary or is secondary to previous therapy with antipsychotic agents. Even if the latter interpretation proves correct, a change in dopamine receptor function in schizophrenia cannot be excluded. The in vitro binding studies thus far performed post mortem in cases of schizophrenia give information about affinity and receptor density but tell us nothing about the responsiveness of the receptor complex. This is true also of the interesting in vivo binding studies now underway in schizophrenic patients, using positron emission tomography. At least one such study tends to support the view that striatal dopamine receptors have an increased density even in non-treated schizophrenic patients (Wong et al. 1986).

The study of dopamine and other neurotransmitters in relation to psychosis has perhaps in the past placed too much emphasis on purely biochemical aspects. The brain is not primarily a chemical factory but rather an extremely complex cell hierarchy, whose function depends on the appropriate communication between billions of nerve cells. Absence, undue presence or inadequacy of synaptic contacts may have devastating functional consequences and yet be very difficult to detect.

The discovery that dopamine is involved in mechanisms underlying severe mental disturbances sprang out of drug research. Pharmacological tools probably still have much to offer in this area. However, for a precise assessment of the role of dopamine in the pathogenesis of psychosis and schizophrenia, more specific pharmacological tools than those available today would be desirable. Such tools may well be sought among dopamine receptor agonists and antagonists with selectivity for special receptor subpopulations.

Dopamine Receptors: A Heterogeneous Family?

Receptors occupy a strategic position as instruments in the chemical transfer of information between cells. Despite considerable technical advances, permitting measurement, for example, of receptor-ligand affinities and of the number of receptor molecules in tissues, important aspects of receptor function are not yet available for precise biochemical assessment. This is true, for instance, of the conformational change believed to be responsible for the activation of the receptor and the subsequent information transfer. To study this phenomenon we have to rely upon secondary biochemical events or classical pharmacology.

Autoreceptors are peculiar in that only one cell appears to be engaged: these receptors are sensitive to the nerve cell's own neurotransmitter. By recording the neurotransmitter concentration in the surrounding extracellular space, they form part of a primitive feedback system, by means of which a nerve cell can monitor the synthesis and release of its own transmitter. Autoreceptors seem to have somewhat different functions in different parts of the nerve cell: stimulation of autoreceptors in the somatodendritic region will inhibit the generation of nerve impulses, whereas in the terminal region it will inhibit the synthesis and reduce the amount of neurotransmitter released by the nerve impulse. Conversely, blockade of autoreceptors will lead to increased firing, release and synthesis of neurotransmitter (for review see Carlsson 1976; Usdin et al. 1984).

From a theoretical standpoint the manipulation of neuronal activity via autoreceptors is an attractive alternative by virtue of its "physiological" character: such manipulation appears to be essentially confined to the release mediated by the nerve impulse (via changes in firing rate, transmitter synthesis and the amount released by each nerve impulse). Moreover, the release of any cotransmitter existing in the neuron (see Donohue et al. 1985) is likely to be influenced in the same way as the main neurotransmitter.

As a sign of postsynaptic dopamine-receptor stimulation, classical dopamine-receptor agonists, such as apomorphine, cause increased motor activity and stereotyped behaviour in experimental animals. These actions are blocked by dopamine-receptor antagonists such as chlorpromazine and haloperidol. However, in lower dosage agonists cause a "paradoxical" response, i.e. the animals appear sedated, with inhibition of spontaneous locomotor activity. Even this paradoxical response can be antagonized by dopamine-receptor antagonists, given in low dosage. It is now generally agreed that this response is due to preferential stimulation of dopamine autorecptors by low doses of apomorphine. Thus, dopamine agonists already in low dosage cause inhibition of firing by dopaminergic nigral neurons as well as of the synthesis and release of dopamine, actions which can all be blocked by dopamine-receptor antagonists (for review see Usdin et al. 1984).

However, dopamine-receptor agonists with a much higher selectivity for autoreceptors than apomorphine have been discovered (for review see Clark et al. 1985 a). For example, the compound B-HT 920 is capable of causing all the paradoxical actions of apomorphine referred to above, but in contrast to apomorphine this agent does not cause the behavioural stimulation characteristic of apomorphine in higher dosage (Andén et al. 1983). In fact, B-HT 920 appears to possess but slight affinity for the postsynaptic dopamine receptors, while being a potent agonist on dopamine autoreceptors controlling, for example, dopamine synthesis, with an intrinsic activity of about 80% B-HT 920 also shows agonist activity on alpha-2-adrenergic receptors, albeit in somewhat higher dosage, leading to a clonidine-like action on blood pressure, etc.

Remarkably enough, there also exist compounds acting as agonists on dopamine autoreceptors but as antagonists on the classical postsynaptic dopamine receptors. Members of this group of agents are (–)-3-PPP [=(–)-3-(3-hydroxyphenyl)-*N-n*-propylpiperidine], (–)-HW 165 [=*trans*-4aS, 10bS-7-hydroxy-1,2,3,4,4a,5,6,10b-octahydrobenzo(*f*)quinoline] and terguride (=*trans*-dihydrolisuride, see Kehr 1984). These agents cause inhibition of spontaneous locomotor activity like apomorphine, but in contrast to the latter they are devoid of stimulatory properties even in very high dosage. Rather, they are capable of blocking such actions of apomorphine and other directly or indirectly acting dopamine agonistis, including amphetamine.

Examination of this group of agents reveals some further, interesting properties. These drugs do not possess full intrinsic activity on the dopamine autoreceptors, controlling, for example, the synthesis of dopamine; the activity ranges between about 70% for HW 165 and (–)-3-PPP and somewhat less than 50% for terguride (Hjorth et al. 1986). On the lactotroph dopamine receptors (causing inhibition of prolactin secretion in the anterior pituitary gland) they act as agonists, apparently with somewhat less then 100% intrinsic activity. They stimulate the emetic dopamine receptors, but seem to be milder than apomorphine in this respect. Most remarkably, on denervated, supersensitive postsynaptic dopamine receptors they act as full agonists, which is in contrast to their apparently pure antagonist action on normosensitive postsynaptic dopamine receptors (Arnt and Hyttel 1984).

In an attempt to explain these variations in receptor responsiveness we have advanced the hypothesis that dopamine receptors (or a component of the "receptor complex") are capable of undergoing long-term adaptive conformational changes in response to a varying agonist occupancy (Carlsson 1983 b). As a consequence, a high occupancy will lead to a low receptor responsiveness and thus to the recognition of a compound such as (–)-3-PPP as a pure antagonist – this would correspond to the condition of the normal postsynaptic receptors – whereas a low occupancy, as after denervation, will lead to a high responsiveness, enabling the receptor to recognize (–)-3-PPP as a full agonist. Autoreceptors, lactotroph receptors and emetic receptors are suggested to have an intermediate degree of physiological agonist occupancy; they would thus recognize (–)-3-PPP as a partial agonist (for review see Clark et al. 1985 b). A varying receptor responsiveness can also be expressed in terms of "spare receptors", that is, a high responsiveness corresponds to a high percentage of spare receptors and vice versa (see Meller et al. 1986).

Subclassification of Dopamine Receptors: Functional Significance

Various subclassifications of dopamine receptors have been proposed, mainly on the basis of in vitro data. The most widely accepted subclassification is the D1, D2 dichotomy proposed by Kebabian and Calne (1979). D1 receptors are characterized by their coupling to adenylate cyclase, which is activated by D1 receptor agonists. D2 receptors are identified by means of in vitro binding techniques, e.g. by displacement of tritiated spiroperidol. Activation of D2 receptors may have an inhibitory influence on adenylate cyclase (Stoof and Kebabian 1981), a finding which is at present difficult to reconcile with some of the functional in vivo data, which rather indicate a cooperation between the two types of receptor (see below). D1 receptors can also be recognized by means of binding techniques, using appropriate ligands.

At first, all major dopaminergic functions appeared to be mediated via D2 sites, and the functional significance of D1 sites remained obscure. With the advent of selective D1 agonists and antagonists this picture has changed. It appears that the two receptor subtypes have to cooperate in order to elicit the classical dopaminergic behavioural response. Thus, both selective D1 and D2 antagonists inhibit motor functions and induce catalepsy. Moreover, the hyperactivity and stereotypies induced by selective D2 agonists can be blocked either by a D1 or a D2 antagonist. Reserpine or alpha-methyltyrosine antagonizes the stimulatory effects of D2 agonists, perhaps by reducing the availability of endogenous dopamine at D1 sites (review by Arnt 1986; Barone et al. 1986; Waddington 1986; Robertson and Robertson 1986; Goldstein et al. 1986). The most commonly used D1 agonist, i.e. SKF 38393, does not induce the full-blown dopaminergic behavioural syndrome; increased grooming is the most striking behavioural response to this agent. However, SKF 38393 is capable of potentiating the action of D2 agonists under certain conditions.

Following degeneration of dopaminergic pathways by means of 6-hydroxy-dopamine and development of receptor supersensitivity, the coupling between D1 and D2 receptors is no longer evident. Dopamine-receptor stimulation, showing up, for example, as rotation following a unilateral lesion, can now be produced by either a D1 or a D2 agonist and can be blocked only by a D1 and D2 antagonist respectively (see Arnt 1986). The molecular mechanism underlying the coupling between the two receptor types under normal conditions and their uncoupling following denervation is not yet understood.

Interestingly, none of the apparently extrasynaptic or non-synaptic dopamine receptors appear to exhibit the coupling between D1 and D2 receptors; they seem to be essentially of the D2 type. This is true of the autoreceptors, the lactotroph receptors and the emetic receptors. The thermolytic dopamine receptors appear to occupy an intermediate position.

Thus, the normosensitive postsynaptic dopamine receptors are apparently unique among the various members of the dopamine receptor family. Whether the coupling between D1 and D2 receptors represents another aspect of the adaptive properties of dopamine receptors, remains to be clarified. In any event, the presence or absence of D1 receptor function in the different dopaminergic sites opens up interesting, as yet unexplored possibilities for selective dopamine receptor manipulation.

Beyond the Receptors

The interaction between the receptors and other molecules in the cell membrane is now being intensively investigated. Receptor molecules appear to interact with other receptor molecules as well as with molecules serving other functions in the information transfer. Thus, the responsiveness of the "receptor complex" depends not only on the conformational properties of the receptor molecule itself but also on very complicated interactions, which appear to add up to a virtual "sociology" of the cell-membrane molecules.

Beyond the receptors the responses of cells seem to be largely mediated via protein phosphorylation. Among neuronal phosphoproteins, DARPP-32 appears to be of special interest in the present context, since it seems to be specific for neurons receiving dopaminergic innervation. The state of phosphorylation of this protein is increased by dopamine and cAMP analogues (see Nestler and Greengard 1984).

Recently interest has also been focussed on phosphodiesterase isoenzymes, which can apparently be selectively inhibited. One such inhibitor, rolipram, appears to have antidepressant properties. Although its major activities appear to be located outside dopaminergic neurons, it is interesting to note that rolipram is capable of stimulating dopamine synthesis, even beyond the threefold stimulation induced by gamma-butyrolactone pretreatment. On the other hand, the utilization of dopamine, studied following pretreatment with alpha-methyltyrosine, is retarded by rolipram. These data support the view that cAMP exerts a stimulatory influence on tyrosine hydroxylase in dopaminergic nerve terminals, perhaps via phosphorylation of the enzyme (Kehr et al. 1985). If this is so, the inhibitory influence of dopamine autoreceptor stimulation on the synthesis of dopamine might be due to inhibition of adenylate cyclase; this is in agreement with in vitro data showing an inhibitory action of dopamine D2 agonists on this enzyme (see above).

Opening of calcium channels is generally believed to form an important aspect of cell stimulation. Data are as yet meagre as to the effect of calcium-channel blockers on neuronal activity. Nimodipine, a calcium-channel blocker of dihydropyridine type, has, however, been found to cause moderate inhibition of the synthesis and metabolism of dopamine in mouse brain in vivo (Pileblad and Carlsson 1986). Earlier it had been proposed, on the basis of in vitro binding data, that certain antipsychotic drugs, besides blocking dopamine receptors, might act by blocking calcium channels; examples of such agents are pimozide and thioridazine (Murphy et al. 1983; Gould et al. 1983). Whether calcium channel manipulation will become a useful principle in psychopharmacology remains to be seen.

Possible Utility of Dopamine-Receptor Agonists in Schizophrenia Research and Treatment

Since all the major groups of antipsychotic agents possess antidopaminergic properties, a dopamine autoreceptor agonist would be expected to be antipsychotic. Clinical trials on selective dopamine autoreceptor agonists in schizophrenia are now underway. No definite results are available so far. Apomorphine appears to act as a sedative in man and has been reported to alleviate psychotic symptoms in schizophrenia and schizoaffective conditions (Corsini et al. 1977 a, b; Smith et al. 1977; Tamminga et al. 1983; see, however, Angrist et al. 1980; Ferrier et al. 1984). Apomorphine is not an adequate drug for more extensive clinical trials, in view of its poor pharmacokinetic properties.

The available animal data indicate that $(-)$-3-PPP and HW 165 possess rather high selectivity for dopamine receptors. They might thus prove useful as clinical probes for the examination of dopaminergic mechanisms. In this context terguride and B-HT 920 have the drawback of acting rather strongly on alpha-adrenergic receptors as well. From a therapeutic point of view, however, additional inhibition of adrenergic systems may not only cause side effects but also lead to increased antipsychotic efficacy.

The hypothesis has been advanced that dopamine receptors in the brains of schizophrenic patients are supersensitive (see Introduction). The evidence in favour of this hypothesis is not conclusive, however. If such supersensitivity exists and is similar in nature to denervation supersensitivity, one might expect an unfavourable effect of (−)-3-PPP and other agents with mixed agonist-antagonist properties in schizophrenia (cf above). These agents might thus serve as probes for testing the supersensitivity hypothesis. In this context some observations on the action of terguride in Parkinson's disease are of interest. In preliminary trials this agent has been found to possess anti-Parkinson activity (Corsini et al. 1984; Brücke et al. 1985; Agnoli, personal communication). This would be in line with expectation, given the fact that the extensive loss of dopamine neurons in Parkinson's disease should result in denervation supersensitivity of dopamine receptors.

The fact that apomorphine appears capable of alleviating rather than worsening psychotic symptoms, at least in a subgroup of schizophrenic patients, does not favour the hypothesis of supersensitivity of postsynaptic dopamine receptors in this disorder. Needless to say, however, more adequate tools are necessary to settle this point.

If we can disregard dopamine-receptor supersensitivity of the type developing after denervation, (−)-3-PPP and other dopamine-receptor agonists with mixed agonist-antagonist properties should have beneficial effects in psychotic conditions such as schizophrenia. The fact that the agonist effects of these agents on dopamine autoreceptors are combined with an antagonist action on postsynaptic dopamine receptors, at least in higher dosage, should contribute to the therapeutic response. In this context it is interesting to note that subchronic treatment of rats with dopamine-receptor-blocking neuroleptics, in contrast to reserpine and denervation by local 6-hydroxydopamine treatment, did not result in an increased intrinsic activity of (−)-3-PPP on dopamine receptors in the forebrain (Arnt and Hyttel 1984). (Possibly the interruption of dopaminergic transmission was less complete during the treatment with dopamine-receptor-blocking agents.) Previous treatment with neuroleptics should thus not represent an obstacle in trials with (−)-3-PPP and similar agents. *Simultaneous* treatment with autoreceptor agonists and neuroleptics may, however, prevent the action of the former agents.

Why Is (−)-3-PPP Devoid of Cataleptogenic Activity?

Dopamine-autoreceptor agonists inhibit motor activity, though less completely than the classical neuroleptics. Unlike the latter, they are devoid of cataleptogenic activity. As a possible explanation, dopamine-autoreceptor stimulation may be unable to overcome the negative feedback mechanism activated by the inhibition of dopamine neurons within the nigrostriatal system: in the limbic dopamine system this feedback seems to be less well developed, and thus the dopamine-autoreceptor stimulation within this system may lead to inhibition of motor activity. However, (−)-3-PPP and the other dopaminergic mixed agonist-antagonists act as almost pure antagonists on postsynaptic normosensitive dopamine receptors; for example, they antagonize apomorphine and amphetamine and are unable to counteract the akinesia and catalepsy induced by reserpine. They might thus be expected to be cataleptogenic per se. In fact, terguride is cataleptogenic, whereas (−)-3-PPP and HW 165 are devoid of such activity. In in vivo binding experiments, (−)-3-PPP has been found capable of displacing a dopamine-receptor agonist (N-dipropyl-5,6-ADTN) from striatal dopamine-receptor sites in the rat brain almost as efficiently as haloperidol (Carlsson and Löfberg 1985). A possible explanation for the lack of cataleptogenic activity of (−)-3-PPP is that there exists a small population of dopamine receptors in the striatum, which remain uninhibited even after large doses of (−)-3-PPP (perhaps they are even stimulated) and which have to be blocked to induce catalepsy. Further work is obviously needed to clarify this issue.

In this context the "jerks" induced by dopamine-receptor agonists in reserpine-treated rats are of interest. Such jerks are induced not only by classical dopamine agonists in low dosage but also by B-HT 920, which is unable to induce the classical dopaminergic behavioural syndrome (Grabowska-Andén and Andén 1983), and by (−)-3-PPP and HW 165, which act as antagonists on the intact postsynaptic dopamine receptors. The jerks are blocked by haloperidol and by other neuroleptics and may thus be due to stimulation of a population of D2 receptors. Apparently this population, although postsynaptically located, has autoreceptor-like properties. The possibility that blockade of this receptor population is required for cataleptogenic action can at this time only be a matter for speculation.

The D1 receptor antagonist SCH 23390 is capable of blocking both D1 and D2 agonist actions. Interestingly, (−)-3-PPP has been found capable of antagonizing dopamine-induced activation of adenylate cyclase in vitro, albeit in relatively high concentration (for references see Clark et al. 1985a). Thus, the possibility exists that (−)-3-PPP does indeed stimulate postsynaptic D2 receptors, but that the behavioural expression of this effect is antagonized by a D1 antagonistic action.

In any event, the absence of cataleptogenic properties is promising, since catalepsy is a good predictor of extrapyramidal side effects. (−)-3-PPP and similar agents are thus not likely to cause extrapyramidal side effects, including tardive dyskinesia. On the other hand, it remains to be seen whether the relatively mild antidopaminergic profile of these agents is sufficient to induce a powerful antipsychotic response. Clinical trials in the not too distant future will hopefully answer this question.

The Mechanism Underlying Tardive Dyskinesia

For many years tardive dyskinesias were believed to be caused by dopamine-receptor supersensitivity. More recently, evidence for a deficiency in the striatonigral GABA pathway, possibly induced by chronic understimulation of this pathway as a consequence of dopamine-receptor blockade by neuroleptics, has been reported to occur in experimental tardive dyskinesia and proposed to be the underlying cause of this disturbance (Gunne and Häggström 1985).

Both the (−)- and the (+)-forms for 3-PPP have been found to counteract dyskinesia in Cebus monkeys, without inducing the dystonias characteristic of classical neuroleptics (Häggström et al. 1983). The (−)-form was found to be more efficient than its enantiomeric twin; it may be recalled that following induction of denervation supersensitivity, (−)-3-PPP acts as a full agonist. The observations with 3-PPP enantiomers are thus not in favour of receptor supersensitivity as a cause of tardive dyskinesia; it should, however, be recalled that following subchronic treatment with receptor-blocking neuroleptics the postsynaptic dopamine receptors were still unable to recognize (−)-3-PPP as an agonist.

Selective Dopamine-Autoreceptor Antagonists: A Novel class of Agents with Therapeutic Potential in Neuropsychiatry

The classical neuroleptics are capable of blocking both dopamine autoreceptors and postsynaptic receptors, although some preference of certain neuroleptics for one or the other type of receptor has been suggested. In an extensive study on the structure-activity relationships within a series of aminotetralins we have recently discovered a number of dopamine-receptor antagonists with selectivity for dopamine autoreceptors; over a wide dosage range these agents are capable of blocking dopamine autoreceptors without showing any clear-cut sign of postsynaptic dopamine-receptor blockade (Svensson et al. 1986). This was especially true of the compound   N-n-propyl-cis-(+)-(1S,2R)-5-methoxy-1-methyl-2-aminotetralin. The behavioural result in rats is a stimulation of motor activity, accompanied by but mild stereotypies (occasional sniffings). Biochemically the blockade of dopamine autoreceptors shows up, for instance, as a pronounced stimulation of dopamine synthesis.

These novel, selective dopamine-autoreceptor antagonists open up a new and comparably "physiological" method for stimulation of dopaminergic mechanisms; blockade of the dopamine autoreceptors causes the dopamine neurons to increase their physiological activity. Previous agents have acted further downstream, at least partly beyond the control of the nerve impulses, i.e. by inducing excessive synthesis followed by release (L-DOPA) or by a more direct action on release (amphetamine) of dopamine, or by stimulating postsynaptic dopamine receptors directly (apomorphine). The new class of dopaminergic agents will thus probably prove useful in the study of dopamine functions. Moreover, they may have therapeutic utility.

The selective dopamine-autoreceptor antagonists seem to have advantages over the previous types of dopaminergic agents in causing a lower risk of excessive dopamine-receptor stimulation: in larger dosage they have a moderate blocking action on the postsynaptic dopamine receptors, implying a built-in self-limitation of their stimulating action.

In schizophrenia research the new class of dopaminergic agents may help to answer some important questions. The administration of such a drug to a schizophrenic patient with positive symptomatology would be expected to worsen the condition. However, a schizophrenic patient with negative rather than positive symptomatology might be improved: it has been proposed that such patients actually suffer from a deficiency in dopamine (see Wyatt 1985). The new class of agents might serve as probes to test this hypothesis.

An Evolutionary Perspective

Perhaps we generally tend to look upon the human brain as a wonder of perfection. However, this organ has undergone a dramatic evolution, which is perhaps still ongoing. Has sufficient time been allowed for a "final polish" (see Dobzhansky 1962)?

When a new, favourable mechanism evolves, a variety of complications may arise. Previous mechanisms serving a similar purpose, though less well, may become redundant. The evolutionary process does not seem to be very efficient in getting rid of redundancies, which may thus occur abundantly in a rapidly evolving organ such as the brain. The slowness of redundancy elimination may explain the existence of a number of "mismatches" between neurotransmitters and receptors. In some instances there is morphological evidence that transmitters and their receptors do not show the appropriate regional coexistence (Kuhar 1986; Schultzberg and Hökfelt 1986), while in other cases pharmacological evidence is suggestive of a mismatch; for example, specific receptor antagonists, such as adrenergic beta-blockers and opiate-receptor antagonists, cause but subtle changes in brain function of doubtful significance, even though they have obviously been given in doses sufficient to block receptors in the CNS. Such observations raise doubt as to the occurrence of adequate amounts of endogenous agonists at receptor sites.

However, the evolutionary process may face more serious problems. Newly evolving structures/mechanisms, though more powerful than the pre-existing ones, may lead to imbalances, which may explain why the rapidly evolving central nervous system plays such a prominent role in human pathology. For example, the functional integration between the evolving neocortex (and neostriatum) and older subcortical structures should be a complicated and vulnerable process. Judging by its position and connections the neostriatum (including the nucleus accumbens and related structures) plays a key role in this integration. This, in turn, may account for the critical role of dopaminergic systems in the pathogenesis of psychoses.

Conclusions

Dopaminergic neurons appear to possess a highly complex intrinsic control machinery. They play an important modulatory role in a variety of mental, motor, endocrine and autonomic functions. As newcomers in the evolutionary process the dopmainergic systems appear to be involved in the functional integration of recent cortical with older subcortical structures.

The "dopamine hypothesis of schizophrenia", in its original, simplistic version, may have to be amended, taking into account our present knowledge of the complexity of dopaminergic mechanisms. Psychosis may not necessarily be due to dopaminergic hyperfunction; it may well be caused by a more subtle dopaminergic dysfunction, or by an imbalance between dopaminergic and other systems.

Recent progress in dopamine research has opened up new approaches for manipulation of dopaminergic mechanisms and may form the basis for novel therapeutic approaches.

References

Andén NE, Golembiowska-Nikitin K, Nilsson H, Ros E, Thornström U (1983) Effects of two azepine derivatives (B-HT 920 and B-HT 933) on pre- and postsynaptic dopamine receptors in the brain. Acta Pharm Suec [Suppl] 1:154–164

Angrist B, Rotrosen J, Gershon S (1980) Responses to apomorphine, amphetamine and neuroleptics in schizophrenic subjects. Psychopharmacology (Berlin) 67:31–38

Arnt J (1987) Behavioral studies of dopamine receptors: evidence for regional selectivity and receptor multiplicity. In: Creese I, Fraser C (eds) Structure and function of dopamine receptors. Liss, New York (in press)

Arnt J, Hyttel J (1984) Postsynaptic dopamine agonistic effects of 3-PPP enantiomers revealed by bilateral 6-hydroxy-dopamine lesions and by chronic reserpine treatment in rats. J Neural Transm 60:205–223

Barone P, Davis TA, Braun AR, Chase TN (1986) Dopaminergic mechanisms and motor function: characterization of D-1 and D-2 dopamine receptor interactions. Eur J Pharmacol 123:109–114

Brücke T, Danielzyk W, Simanyi M, Sofic E, Riederer P (1987) Terguride: Partial dopamine agonist in the treatment of Parkinson's disease. In: Yahr MD, Bergmann KJ (eds) Advances in neurology, vol 45. Raven Press, New York, pp 573–577

Carlsson A (1976) Dopaminergic autoreceptors. In: Almgren O, Carlsson A, Engel J (eds) Chemical tools in catecholamine research, vol II. North-Holland, Amsterdam, pp 219–224

Carlsson A (1978) Antipsychotic drugs, neurotransmitters and schizophrenia. Am J Psychiatry 135(2):164–173

Carlsson A (1980) Psychopharmacology: basic aspects. In: Kisker KP, Meyer J-E, Müller C, Strömgren E (eds) Psychiatrie der Gegenwart, vol I/2 2nd edn. Springer, Berlin Heidelberg New York, pp 197–242

Carlsson A (1983a) Dopamine receptor agonists; intrinsic activity vs state of the receptor. J Neurol Transm 57:309–315

Carlsson A (1983b) Antipsychotic agents: elucidation of their mode of action. In: Parnham MJ, Bruinvels J (eds) Psycho- and neuropharmacology. Elsevier, Amsterdam, pp 197–206 (Discoveries in pharmacology, vol 1)

Carlsson A (1987) Perspectives on the discovery of central monoaminergic neurotransmission. Ann Rev Neurosci 10:19–40

Carlsson A, Löfberg L (1985) In vivo displacement by 3-PPP enantiomers of N,N-dipropyl-5,6-ADTN from dopamine-receptor binding sites in rat striatum. J Neural Transm 64:173–185

Clark D, Hjorth S, Carlsson A (1985a) Dopamine receptor agonists: mechanisms underlying autoreceptor selectivity. I. Review of the evidence. J Neural Transm 62:1–52

Clark D, Hjorth S, Carlsson A (1985b) Dopamine receptor agonists: mechanisms underlying autoreceptor selectivity. II. Theoretical considerations. J Neural Transm 62:171–207

Corsini GU, Del Zompo M, Manconi S, Cianchetti C, Mangoni A, Gessa GL (1977a) Sedative, hypnotic and antipsychotic effects of low doses of apomorphine in man. Adv Biochem Psychopharmacol 16:645–648

Corsini GU, Del Zompo M, Piccardi MP, Onali PL, Mangoni A (1977 b) Evidence for dopamine receptors in the human brain mediating sedation and sleep. Life Sci 20:1613–1618

Corsini GU, Horowsky R, Rainer E, Del Zompo M (1984) Treatment of Parkinson's disease with a dopamine partial agonist. Clin Neuropharmacol 7 [Suppl 1]:950–951

Dobzhansky T (1962) Mankind evolving. Yale University Press, New Haven

Donohue TL, Millington WR, Handelmann GE, Contreras PC, Chronwall BM (1985) On the 50th anniversary of Dale's law. Multiple neurotransmitter neurons. Trends Pharmacol Sci 6:305–308

Ferrier IN, Johnstone EC, Crow TJ (1984) Clinical effects of apomorphine in schizophrenia. Br J Psychiatry 144:341–348

Goldstein M, Lieberman A, Meller E (1986) Reply. Trends Pharmacol Sci 7:225

Gould RJ, Murphy KMM, Reynolds IJ, Snyder SH (1983) Antischizophrenic drugs of the diphenylbutylpiperidine type act as calcium channel antagonists. Proc Natl Acad Sci USA 80:5122–5125

Grabowska-Andén M, Andén N-E (1983) Stimulation of postsynaptic DA_2 receptors produces jerks in reserpine-treated rats. J Pharm Pharmacol 35:543–545

Gunne LM, Häggström J-M (1985) Pathophysiology of tardive dyskinesia. In: Casey DE, Chase TN, Christensen AV, Gerlach J (eds) Dyskinesia: research and treatment. Springer, Berlin Heidelberg New York Tokyo, pp 191–193

Häggström J-E, Gunne LM, Carlsson A, Wikström H (1983) Antidyskinetic action of 3-PPP, a selective dopaminergic autoreceptor agonist, in Cebus monkeys with persistent neuroleptic-induced dyskinesias. J Neural Transm 58:135–142

Hjorth S, Svensson K, Carlsson A, Wikström H, Andersson B (1986) Central dopaminergic properties of HW-165 and its enantiomers; trans-octahydrobenzo(f)quinoline congeners of 3-PPP. Naunyn Schmiedebergs Arch Pharmacol 333:205–218

Kebabian JW, Calne DB (1979) Multiple receptors for dopamine. Nature 277:93–96

Kehr W (1984) Transdihydrolisuride, a partial dopamine receptor antagonist: effects on monoamine metabolism. Eur J Pharmacol 97:111–119

Kehr W, Debus G, Neumeister R (1985) Effects of rolipram, a novel antidepressant, on monoamine metabolism in rat brain. J Neural Transm 63:1–12

Kuhar MJ (1986) The mismatch problem in receptor mapping studies. Trends in Neurosci 8:190–191

Meller E, Helmer-Matyjek E, Bohmaker K, Adler CH, Friedhoff AJ, Goldstein M (1986) Receptor reserve at striatal dopamine autoreceptors: implications for selectivity of dopamine agonists. Eur J Pharmacol 123:311–314

Murphy KMM, Gould RJ, Larger BL, Snyder SH (1983) A unitary mechanism of calcium antagonist drug action. Proc Natl Acad Sci USA 80:860–864

Nestler EJ, Greengard P (1984) Protein phosphorylation in nervous tissue. In: Usdin E, Carlsson A, Dahlström A, Engel J (eds) Catecholamines. Part A: Basic and peripheral mechanisms. Liss, New York, pp 9–22

Pileblad E, Carlsson A (1986) In vivo effects of the Ca^{2+}-antagonist nimodipine on dopamine metabolism in mouse brain. J Neural Transm 66:171–187

Robertson HA, Robertson GS (1986) The antiparkinson action of bromocriptine in combination with levo-dopa. Trends Pharmacol Sci 7:224–225

Schultzberg M, Hökfelt T (1986) The mismatch problem in receptor autoradiography and the coexistence of multiple messengers. Trends Neurosci 9:109–110

Smith RC, Tamminga CA, Davis JM (1977) Effect of apomorphine on schizophrenic symptoms. J Neural Transm 40:171–176

Stoof JC, Kebabian JW (1981) Opposing roles for D-1 and D-2 dopamine receptors in efflux of cyclic AMP from rat neostriatum. Nature 294:366–368

Svensson K, Carlsson A, Johansson AM, Arvidsson L-E, Nilsson JLG (1986) A homologous series of N-alkylated cis-(+)-(1S,2R)-5-methoxy-1-methyl-2-aminotetralins: central DA receptor antagonists showing profiles ranging from classical antagonism to selectivity for autoreceptors. J Neural Transm 65:29–38

Tamminga CA, Gotts MD, Miller MR (1983) N-propyl-norapomorphine in the treatment of schizophrenia. Acta Pharm Suec [Suppl] 2:153–158

Usdin E, Carlsson A, Dahlström A, Engel J (eds) (1984) Catecholamines. Part B: neuropharmacology and central nervous system theoretical aspects. Liss, New York, pp 3–46

Waddington JL (1986) Bromocriptine, selective D-2 dopaminergic receptor agonists and D-1 dopaminergic tone. Trends Pharmacol Sci 7:223–224

Wong DF, Wagner, HN, Jr, Tune LE, Dannals RF, Pearlson GD, Links JM, Tamminga CA, Brousolle EP, Ravert HT, Wilson AA, Toung JKT, Malat J, Williams JA, O'Tuama LA, Snyder SH, Kuhar MJ, Gjedde A (1986) Positron emission tomography reveals elevated D2 dopamine receptors in drug-naive schizophrenics. Science 234:1558–1563

Wyatt RJ (1985) The dopamine hypothesis: variations on a theme. In: Cancro R, Dean SR (eds) Research in the schizophrenic disorders. The Stanley R. Dean Award Lectures, Vol II. Spectrum, New York, pp 225–247

Postmortem Neurochemical Studies in Schizophrenia

G. P. REYNOLDS

The search for a biochemical abnormality in schizophrenia has classically involved the analysis of body fluids. Although we have presupposed the dysfunction to occur within the brain, practical limitations have, in the past, necessitated
biochemical studies outside the brain. Nevertheless, changes within the brain can
be reflected in the periphery; for example, gross variations in central noradrenaline function can be monitored by measuring plasma and urine metabolites of
noradrenaline. However, the reverse is not necessarily true: changes in these peripheral markers may be due to other events, such as changes in diet or activity,
that would mask any possible variation due to brain function. In addition, these
parameters reflect the biochemistry of the whole brain, within which the subtle
changes due to malfunction of a specific brain region may be lost. Nevertheless,
neurochemical investigations still remain a major approach to the identification
of possible malfunctioning neuronal systems in these diseases. Thus, the recent
increasing use of brain tissue taken post mortem has provided a more specific
means of testing the various neurochemical hypotheses. The most rigorously investigated of these is that the symptoms of schizophrenia derive from a hyperactivity of dopamine neurotransmission. Few conclusive results in support of this
have been reported, although the "dopamine hypothesis" continues to attract the
most interest. This reflects the fact that despite the paucity of evidence for its primary importance in schizophrenia, dopamine does seem to play a central role in
antipsychotic drug action. The neuroleptic drugs effective in schizophrenia have
many neurochemical actions, but of these it is the ability to bind to dopamine D2
receptors, thereby blocking doppaminergic activity, which best correlates with
clinical antipsychotic dosage (Seeman et al. 1976).

In investigating the dopamine hypothesis of schizophrenia much effort has
been expended on measuring concentrations of the transmitter, its metabolites
and associated enzymes in postmortem brain tissue, albeit with few conclusive results. Recently attention has focused on a more consistently reported finding.
First reported in 1978 (Owen et al. 1978) there has since been substantial confirmation that dopamine D2 receptors are increased above control levels in several
brain regions of schizophrenic patients (Mackay et al. 1982; Reynolds et al. 1981;
Seeman et al. 1984).

However, animal studies have shown us that dopamine receptors increase in
number after chronic treatment with neuroleptics (Clow et al. 1980), a treatment

Department of Pathology, University of Nottingham Medical School, Queen's Medical Centre,
Nottingham NG7 2UH, United Kingdom

which most schizophrenics inevitably receive. Thus it seems quite possible that medication is responsible for these findings. The original publications refute this, identifying one or two unmedicated patients who also have increased numbers of D2 receptors. On the other hand, there are now several reports showing no increase in small groups of unmedicated schizophrenics (Mackay et al. 1982; Reynolds et al. 1981).

Using a gamma-emitting ligand for the dopamine receptors, a very recent study has attempted to assess relative dopamine receptor number in vivo in schizophrenic patients (Crawley et al. 1986). The patients studied were all free of neuroleptic drugs for at least 6 months and only a very small (11%) increase in the relative number of receptors was observed in the schizophrenic group. Thus, despite substantial efforts to solve this problem, by, for example, assessing receptor numbers in non-schizophrenic neuroleptic-treated groups of patients, it remains a point of considerable controversy whether the increase in receptors in postmortem brain tissue bears any relation to the disease process per se.

It is notable that these and other investigations into the possible involvement of dopamine systems in schizophrenia using postmortem brain tissue have concentrated on the heavily dopamine-innvervated striatum. However, the terminal regions of the mesolimbic and mesocortical dopaminergic pathways have received little attention in spite of their being particularly implicated in psychosis and antipsychotic drug action (Stevens 1973; Hornykiewicz 1978).

These pathways have their cell bodies in the ventral tegmental area (VTA) and recurrent electrical stimulation ("kindling") of the VTA has been found to elicit behavioural changes in the cat which are reminiscent of psychotic behaviour (Stevens and Livermore 1978). These are reported to be dependent on intact dopaminergic function. One limbic structure in the medial temporal lobe, the amygdala, receives dopaminergic innervation, and kindling of the amygdala, too, can evoke a range of behavioural changes (Post et al. 1982). Thus the amygdala would certainly seem to be a better candidate for the pathophysiological site in schizophrenia than the striatal regions.

Recent postmortem studies have identified a highly specific neurochemical abnormality in schizophrenia (Reynolds 1983). Table 1 summarises these results and indicates an increase in amygdala dopamine in the schizophrenic group; an increase which is not reflected by any changes in a range of markers for other neurotransmitter systems. Most notable, however, is the lateralisation of the dopamine increase; it is restricted to the left hemisphere.

This dopamine asymmetry in the amygdala in schizophrenia is also regionally specific; no such asymmetry was found in the caudate nucleus, nucleus accumbens, hippocampus or frontal cortex in this study.

We have recently replicated the finding of asymmetry in the amygdala with a new series of postmortem brain tissues from schizophrenics and age-matched controls. In this somewhat larger series a laterality of homovanillic acid (HVA), the major dopamine metabolite, is also apparent, again with an increase in the left amygdala in the schizophrenic group (Table 2). Other regions did not show this effect. HVA in frontal cortex in schizophrenia did appear to be increased.

These results are interesting in the light of a previous report which identified increases in HVA in cortical regions, but not in the putamen or nucleus ac-

Table 1. Concentrations of neurotransmitters and metabolites in the amygdala. (Data from Reynolds et al. 1983, 1986)

	Controls		Schizophrenics	
	Left	Right	Left	Right
Dopamine	57.3	50.8	96.1[a]	55.7
Noradrenaline	54.2	63.2	58.7	61.8
5-HT	243	206	270	251
GABA	20.7	18.7	19.8	17.6
HVA	948	986	1102	1028
5-H1AA	1118	1080	1046	1041

Geometric means in ng/g tissue (except GABA, µmol/g protein) from 16 schizophrenia and 14 control brains.
[a] $p < 0.001$ vs right side by paired t-test of logarithmically transformed data.

Table 2. Dopamine and homovanillic acid (HVA) concentrations in brain tissue

	Dopamine		HVA	
	Left	Right	Left	Right
Amygdala				
Schizophrenics	87.4[a]	53.4	1168[b]	1023
Controls	36.4	31.1	863	869
Caudate				
Schizophrenics	2399	2143	3960	3845
Controls	2118	2341	4060	4155
Temporal cortex				
Schizophrenics	3.2	3.9	173	180
Controls	3.8	5.3	154	178
Frontal cortex				
Schizophrenics	0.44	0.62	94.2	98.3
Controls	0.46	0.27	73.2	73.8

Geometric means in ng/g tissue from 19 schizophrenic and 11 control brains.
[a] $p < 0.01$ vs control L and schizophrenic R; [b] $p < 0.01$ vs schizophrenic R.

cumbens, of postmortem brain tissue from neuroleptic-treated schizophrenic patients (Bacopoulos et al. 1979). Patients not receiving antipsychotic treatment had HVA concentrations in the control range. These results are very similar to those obtained in animal experiments in which a tolerance to the effects of antipsychotic drugs on HVA concentrations develops in subcortical, but not cortical regions (Bacopoulos et al. 1978).

Since many of the schizophrenic patients studied will inevitably have received neuroleptic treatment, it seems probable that some of the changes we observed are an effect of that treatment. This raises the question of whether the amygdala asymmetry is possibly also a result of prior drug treatment. While no neurochemical asymmetry deriving from psychiatric medication has so far been identified, a laterality of the effects of dopamine infused into the rat amygdala has recently been described in which hyperactivity is dependent on the laterality of both the amygdala perfused and the turning preference of the animal studied (Bradbury et al. 1985).

Other indications of lateral asymmetries have also been found (reviewed in Reynolds 1983). Left-right differences in dopamine concentrations can be found normally in the cortex and basal ganglia of rat brain. Notable is the increase in contralateral dopamine in rats trained to turn in one direction which presumably reflects a change in dopaminergic activity. Of particular importance to an understanding of the effects of neuroleptic drugs is the observation that D2 receptors are lateralised in the rat brain, this asymmetry differing between striatal and limbic structures (Schneider et al. 1982). Along with the observations on response to amygdala dopamine infusion, these reports provide evidence for functional asymmetries of both nigrostriatal and mesolimbic dopamine systems, thereby providing a mechanism for an asymmetric response to a bilateral influence such as neuroleptic drug administration. Whether the dopamine asymmetry is an effect of drug treatment remains to be found. However, it does provide the first neurochemical evidence in support of a left temporal lobe disorder in schizophrenia.

This hypothesis, originally proposed by Flor-Henry (1969), derives from the association of schizophreniform psychosis with left-sided temporal lobe epilepsy, an observation which has had strong support from a recent study (Perez et al. 1985). In addition, a wide range of psychological and neurophysiological observations, including studies of skin conductance and evoked potentials wave, implicated a left hemisphere disorder in schizophrenia (reviewed by Gruzelier 1981; Newlin et al. 1981).

There is also a fast-increasing body of evidence which indicates the presence of anatomical abnormalities of the brain in schizophrenia. Certainly some of these, employing imaging techniques, have pointed to asymmetric structural changes. Morphological study of post-mortem brain tissue has supported the suggestion of atrophic changes in schizophrenia in temporal/limbic regions (Bogerts et al. 1985) and particularly in the parahippocampal gyrus, this latter effect being significantly greater in the left hemisphere (Brown et al. 1986).

It is difficult to integrate all these various observations. Clearly several different aetiological factors may contribute to a collection of diseases described as schizophrenia. Developmental effects such as perinatal injury or viral infection have been proposed; subsequent neuronal loss could perhpas result in a relative increase in dopamine function in the amygdala, if only via a selective atrophy of another neuronal system. Whether the mechanism responsible for the dopaminergic asymmetry is physiological or pharmacological, it is certainly an observation which deserves further investigation.

References

Bacopoulos NG, Bustos G, Redmond DE, Baulu J, Roth RH (1978) Regional sensitivity of primate brain dopaminergic neurons to haloperidol: alterations following chronic treatment. Brain Res 157:396–401

Bacopoulos NC, Spokes EG, Bird ED, Roth RH (1979) Antipsychotic drug action in schizophrenic patients: effects on cortical dopamine metabolism after long-term treatment. Science 205:1405–1407

Bogerts B, Meertz E, Schonfeldt-Bausch R (1985) Basal ganglia and limbic system pathology in schizophrenia: a morphometric study. Arch Gen Psychiatry 42:784–791

Bradbury AJ, Costall B, Domeney AM, Naylor RJ (1985) Laterality of dopamine function and neuroleptic action in the amygdala in the rat. Neuropharmacology 24:1163–1170

Brown R, Colter N, Corsellis JAN, Crow TJ, Frith CD, Jagoe R, Johnstone EC, Marsh L (1986) Postmortem evidence of structural brain changes in schizophrenia. Arch Gen Psychiatry 43:36–42

Clow A, Theodorow A, Jenner P, Marsden CD (1980) Changes in rat striatal dopamine turnover and receptor activity during one year's neuroleptic administration. Eur J Pharmacol 63:135–144

Crawley JCW, Crow TJ, Johnstone EC, Oldland SRD, Owen F, Owens DGC, Poulter M, Smith T, Veall N, Zanelli GD (1986) Dopamine D2 receptors in schizophrenia studied in vivo. Lancet 11:224–225

Flor-Henry P (1969) Psychosis and temporal lobe epilepsy: a controlled investigation. Epilepsie 10:363–395

Gruzelier JH (1981) Cerebral laterality and psychopathology: fact and fiction. Psychol Med 113:219–227

Hornykiewicz O (1978) Psychopharmacological implications of dopamine and dopamine antagonists. Neurosci 3:773–783

Mackay AVP, Iversen LL, Rossor M, Spokes E, Bird E, Arregui A, Creese I, Snyder SH (1982) Increased brain dopamine and dopamine receptors in schizophrenia. Arch Gen Psychiatry 39:991–997

Newlin DB, Carpenter B, Golden CJ (1981) Hemispheric asymmetries in schizophrenia. Biol Psychiatry 16:561–582

Owen F, Crow TJ, Poulter M, Cross AJ, Longden A, Riley GJ (1978) Increased dopamine-receptor sensitivity in schizophrenia. Lancet 11:223–225

Perez MM, Trimble MR, Murray NMF, Rieder R (1985) Epileptic psychosis: an evaluation of PSE profiles. Br J Psychiatry 146:155–163

Post RM, Unde TW, Ballenger JC, Bunney WE (1982) Carbamazepine, temporal lobe epilepsy and manic-depressive illness. Adv Biol Psychiatry 8:117–156

Reynolds GP (1983) Increased concentrations and lateral asymmetry of amygdala dopamine in schizophrenia. Nature 305:527–529

Reynolds GP (1986) Amygdala dopamine asymmetry in schizophrenia. In: Woodruff GN, Poat JA, Roberts PJ (eds) Dopaminergic systems and their regulation. Macmillan, London, p 285

Reynolds GP, Riederer P, Jellinger K, Gabriel E (1981) Dopamine receptors and schizophrenia: the neuroleptic drug problem. Neuropharmacology 20:1319–1320

Schneider LH, Murphy RB, Coons EE (1982) Lateralisation of striatal dopamine (D2) receptors in normal rats. Neurosci Lett 33:281–284

Seeman P, Lee T, Chau-Wong M, Wong K (1976) Antipsychotic drug doses and neuroleptic/ dopamine receptors. Nature 261:717–719

Seeman P, Ulpian C, Bergeron C, Riederer P, Jellinger K, Gabriel E, Reynolds GP, Tourtellotte WW (1984) Bimodal distribution of dopamine receptor densities in brains of schizophrenia. Science 225:728–731

Stevens JR (1973) An anatomy of schizophrenia? Arch Gen Psychiatry 29:177–189

Stevens JR, Livermore A (1978) Kindling of the mesolimbic dopamine systems. Animal model of psychosis. Neurology 28:36–46

Biochemical and Neuropathological Indices for the Aetiology of Schizophrenia

H. Beckmann[1], W. F. Gattaz[2], and H. Jakob[3]

Cerebrospinal Fluid Studies

Neurochemical investigations of the cerebrospinal fluid (CSF) are frequently used as an indirect approach to the evaluation of the neuronal activity in the brain. A large number of CSF studies of the concentrations of substances presumably related to the central neuronal activity in schizophrenia have been published, but results are in part still controversial (van Kammen et al. 1986). This might stem from the possibility that a functional abnormality in schizophrenia is not localised to one isolated neurotransmitter system but rather is involved in the interrelationship among the different systems in the brain.

To investigate the interrelationship among the major neurotransmitter systems in schizophrenia as well as the possible effects of neuroleptic drugs on them, we concomitantly determined the concentrations of several substances in the CSF of schizophrenic patients (off and on neuroleptics) and healthy controls.

Patients and Methods

The study involved 28 paranoid schizophrenic patients (all males, mean age 30.6 ± 8.0 years) and 16 controls (14 males and 2 females, mean age 35.0 ± 15.7 years). Patients were diagnosed according to the Research Diagnostic Criteria (Spitzer et al. 1978). Two experienced psychiatrists independently evaluated the patients' psychological state by means of the Brief Psychiatric Rating Scale (BPRS). Fifteen patients were under treatment with neuroleptic drugs (butyrophenones and phenothiazines) for at least 3 weeks (mean dose $\pm$ SD in chlorpromazine equivalents $= 585 \pm 755$ mg/day). Thirteen patients did not take any drugs for a period of at least 4 weeks prior to the study. Controls were subjects with nonspecific neurological symptomatology (headaches, dizziness, etc.) in whom a lumbar puncture was necessary for diagnostic purposes. They were not under drug treatment at the time of the lumbar puncture. CSF was obtained by lumbar puncture between 9 and 10 a.m. The biochemical determinations were performed blind to the origin of each sample.

[1] Department of Psychiatry, University of Würzburg, Füchsleinstr. 15, 8700 Würzburg, Federal Republic of Germany
[2] Central Institute of Mental Health, P.O. Box 5970, 6800 Mannheim, Federal Republic of Germany
[3] Am Götzenberg 8, 6900 Heidelberg, Federal Republic of Germany

Noradrenalin and MHPG

Noradrenalin (NA) and its major metabolite 3-methoxy-4-hydroxyphenylglycol (MHPG) have been reported to be increased in the CSF of schizophrenic patients and in the brains of deceased schizophrenics (Gomes et al. 1980; Farley et al. 1978). It has been postulated that an increased noradrenergic activity could play a significant role in the etiology of the disease. We determined the CSF concentrations of NA and MHPG, its major metabolite in the brain (Gattaz et al. 1982; Gattaz et al. 1983 a).

No significant difference in the NA concentration was found between patients not receiving neuroleptics and controls (Table 1). Conversely, patients under neuroleptic therapy showed significantly higher CSF concentrations of NA than controls ($P<0.01$). Further significant differences could be detected in the CSF concentrations of MHPG among patients receiving and those not receiving neuroleptics and controls. This finding does not simply support the hypothesis of a disturbed noradrenergic function in schizohrenia per se. It indicates further that neuroleptic treatment might enhance the concentrations of NA in the CSF. Findings of increased NA in the CSF and brain areas of deceased schizophrenics, as described in the literature, could be due to the chronic intake of neuroleptic drugs.

Table 1. Concentrations of 17 substances in the cerebrospinal fluid of 28 schizophrenic patients (13 off drugs and 15 on drugs) and 16 controls. Mean ± SD (median)

	Controls	Patients on drugs	Patients off drugs	
Glutamate	18.9± 5.6 (19.4)	25.2± 5.8 (26.6)[a]	20.5± 4.0 (19.4)	(nmol/m
Dopamine	207.0±263.0 (119.0)	524.0±549.0 (286.0)[a]	200.0±124.0 (151.0)	(pg/ml)
Noradrenaline	133.0± 37.0 (124.0)	210.0± 73.0 (224.0)[a]	163.0± 44.0 (148.0)	(pg/ml)
Adrenaline	159.0± 85.0 (85.0)	325.0±246.0 (330.0)[a]	225.0±118.0 (230.0)	(pg/ml)
HVA	33.9± 18.1 (18.1)	39.0± 15.1 (39.6)	37.3± 20.2 (32.9)	(ng/ml)
MHPG	16.2± 4.9 (16.7)	14.6± 3.4 (14.4)	17.8± 4.8 (18.7)	(ng/ml)
HIAA	15.3± 4.4 (16.3)	9.9± 3.7 (8.6)[a]	11.8± 4.6 (11.3)[a]	(ng/ml)
PAA (free)	22.2± 11.8 (21.2)	14.5± 10.4 (12.8)	11.5± 5.7 (10.8)[a]	(ng/ml)
PAA (conj.)	23.6± 20.8 (23.6)	14.8± 7.8 (13.8)	20.4± 19.8 (18.2)	(ng/ml)
Cyclic AMP	15.2± 4.2 (14.5)	11.3± 4.3 (9.2)[a]	10.4± 9.4 (7.5)[a]	(pmol/m
Cyclic GMP	4.0± 1.2 (4.2)	2.8± 1.2 (2.6)[a]	2.6± 0.9 (2.5)[a]	(pmol/m
Prolactin	4.8± 2.7 (5.0)	7.1± 2.6 (6.2)[a]	4.2± 2.0 (4.3)	(nmol/l
Cortisol	14.0± 9.0 (11.8)	19.8± 15.1 (12.8)[a]	8.3± 7.1 (5.1)	(nmol/l
Calcium	2.0± 0.4 (2.1)	2.1± 0.3 (2.3)	2.3± 0.2 (2.3)	(mEq/l)
Magnesium	2.0± 0.3 (2.2)	2.0± 0.4 (2.2)	2.2± 0.1 (2.3)	(mEq/l)
Zinc	2.4± 0.4 (2.4)	2.8± 0.9 (2.9)	2.6± 0.4 (2.6)	(mEq/l)
Oxytocin	7.5± 4.9 (6.7)	13.4± 6.1 (13.0)[a]	10.0± 4.1 (9.3)	(pg/ml)

HVA, homovanillic acid; *MHPG*, 3-methoxy-4-hydroxyphenylglycol; *HIAA*, hydroxyindole-acetic acid; *AMP*, adenosine 5'-monophosphate; *GMP*, guanosine 3',5'-monophosphate; *PAA*, phenylacetic acid.
[a] Significant differences from controls.

Dopamine, Homovanillic Acid and Prolactin

We determined the CSF concentrations of dopamine (DA) its major metabolite homovanillic acid (HVA) and of prolactin. No significant differences in DA concentration were found between patients not receiving neuroleptics and controls (Table 1). Patients on neuroleptics had significantly higher DA than controls ($P<0.001$) and patients not receiving neuroleptics ($P<0.01$). No significant differences in HVA concentration were found among the subgroups.

These results are not in favour of the hypothesis of an increased DA turnover in schizophrenic patients. On the other hand the finding of increased DA concentrations in patients on neuroleptics is in line with animal experiments and could provide a rationale for at least part of the reports on increased DA concentrations in the brains of deceased schizophrenic patients. In addition, our finding of normal concentrations of prolactin in schizophrenics without drugs indicates that a hyperdopaminergic state in schizophrenia, so far as it exists, does not affect the tuberoinfundibular dopaminergic pathway.

In conclusion, our results from the determinations of DA, HVA and prolactin do not simply support the hypothesis of an altered DA turnover in schizophrenia. The possibility that a hyperdopaminergic function in this diseases is caused by an increase in the number of DA receptors or an enhanced DA receptor sensitivity has been investigated by other authors with inconclusive results (Reynolds 1985).

Functional Balance Between the Cholinergic and Dopaminergic Function?

A functional relationship between the cholinergic and the dopaminergic system has been suggested (Janowsky et al. 1973). The short half-life of acetylcholine (ACH) in body fluids makes it awkward to measure the concentrations of this transmitter in the CSF. One way out of this difficulty may be to determine the concentrations of cyclic guanosine 3'5'-monophosphate (cGMP), which has been shown to reflect to some extent central cholinergic activity (Bloom 1976).

The CSF concentrations of cGMP were significantly reduced in the subgroup of patients not receiving neuroleptics as compared to controls ($P<0.01$) (Gattaz et al. 1983 b). In the group of patients under neuroleptic therapy, this difference was just below the level of significance ($P=0.04$, Table 1). The finding of reduced cGMP could suggest a reduced cholinergic activity in these patients. Thus, even given a normal dopaminergic activity in schizophrenia, a reduced cholinergic activity would result in a relative hyperfunction of the dopaminergic system. In this context, the tendency shown by neuroleptics to increase cGMP concentrations observed in our and other studies could be understood as a restoration of the cholinergic-dopaminergic balance through cholinergic stimulation and dopaminergic blockade.

5-HIAA

Schizophrenic patients showed lower concentrations of 5-hydroxyindole acetic acid (5-HIAA) than controls ($P < 0.005$). No differences were found in the levels of the metabolite between patients with and without neuroleptics (Table 1). The changes correlated positively with the items "grandiosity" ($P < 0.05$) and hallucinatory behaviour ($P < 0.01$) from the score "thought disturbances". Our finding of reduced 5-HIAA in schizophrenic patients is in agreement with some investigations but not with others (Gattaz et al. 1982). The possibility that our results reflect a decrease in synthesis of serotonin is supported by the findings of Winblad et al. (1979) of diminished levels of this amine in brain tissues of deceased schizophrenics.

Vasopressin and Oxytocin

Vasopressin and oxytocin seem to be involved in the process of learning and memory in animals and probably also in man (Ader and de Wied 1972; Walter et al. 1978). They appear to have opposite effects in that vasopressin improves memory processes and oxytocin produces amnesic affects.

There were no significant differences in vasopressin concentrations between schizophrenics and controls (Beckmann et al. 1985). No influence of neuroleptic treatment on vasopressin concentrations was detected (Table 1). In contrast, concentrations of oxytocin were increased in all schizophrenic patients and were higher in those receiving neuroleptic treatment. In addition, oxytocin concentrations increased after 3 weeks' neuroleptic treatment. Drug-induced increase of oxytocin concentrations may be of significance in the clinically observed amnesic syndromes sometimes occurring in schizophrenics treated chronically with neuroleptic drugs.

Angiotensin-Converting Enzyme

Angiotensin-converting enzyme (ACE) was present in the CSF of paranoid schizophrenic patients and psychiatrically healthy controls. Both schizophrenics under neuroleptic treatment and those drug free had low cerebrospinal enzyme activity when compared with controls (Table 1). No correlation existed with the scores of the BPRS (Beckmann et al. 1984). In addition to angiotensin II formation, ACE is involved in the metabolism of other neuropeptides, notable bradykinin and opioid peptides (Soffer 1976). Thus, alterations in ACE activity may represent abnormalities in neuropeptide metabolism other than angiotensin II. It is important to note that the central source (s) of CSF ACE has not been determined. The enzyme could have originated from the choroid plexus or, at least in part, from brain areas rich in enzyme activity. ACE is low in the substantia nigra in schizophrenics (Arregui et al. 1979), but this area as well as the caudate nucleus, in the rat, are devoid of angiotensin II receptors, implicating neuropeptides other than angiotensin II in these alterations. The nigrostriatal pathway contains opioid peptides, including enkephalins (Yang et al. 1979). Since ACE is one of the enzymes involved in enkephalin metabolism, our results could also represent an alteration in central enkephalin metabolism in schizophrenia. In addition, an increased concentration of bradykinin may be another sequela of low central ACE activity. However, clarification of these relationships requires additional studies.

Evaluation of 17 CSF Parameters Through Multidimensional Scaling

We hypothesise that the simultaneous evaluation of all variables together should provide more information than each of them taken alone could. This assumption may be evaluated by obtaining a two-dimensional representation through multidemensional scaling (MDS) of the subjects represented in a high-dimensional space of 17 biochemical parameters (Table 1). These statistical methods have been described in detail elsewhere (Gasser and Möcks 1983). Briefly, in order to make the 17 biochemical parameters comparable, they were standardized for all subjects such that the standard deviation with respect to the control group became 1. The full data set can be regarded as a cloud of points consisting of the 44 subjects in the 17-dimensional parameter space. MDS seeks a two-dimensional

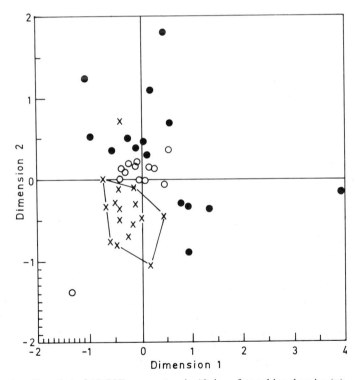

Fig. 1. Multidimensional scaling plot of 17 CSF parameters in 13 drug-free schizophrenics (o), 15 schizophrenics on drugs (●) and 16 controls (x)

representation of this 17-dimensional cloud of points while retaining as far as possible the distance between subjects. The MDS algorithm is based on the ranking of the distances, and this lowers the influence of an aberrant value in some dimension. To characterise the normative region occupied by the control group (1-p) convex hulls were introduced. A convex hull of a two-dimensional cloud of points is the region defined by its extreme points and the straight lines between them.

Figure 1 provides the two-dimensional representation of all 44 subjects for 17 CSF biochemical parameters obtained by MDS. The normative region, defined by the 15/16 convex hull of the control group, is quite compact and does not contain a single schizophrenic subject. There is one subject of the control group lying amid schizophrenic subjects. With one exception, all untreated schizophrenic patients are close together, separated from the normative region with respect to dimension 2. The group of schizophrenics on neuroleptics, on the other hand, is on the average more distant from the normative region and shows a very wide scatter, indicating a substantial heterogeneity with regard to the CSF parameters.

The two-dimensional reduction of 17 CSF parameters via MDS followed by the introduction of (1-p) convex hulls (Fig. 1) correctly separated 15 out of 16 controls from the schizophrenic subjects. This indicates that a biological heterogeneity between schizophrenic and nonschizophrenic subjects can be detected by the simultaneous analysis of the CSF concentrations of substances related directly or indirectly to the neuronal activity in the brain.

Neuropathological Studies

Jakob and Beckmann (1984, 1986 a, b) reported on pathomorphological findings in 64 unselected cases of definite schizophrenia retrospectively diagnosed according to the Research Diagnostic Criteria and International Classification of Diseases. Material and methods have been described elsewhere.

In 20 of the cases, the histological examination of coronal sections through the temporal lobe revealed cytoarchitectonic disturbances in two limbic regions, namely in the ventral part of the insular and the rostral part of the entorhinal cortex lying at the base of the hemisphere in the parahippocampal gyrus. In 22 cases the findings of the cytoarchitectonic pattern were equivocal, perhaps because of an unfavourable section plane. All these brains also had gross abnormalities: either definite deviations of the sulcogyral pattern of the temporal lobe or an abnormal, gross configuration with a tendency towards micrencephaly, but without atrophy. Histologically a poor development of the four upper layers in the entorhinal region was detected as a rule. However, the most important changes were found in the layer II (pre-α). In this layer, mainly in the central and lateral fields, the nerve cells normally lie in nodules with a characteristic architecture (Braak 1980). In our cases the nerve cells lie in these regions often in an irregular structure in a double row, not in nodules as is normal. Heterotopic groups of nerve cells belonging to layer II pre-α lie in the layer III pre-β (Fig. 2). The number of neurons in the layer III pre-β and IV pre-α was often reduced. Furthermore, in the ventral insular, the number of nerve cells in layers II and III were, compared

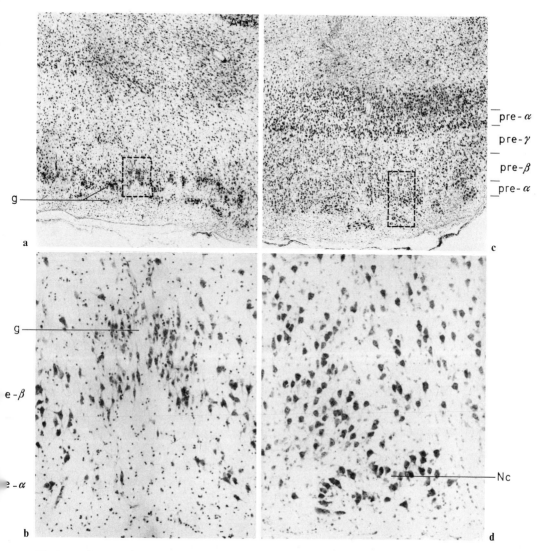

Fig. 2 a–d. Coronal sections through the left temporal lobe, showing the surface of the parahippocampal gyrus. **a** Rostral part of the entorhinal region at the level of the amygdaloid nucleus, medial and central fields. Poorly developed layers and disturbed structure of the layer II *pre-α*. *Am*, amygdaloid nucleus; *g*, double row and heterotopic groups of nerve cells. Nissl (20 μ thick × 25). **b** Magnification of the rectangle in **a**. Disarranged layer *pre-α*. The island structure of nerve cells in layer II pre-α is lacking. Note the diminution of the nerve cell population and the heterotopic group of nerve cells (*g*) in layer *pre-β*. Nissl (20μ thick × 100). **c** Control of the cytoarchitecture at the same level. Designation of the layers according Rose (1927 a, b). Nissl (20 μ thick × 25). **d** Control case. Magnification of the rectangle in **c**. The layers *pre-α* and *pre-β* with normal structure. Note the island structure of nerve cells (*Nc*) in *pre-α*. Nissl (20 μ × 100)

with the controls, considerably reduced. Generally, it is noteworthy that the disturbances of the cytoarchitectonic structure lie within narrow and exactly defined limits of the two allocortical regions in all 20 cases, deviating only slightly. In serial sections, the deviations of the basal entorhinal region cannot be found across the limit frontal to the prepiriform and occipital to the level of the hippocampal region.

These findings may indicate an abnormal ontogenetic development of the entorhinal region towards the end of the migration within the cerebral cortex, during the 4th to 5th fetal month. The nerve cells migrate from the subependymal ventricular matrix to the surface of the cortex. First layers V and VI are formed, the superficial layers last (Berry and Rogers 1965). The migration is essentially complete by the end of the 5th fetal month. If nerve cells are prevented from their migration towards the surface, some would probably remain as heterotopic islands and cause a poorly developed, disorganised architecture in the upper layers of the cortex. Further, the reduced number of nerve cells in the lower insular cortex seems to be related to the suggested migration disorder. These two regions are small but of great functional significance in the limbic system.

We would assume a genetically induced malformation in the rostral entorhinal region and probably in the ventral insular area as contributory to schizophrenia. However, one cannot exclude that other environmental conditions would play a role during development. Interestingly, neuropathological changes were found in all hebephrenic cases and in the majority of the undifferentiated and residual subtypes.

References

Ader R, de Wied D (1972) Effect of lysine vasopressin on passive avoidance learning. Psychonorm Sci 29:46–48

Arregui A, Mackay AVP, Iversen LL, Spokes EG (1979) Reduction of angiotensin-converting enzyme in substantia nigra in early onset schizophrenia. N Engl J Med 300:503

Beckmann H, Saavedra JM, Gattaz WF (1984) Low angiotensin-converting enzyme activity (kininase II) in cerebrospinal fluid of schizophrenics. Biol Psychiatry 19, 5:679–684

Beckmann H, Lang RE, Gattaz WF (1985) Vasopressin-oxytocin in cerebrospinal fluid of schizophrenic patients and normal controls. Psychoneuroendocrinology 10(2):187–191

Berry M, Rogers AW (1965) The migration of neuroblasts in the developing cerebral cortex. J Anat 99:691–709

Bloom FE (1976) The role of cyclic nucleotides in central synaptic function. In: Costa E, Giacobini E, Paoletti R (eds) Advances in biochemical psychopharmacology, vol 15. Raven, New York, pp 273–282

Braak H (1980) The allocortex. The entorhinal region. In: Braitenberg V(ed) Studies of brain function. Architectonics of the human telencephalic cortex, vol 4. Springer, Berlin Heidelberg New York, pp 37–48

Farley IF, Price KS, McCollough E, Deck JHN, Hordynski W, Hornykiewicz O (1978) Norepinephrine in chronic paranoid schizophrenia: above-normal levels in limbic forebrain. Science 200:456

Gasser R, Möcks J (1983) Graphical representation of multidimensional EEG data and classificatory aspects. Electroencephalogr Clin Neurophysiol 55:609–612

Gattaz WF, Waldmeier P, Beckmann H (1982) CSF monoamine metabolites in schizophrenic patients. Acta Psychiatr Scand 66:350–360

Gattaz WF, Riederer P, Reynolds GP, Gattaz D, Beckmann H (1983a) Dopamine and nor-adrenalin in the cerebrospinal fluid of schizophrenic patients. Psychiatry Res 8:243–250

Gattaz WF, Cramer H, Beckmann H (1983b) Low CSF concentrations of cyclic GMP in schizophrenia. Br J Psychiatry 142:288–291

Gattaz WF, Cramer H, Beckmann H (1984) Haloperidol increases the cerebrospinal fluid concentrations of cyclic GMP in schizophrenic patients. Biol Psychiatry 19(8):1229–1235

Gattaz WF, Gasser T, Beckmann H (1985) Multidimensional analysis of the concentrations of 17 substances in the CSF of schizophrenics and controls. Biol Psychiatry 20:360–366

Gomes UCR, Shanley BC, Potkieter L, Roux JT (1980) Noradrenergic overactivity in chronic schizophrenia: evidence based on cerebrospinal fluid noradrenalin and cyclic nucleotide concentrations. Br J Psychiatry 137:346

Jakob H, Beckmann H (1984) Clinical and neuropathological studies of developmental disorders in the limbic system in chronic schizophrenia. In: Schizophrenia: an integrative view. XIV Collegium Internationale Neuropsychopharmacologicum. Ricerca Scient. Educazione Permante, [Supp] 39:81 (Abstract)

Jakob H, Beckmann H (1986a) Prenatal developmental disturbances in the limbic allocortex in schizophrenia. In: Shagass CH, Josiassen RC, Bridger WH, Weiss KJ, Stoff D, Simpson GM (eds) Biological Psychiatry 1985. Elsevier, Amsterdam

Jakob H, Beckmann H (1986b) Prenatal developmental disturbances in the limbic allocortex in schizophrenics. J Neural Transm 65:303–326

Janowsky DS, Khaled El-Yousef M, Davis JM, Sekerke HJ (1973) Parasympathetic suppression of manic symptoms by physostigmine. Arch Gen Psychiatry 28:542–547

Overall LE, Gorham DR (1962) The brief psychiatric rating scale. Psychol Rep 19:799–812

Reynolds GP (1985) Receptors, neuroleptics and dopamine concentrations in schizophrenia – postmortem studies of human brain tissue. In: Beckmann H, Riederer P (eds) Pathochemical markers in major psychoses. Springer, Berlin Heidelberg New York, pp 29–34

Rose M (1927a) Der Allocortex bei Tier und Mensch, part 1. J Psychol Neurol 34:1–111

Rose M (1927b) Die sog. Riechrinde beim Menschen und beim Affen: II. Allocortex bei Tier und Mensch. J Psychol Neurol 34:261–401

Soffer RL (1976) Angiotensin-converting enzyme and the regulation of vasoactive peptides. Ann Rev Biochem 45:73–94

Spitzer RL, Endicott J, Robins E (1978) Research diagnostic criteria: rationale and reliability. Arch Gen Psychiatry 35:773–782

Van Kammen DP, Peters J, Pleak R (1986) Cerebrospinal fluid monoamine metabolism in schizophrenia: an uptdate. In: Burrows GD, Norman TR, Rubinstein G (eds) Handbook of studies on schizophrenia, part 2. Elsevier, Amsterdam, pp 219–242

Walter R, VanRee JM, DeWied D (1978) Modification of conditioned behavior of rats by neuro-hypophyseal hormones and analogues. Proc Natl Acad Sci USA 75:2493–2496

Winblad B, Bucht G, Gottfries CG, Roos BE (1979) Monoamines and monoamine metabolites in brains from demented schizophrenics. Acta Psychiatr Scand 60:17–28

Yang HYT, Hong IS, Fratta W, Costa E (1979) Dynamics of (Met^5)-enkephalin storage in rat striatum. In: Usdin E, Bunney WE, Kline NS (eds) Endorphins in mental health research. Oxford University Press, New York, p 235

Structural Brain Abnormalities in Schizophrenia: An Integrative Model

W. F. Gattaz, K. Kohlmeyer, and T. Gasser

Introduction

At the beginning of this century Emil Kraepelin (1971) dedicated the Chap. 8 of his book *Dementia Praecox and Paraphrenia* to the topic of morbid anatomy. Reviewing the available literature on neuropathological studies in dementia praecox he stated that "... in the cortex we have to do with severe and widespread disease of the nerve tissue", and further, "... diffuse loss of cortical cells could be established."

Not many years later, pneumoencephalography (PEG) was introduced by Dandy (1918) and provided the first possibility of studying the brain structures during life. Jacobi and Winkler (1927) carried out the first PEG study in schizophrenia and reported "hydrocephalus internus" in 18 of 19 chronic schizophrenics investigated. This striking result was followed by over 35 studies which to a considerable extent confirmed the findings of ventricular enlargement in schizophrenia.

In a series of studies, Huber (1957) and collaborators systematically searched for clinical correlates of the PEG findings in schizophrenia. They found that enlargement of the third ventricle occurs predominantly in chronic, unremitting schizophrenics, and that the atrophic findings correlate with the "reduction of the energetic potential", something in part related to the present "negative symptoms". In a follow-up study over 20 years, Huber (1975) confirmed his earlier findings of an association between ventricular enlargement and the "pure residual syndromes" with poor prognosis.

However, caution has been recommended for the interpretation of PEG findings in schizophrenia because of methodological problems inherent in this neuroradiological procedure. Weinberger and collaborators (1979) pointed out that many studies used biased patient and control selection, unspecified diagnostic criteria and inadequately validated standards for normal ventricular size.

Computerized Axial Tomography in Schizophrenia

The introduction of computerized axial tomography (CAT) provided a more reliable and noninvasive neuroradiological method of studying the brain structures. The results of the first investigation in schizophrenic patients were published

Central Institute of Mental Health, P.O. Box 5970, 6800 Mannheim 1, Federal Republic of Germany

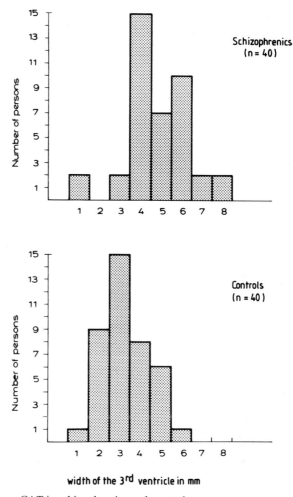

Fig. 1. Width of the third ventricle on CAT in schizophrenics and controls

10 years ago by Johnstone and collaborators (1976), who found increased cerebral ventricular size in 17 schizophrenics as compared to eight age-matched controls. These initial findings have been supported by a large number of subsequent studies, although negative findings have also been reported (see reviews in Seidman 1983; Weinberger et al. 1983).

In a CAT study we compared the width of the third ventricle in 40 schizophrenic patients with that in 40 sex- and age-matched controls (Gattaz et al. 1981) (Fig. 1). Although our patients did have significantly larger ventricles than the controls, the mean ventricular width from the schizophrenic group as a whole was still within the normal range. Similar findings have been obtained in other CAT studies (Weinberger et al. 1979) and suggest that the magnitude of the ventricular enlargement in schizophrenics might not be so dramatic as described in some PEG studies but rather mild or moderate.

Beside ventricular enlargement, CAT studies in schizophrenia have revealed other structural brain abnormalities such as cortical and cerebellar atrophy, decreased cerebral density and reversed cerebral asymmetry. To investigate the interrelationship between these different CAT findings in schizophrenia, Coffman and Nasrallah (1985) compared the results of density measurements with area and linear measurements of ventricular size and radiological assessments of cortical and cerebellar atrophy and found that abnormalities in one CAT parameter are not necessarily related to changes in another. These findings suggest that the atrophic changes in schizophrenia are not circumscribed to determined structures but are instead diffuse, affecting different brain areas independently. This indicates that a simultaneous evaluation of different CAT parameters might be necessary to delineate more precisely the subgroups of schizophrenics with and without brain atrophy.

Seidman (1983), in his excellent review of the literature, observed that in spite of qualitatively consistent results, the prevalence of atrophic findings in schizophrenia varies widely between studies. For instance, the frequency of ventricular enlargement – the most common finding in schizophrenia – varies from 6%–60%. Although methodological differences could account for such disparities, these figures indicate that the majority of schizophrenics probably do *not* have CAT abnormalities.

Furthermore, the atrophic findings in schizophrenia are not specific for this disease and do not have per se clinical relevance. A number of studies concentrated on the search for clinical and functional correlates of these findings and reported, in line with the earlier PEG studies, that CAT abnormalities were found more frequently in patients with chronic schizophrenia and correlated with variables such as poor premorbid adjustment, prominent negative symptoms and poor response to neuroleptic therapy. Conversely, acute schizophrenics were not found to show radiological evidence of brain atrophy. Crow (1980) postulated that the structural brain abnormalities could be seen as the pathological process underlying the type II syndrome.

We are presently investigating these clinical correlations with eight linear CAT parameters in schizophrenia. As noted above, we assumed that the simultaneous analysis of multivariate CAT data could provide a more accurate separa-

Table 1. Eight linear CAT parameters in schizophrenics and controls

	Patients ($n=19$)	Controls ($n=19$)
Sylvian fissure R	2.9 ± 1.4	2.9 ± 1.1
Sylvian fissure L	2.8 ± 1.8	2.9 ± 1.2
3rd ventricle	4.3 ± 1.3	3.4 ± 0.9
Huckmann number	45.0 ± 8.0	44.2 ± 5.1
Cella media index	4.8 ± 0.6	5.0 ± 0.8
Sulcal index	4.5 ± 5.2	3.2 ± 5.0
Interhemispheric fissure	3.1 ± 2.2	3.2 ± 2.2

tion of patients with and without brain atrophy. We wish to present here the preliminary data from the first 19 patients in order to illustrate the approach used in this study. Patients were diagnosed according to the Research Diagnostic Criteria and their psychopathological state was evaluated by means of the Brief Psychiatric Rating Scale (BPRS). Their mean age was 29 ± 10 years and the mean duration of the disease was 5 ± 7 years. Nineteen controls were matched to the patients by age and sex. The comparisons for each parameter are summarized in Table 1. Compared to controls, schizophrenics showed a trend towards larger third ventricle and higher sulcal index, which is the sum of the largest sulci in the frontal, temporal and parietal areas. Moreover, the width of the third ventricle, as well as the sulcal index and the interhemispheric fissure, correlated positively with the duration of the disease ($r_s = 0.38$, $p = 0.05$; $r_s = 0.43$, $p < 0.05$; and $r_s = 0.42$, $p < 0.05$ respectively).

To separate the patients into those with and without CAT deviations in regard to the controls we analysed the data through multidimensional scaling (MDS). To ensure comparability, the eight CAT parameters were standardized for all subjects such that the standard deviation with respect to the control group became 1. The full data set can be considered as a cloud of points consisting of the 38 subjects in the eight-dimensional parameter space. MDS seeks a two-dimen-

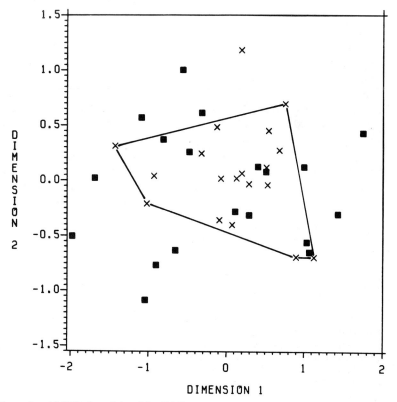

Fig. 2. Two-dimensional MDS plot of the eight CAT parameters. x, controls; □, patients

sional representation of this eight-dimensional cloud of points, while retaining as far as possible the distances between the subjects (Fig. 2).

To characterize the normative region occupied by the control group, a $(1-p)$ convex hull was introduced: a convex hull of a two-dimensional cloud of points is the region defined by its extreme points and the straight lines between them. To obtain the $(1-p)$ convex hull, a proportion p of the most extreme subjects is eliminated, such that the area covered becomes minimized ($p = 1/19$ in the present study).

The normative region defined by the convex hull of the control group allowed the separation of the schizophrenic patients into two subgroups: those within the normative region, and therefore without deviant CAT measures, and those outside the normative region, i.e. with deviant values from the controls in one or more CAT parameters.

This intergroup separation was used for further statistical comparisons. No significant differences were found between patients inside and outside the normative region concerning the individual variables and the baseline BPRS scores. To evaluate the therapeutic response to neuroleptics, some of these patients were treated for 3 weeks with a standard dose of haloperidol (10 mg/day), after which a second psychopathological evaluation was undertaken. BPRS changes are given in Table 2 as percentages of the baseline values. We found that patients lying outside the normative region showed a lower improvement in the BPRS scores "anergia" and, to a lesser extent, "anxiety/depression" than patients within the normative region. These scores are composed of some items closely related to type II schizophrenia, such as emotional withdrawal, motor retardation and blunted affect.

These preliminary findings must be viewed with caution because of the small size of the sample and the fact that the BPRS might not be completely adequate to assess the negative symptoms. However, in spite of these limitations, our findings point in the same direction as the reports of poor response to neuroleptic therapy in schizophrenic patients with CAT abnormalities.

Brain atrophy has also been found to correlate with neurodiagnostic variables indicative of a diffuse brain dysfunction in schizophrenia. These correlations have in part been discussed by Venables and by Cohen and Borst (this volume) and include neuropsychological impairments, attentional and cognitive deficits, elec-

Table 2. Percentage improvement in BPRS scores in schizophrenics inside and outside the normative region

BPRS variable	Inside ($n=4$)	Outside ($n=6$)
Anxiety/depression	54 ± 31	31 ± 32
Anergia	50 ± 14	20 ± 31
Thought disturbance	60 ± 32	63 ± 16
Activation	3 ± 6	19 ± 32
Hostility	54 ± 38	56 ± 18
Total	55 ± 26	45 ± 18

troencephalographic (EEG) abnormalities and the presence of neurological soft signs.

Summarizing up to this point, it seems well established that one subgroup of schizophrenic patients has neuroradiological signs of brain atrophy. This finding is associated with the most deleterious form of the disease and is frequently accompanied by neurological and neuropsychological impairment. However, little is known about the pathogenic mechanisms underlying such abnormalities. Whereas a possible role for birth complications and head injuries has been discussed in the literature, special attention has been concentrated on the investigation of a genetic component to brain atrophy in schizophrenia, but results are still contradictory. Nasrallah and collaborators (1983) compared the frequency of schizophrenia in first-degree relatives of schizophrenics with ventricle/brain ratios (VBR) above and below two standard deviations from the control mean. They found that patients with larger VBR had a significantly higher frequency of history of schizophrenia in a first-degree relative. In line with this finding, DeLisi and collaborators (1986) recently reported a familial component to ventricular size and suggested an association between greater ventricular size and the diagnosis of schizophrenia within the family. However, other studies failed to confirm these findings (Pearlson et al. 1985) or obtained results pointing in the opposite direction, namely a significant association between brain atrophy and *non*-genetic schizophrenia (Revely et al. 1984).

The heterogeneity among the findings of the different studies could be the reflection of a heterogeneous etiology for the brain atrophy in schizophrenia. Nasrallah and collaborators (1983) suggested that "...it is quite possible that while ventricular enlargement in some schizophrenic patients is due to a strong genetic loading, in others it may be related to non-genetic, acquired factors such as viral/immunologic processes, perinatal brain damage or head injury."

Structural Brain Abnormalities and Brain Maturation

We will now discuss one possible model for the development of structural brain abnormalities in schizophrenia in light of experimental data on the processes involved in the maturation of the brain.

The possibility cannot be completely ruled out that the neurodiagnostic abnormalities in chronic schizophrenia are in part a consequence of the chronic disease itself and its treatment. Speaking against this assumption, however, are the following:

1. The earliest PEG findings of brain atrophy as well as EEG abnormalities and neurological impairment in schizophrenic patients were reported before the advent of modern psychiatric therapies (e.g. neuroleptics, ECT).

2. Signs of brain damage were observed in young schizophrenic patients at the first episode of the disease and correlated with poor premorbid personality and social adjustment. These findings suggest that the structural brain abnormalities in schizophrenia are already present before the clinical manifestation of the psychosis and may result from an earlier defect in the maturation of the brain.

The maturation of the central nervous system (CNS) continues long after birth. One essential process in the structural development of the brain is represented by the changes in synaptic density, as described by Huttenlocher and collaborators (1979, 1982). These investigators measured the synaptic density in human brains in relation to age and found that after birth synaptic density (a) increases to an apparent maximum at age 2–3 years, and then (b) declines steeply in late childhood and early adolescence to levels that are maintained until extreme old age. Synaptic elimination is accompanied by a reduction in neuronal density as measured by an increase in the ratio of the volume of cortical grey matter to the volume of cortical neurons (von Economo's index) during the maturation of the brain. This process has also been observed in animals (Sturrock and Rao 1985), and it can be concluded that neuronal loss occurs as a normal developmental event in the CNS. Feinberg (1983) suggested a model to explain the acquisition of more complex forms of behaviour from childhood and adolescence concomitant with the decreased in neuronal density:

The human brain develops all potentially useful neuronal interconnections in the first years of life, since it cannot be specified in advance which connections will actually be needed. However, the excess connections impose a substantial cost on information processing capability, id est too many neuronal connections could make it difficult to distinguish and organize functionally the particular chains required for sustained logical thought and the solution of complex problems. At the end of childhood, when the kinds of neuronal connections required for adaptation have been determined by the individual's interaction with his environment, little-used connections are eliminated.

Based on these data, Feinberg (1983) and more recently Haracz (1985) suggested that schizophrenia might be produced by excessive neuronal loss during the maturation of the CNS. This hypothesis is supported by the results of several neurohistological postmortem studies reporting a neuronal loss in different areas of the brains from schizophrenics (Stevens 1982; Weinberger et al. 1983; Kovelman and Scheibel 1984; Benes et al. 1986). Two recent studies indicate further that the neuronal loss is predominant in the limbic temporal lobe, which has frequently been involved in the etiology of schizophrenia (Bogerts et al. 1985; Brown et al. 1986). Against the possibility that a neuronal degeneration occurs in the schizophrenic cortex are the findings that the neuronal loss is not accompanied by gliosis, indicating thus that the atrophy in schizophrenia results from an accelerated process of neuronal elimination early in life (Bogerts et al. 1985; Benes et al. 1986).

The results of animal experiments indicate that neuronal activity appears to be a factor controlling the rate of synaptic and neuronal elimination during the development of the central nervous system. Whereas environmental factors such as deprivation of stimuli and social isolation early after birth were found to accelerate this process, also biochemical manipulations affecting the neuronal activity in the early developmental period were found to impair the development and maturation of circumscribed areas in the brain (Kalaria and Prince 1985). This was illustrated by the recent report of O'Kusky (1985), who studied the rate of synaptic elimination in the developing visual cortex of normal and dark-reared cats. Visually deprived cats showed a twofold increase in synaptic elimination compared with normally reared animals. Similar effects have been observed in the

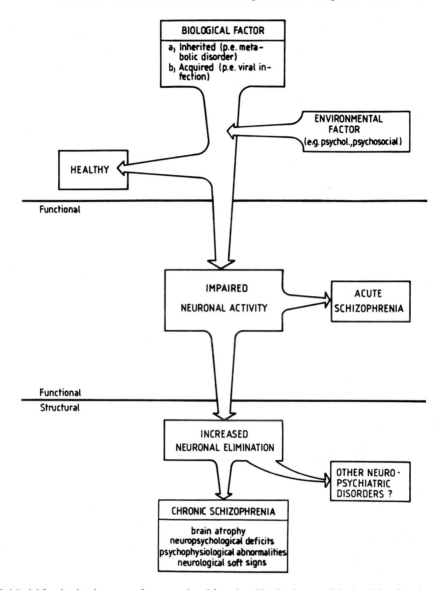

Fig. 3. Model for the development of structural and functional brain abnormalities in schizophrenia

olfactory bulb of animals submitted to odour deprivation during the neonatal period, including neuronal loss and permanent reduction of growth, total cell number and activity of enzymes related to the metabolism of neurotransmitters (Meisami and Firoozi 1985). Conversely, these effects of environmental and biological manipulations on brain structure were attenuated in animals beyond the age of developed maturation.

Based on these data and in the face of the neurodiagnostic findings in schizophrenia, we speculate that inherited or acquired biological abnormalities which impair the neuronal activity during the period of brain maturation accelerate the process of neuronal elimination, resulting in structural and functional brain abnormalities. In some cases, possibly depending on their intensity and/or localization, these abnormalities could underlie the clinical onset of a schizophrenic psychosis. It seems conceivable that the biological effect can be modulated by environmental influences, preventing or reinforcing its pathogenicity (Fig. 3). Depending upon the interaction of both dimensions, the disease could develop as a continuum between two extremes of intensity: At the highest intensity extreme would be those patients in whom massive neuronal loss takes place. They would present irreversible structural brain abnormalities and the clinical picture of chronic, unremitting schizophrenia. At the lowest extreme the opposite could be expected, namely individuals with sporadic functional disturbance not resulting in atrophic changes. They would present the clinical picture of acute, fully remitting schizophrenic episodes.

The present model is an attempt to integrate some current notions on the etiology of schizophrenia by specifying one common mechanism by which different causes could result in the schizophrenic syndrome. It should be seen as hypothetical and it needs experimental verification. We are presently working towards a study of neurodiagnostic and biochemical variables known to affect neuronal function and morphology directly or indirectly. Based on such an approach, it might be possible to accumulate further evidence in favour of or discrepant with the model presented.

References

Benes FM, Davidson J, Bird ED (1986) Quantitative cytoarchitectural studies of the cerebral cortex of schizophrenics. Arch Gen Psychiatry 43:31–35
Bogerts B, Meertz E, Schönfeld-Bausch R (1985) Basal ganglia and limbic system pathology in schizophrenia. Arch Gen Psychiatry 42:784–790
Brown R, Colter N, Corsellis JAN, Crow TJ, Frith CD, Jagoe R, Johnstone EC, Marsh L (1986) Postmortem evidence of structural brain changes in schizophrenia. Arch Gen Psychiatry 43:36–42
Coffman JA, Nasrallah HA (1985) Relationships between brain density, cortical atrophy and ventriculomegaly in schizophrenia and mania. Acta Psychiatr Scand 72:126–132
Crow TJ (1980) Molecular pathology of schizophrenia: more than one disease process. Br Med J 280:66–68
Dandy WE (1918) Ventriculography following the injection of air into the cerebral ventricles. Ann Surg 68:5–7
DeLisi LE, Goldin LR, Hamovit JR, Maxwell ME, Kurtz D, Gershon ES (1986) A family study of the association of increased ventricular size with schizophrenia. Arch Gen Psychiatry 43:148–153
Feinberg I (1983) Schizophrenia: caused by a fault in programmed synaptic elimination during adolescence? J Psychiatr Res 17:319–334
Gattaz WF, Kasper S, Kohlmeyer K, Beckmann H (1981) Die kraniale Computertomographie in der Schizophrenieforschung. Fortschr Neurol Psychiatr 49:286–291
Haracz JL (1985) Neural plasticity in schizophrenia. Schizophr Bull 11:191–229
Huber G (1957) Pneumoencephalographische und psychopathologische Bilder bei endogenen Psychosen. Springer, Berlin

Huber G, Gross G, Schuttler R (1975) A long-term follow-up study of schizophrenia: psychiatric course of illness and prognosis. Acta Psychiatr Scand 52:49–57

Huttenlocher PR (1979) Synaptic density in human frontal cortex – developmental changes and effects of aging. Brain Res 163:195–205

Huttenlocher PR, de Courten C, Garey LJ, Van der Loos H (1982) Synaptogenesis in human visual cortex – evidence for synapse elimination during normal development. Neurosci Lett 33:247–252

Jacobi W, Winkler H (1927) Encephalographische Studien an chronisch Schizophrenen. Arch Psychiatr Nervenkr 81:299–332

Johnstone EC, Crow TJ, Frith CD, Husband J, Kreel L (1976) Cerebral ventricular size and cognitive impairment in chronic schizophrenia. Lancet 11:924–926

Kalaria RN, Prince AK (1985) The effects of neonatal thyroid deficiency on acetylcholine synthesis and glucose oxidation in rat corpus striatum. Dev Brain Res 20:271–279

Kovelmann JA, Scheibel AB (1984) A neurohistological correlate of schizophrenia. Biol Psychiatry 19:1601–1621

Kraepelin E (1971) Dementia praecox and paraphrenia. Krieger, Huntington Ny, pp 213–223

Meisami E, Firoozi M (1985) Acetylcholinesterase activity in the developing olfactory bulb: a biochemical study on normal maturation and the influence of peripheral and central connections. Dev Brain Res 21:115¹24

Nasrallah HA, Kuperman S, Hamra BJ, McCalley-Whitters M (1983) Clinical differences between schizophrenic patients with and without large cerebral ventricles. J Clin Psychiatry 44:407–409

O'Kusky JR (1985) Synapse elimination in the developing visual cortex: a morphometric analysis in normal and dark-reared cats. Dev Brain Res 22:81–91

Pearlson GD, Garbacz DJ, Moberg PJ, Ahn HS, DePaulo JR (1985) Symptomatic, familial, perinatal and social correlated of computerized axial tomography (CAT) changes in schizophrenics and bipolars. J Nerv Ment Dis 173:42–50

Reveley AM, Reveley MA, Murray RM (1984) Cerebral ventricular enlargement in non-genetic schizophrenia: a controlled twin study. Br J Psychiatry 144:89–93

Seidman LJ (1983) Schizophrenia and brain dysfunction: an integration of recent neurodiagnostic findings. Psychol Bull 94:195–238

Stevens JR (1982) Neurophathology of schizophrenia. Arch Gen Psychiatry 39:1131–1139

Sturrock RR, Rao KA (1985) A quantitative histological study of neuronal loss from the locus coeruleus of ageing mice. Neuropathol Appl Neurobiol 11:55–60

Weinberger DR, Torrey EF, Neophytides AN, Wyatt RJ (1979) Lateral cerebral ventricular enlargement in chronic schizophrenia. Arch Gen Psychiatry 36:735–739

Weinberger DR, Wagner RL, Wyatt RJ (1983) Neuropathological studies of schizophrenia: a selective review. Schizophr Bull 9:193–212

The Retrovirus/Transposon Hypothesis of Schizophrenia

T. J. CROW

Introduction

A role for genes in the aetiology of schizophrenia has been established by twin and adoption studies, but the size and nature of the contribution remain in doubt. Only 10% of patients have an affected parent, and concordance in monozygotic twins is probably no greater than 50%. For these reasons most workers have concluded that genes are only one of several contributors to aetiology. Either genes predispose to environmental pathogens or there are both genetic and non-genetic forms of illness.

To identify the non-genetic aetiological factors is the difficulty. Most of the common classes of causative agent can be ruled out. Thus trauma, toxins and neoplasia do not seem to play a role. The known pathology and epidemiology of the disease are inconsistent with a contribution from such factors as ordinarily understood. This leaves immunity and infection as prime suspects, and immune dysfunction is often secondary to infection.

Origins of the Viral Hypothesis

The concept of schizophrenia as an infectious disease goes back to the middle of the nineteenth century, particularly in relation to cases of folie à deux. That the disease might be caused by a virus was first seriously considered by K. Menninger and E. Goodall in the aftermath of the 1918 epidemic of influenza and the outbreak of encephalitis lethargica which succeeded it (and may have been related). Post-influenzal and post-encephalitic psychoses were seen which had schizophrenia-like features. Subsequently there have been reports of schizophrenic illnesses associated with viral infections, although relationships to identified viruses have not been established (Torrey and Peterson 1976; Crow 1978). It is clear that some of the characteristic symptoms of schizophrenia may be provoked by infection, although this appears to be a relatively unusual or at least infrequently recognised event. The question arises of whether schizophrenia itself could be caused either by an atypical response to a common pathogen or by a hitherto unrecognised virus. Genetic factors predispose to some infections, e.g. polio and tuberculosis. Schizophrenia could be due to a virus to which certain individuals are predisposed by their genes.

Division of Psychiatry, Clinical Research Centre, Northwick Park Hospital, Watford Road, Harrow, Middlesex HA1 3UJ, United Kingdom

Recent discussions of epidemiology are relevant. It has been argued that significant changes over time, e.g. an increase in the course of the nineteenth century (Hare 1983), have taken place, and also that there are variations across the populations of the world (Torrey 1980). Such variations are consistent with spread in the manner of an epidemic.

Refutation of the Contagion Theory

If the disease is transmitted from one individual to another this should be seen within families as well as at the population level. Some findings in family studies can be interpreted as consistent with contagion (Crow 1983). For example, concordance rates are generally reported as higher in same-sex than opposite-sex pairs of relatives, and in dizygotic twins than in siblings. In these cases it could be that higher concordance rates are seen in pairs of relatives who are likely to be in closer physical contact. Similarly, in Abe's analysis of onset of illness (Abe 1969), in monozygotic twins the second twin was at increased risk in the 2 years following illness onset in the first twin, the increase in risk being confined to pairs who were together at this time.

A critical test of the contagion hypothesis can be conducted in pairs of siblings. An analysis of age of onset in five reported series reveals a consistent tendency for age of onset to be earlier in younger siblings (Fig. 1) (Crow and Done 1986).

Three explanations must be considered:

1. The disease is transmitted from one sibling to the other, or both are exposed to an exogenous pathogen at the same point in time (the "contagion" or "horizontal transmission" hypothesis).

2. The disease is detected earlier when it is already known to be present in the family ("early detection").

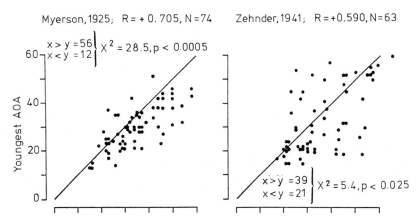

Fig. 1. Age on (first) admission (AOA) in elder sibling plotted against AOA in younger sibling. (From Crow and Done 1986)

262   T.J.Crow

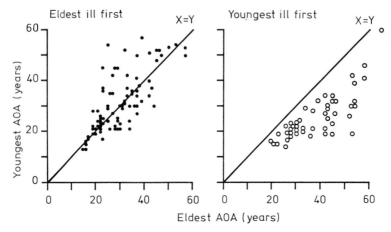

Fig. 2. Age on admission (AOA) in elder sibling plotted against AOA in younger sibling according to which sibling is ill first. (From Crow and Done 1986)

3. Because the data are collected at a particular point in time (e.g. close to onset of illness in one sibling) a bias enters, excluding later onsets of illness in younger siblings ("ascertainment bias").

The first two hypotheses predict that the shift to younger age of onset will be seen in pairs in which the elder sibling is ill first. However, this appears not to be the case (Fig. 2).

In pairs in which the elder sibling becomes ill first, mean age of onset in the siblings is approximately equal. Ascertainment bias, rather than contagion or early detection, accounts for the trend towards younger age of onset in the younger sibling.

When the ascertainment bias is taken into account (as in the elder sibling ill first subsample), age of onset remains highly correlated between siblings but apparently uninfluenced by actual time of onset. The findings not only rule out contagion (at least in adult life) but also discourage the concept that onset of illness is influenced at all by environmental factors of the type that occur at a defined point in time. It is as though a clock is ticking away within the predisposed individual to ensure not only that he will suffer from the illness but that it will occur at a predetermined age.

The findings do not rule out an environmental influence in the prenatal period. Such an influence is suggested by the season of birth effect (Dalen 1975), although whether this reflects an event at birth or earlier is uncertain. It is also unclear how events at this stage of life can influence the onset of illness 20 or 30 years later.

A hypothesis (Crow 1984, 1986a) that attempts to account for the season of birth effect as well as onset of illness in adult life is as follows:

The disease is due to a potential pathogen (e.g. a retrovirus or other mobile genetic element) in the human genome that can be expressed to cause disease either because it is inherited (in its pathogenic form) direct from an affected or predisposed parent or because it acquires this form as a result of a genetic rearrangement (e.g. a transposition or replication event) occurring early in development (e.g. at meiosis or fertilisation).

According to this hypothesis the season-dependence of such events is responsible for the deviation of birth dates of psychotic patients from expectation for the general population.

Location of the Element in the Genome

Evidence from electrophysiological, CT scan and postmortem studies suggests that the schizophrenic process has a predilection for the left or dominant hemisphere (Crow 1986a). This is difficult to understand if the disease is due to an exogenous pathogen, but might be explained if the pathogen is integrated in association with a gene which is expressed preferentially in the left hemisphere. An asymmetry of cerebral structure is present in the planum temporale, this region being of greater extent on the left side of the brain in most individuals. The asymmetry develops early. Presumably it is due to the differential expression of a growth factor (the "cerebral dominance gene"). Selectivity for the left hemisphere might be explained if the "virogene" were integrated close to the cerebral dominance gene and expressed in association with it.

Nature of the Element

Agents of the retrovirus class sometimes become associated with cellular growth factors and may be responsible for aberrations of cellular development. Other types of retrotransposon (e.g. LINE elements) may do likewise.

A number of types of retrovirus sequence have been identified in the human genome. These include the HLM-2 group of sequences identified by hybridisation to mouse mammary tumour virus (Callahan et al. 1985) and another group identified by hybridisation to retroviral sequences in an African green monkey genomic library (Steele et al. 1984). There are approximately 50 copies of each of these sequences in the human genome. About 800–1000 copies of a retrovirus-like sequence originally identified in the β-globin gene cluster (Mager and Henthorn 1984) are also present. Whether any of these sequences are transcribed in normal or pathological circumstances remains to be established. In addition, a 2- to 3-kb transposon-like element has been found which is also present in extrachromosomal circular DNA (Paulson et al. 1985).

Mode of Transmission

If the determinants of schizophrenia are, as argued above, primarily genetic, the persistence of the disease at a relatively high prevalence in the populations of the world in the face of reduced fertility in affected individuals remains to be explained.

One possibility is that the gene confers advantages on individuals who carry the gene but are unaffected by the disease. However, such individuals and the nature of the advantage have not been identified. Another possibility arises if the pathogen is an element which is mobile within the genome. As pointed out by Hickey (1982), such an element might replicate between haploid genomes to circumvent the laws of mendelian genetics, and spread within the population even though it reduced fitness. The agent would thus be horizontally transmitted not at a time close to disease onset but at gamete formation. It is not clear, however, whether an equilibrium state such as is observed in schizophrenia could be set up in this manner.

An alternative explanation is that schizophrenia is but a part of a wider genetic spectrum. There is a case that schizophrenia and manic-depressive psychosis, rather than representing distinct disease entities, are points on a continuum extending from unipolar through bipolar affective illness to schizoaffective psychosis and schizophrenia with increasing severities of defect. The case is argued on the basis of the failure of attempts to demonstrate a bimodal distribution of scores on a discriminant function of symptoms, on the overlap in family studies of schizoaffective psychosis with both of the prototypical psychoses and on evidence for an excess of individuals with schizoaffective disorders and schizophrenia amongst the descendants of patients with affective disorders (Crow 1986 b). The hypothesis generates the prediction that the gene responsible for psychosis is itself variable, the presence of the gene in a pathogenic form increasing risk of disease of greater severity. Such increases in severity might be due to replications within the genome, e.g. the generation of tandem repeats.

The concept leads to the suggestion that the reason for the persistence of the schizophrenia gene lies elsewhere on the continuum. There is evidence, for example, for an association between affective illness and creativity (Jamison 1986) and also for particular achievement in the relatives of patients with schizophrenia (Karlsson 1984). In a study in Norway amongst those with occupations in the professional services (Noreik and Ødegaard 1966), admissions for manic-depressive psychosis were increased and those for schizophrenia decreased with respect to the general population. This suggests that the relationship of achievement to affective illness may be closer than that to schizophrenia. However, while fertility is certainly decreased in schizophrenia it is far from clear that fertility is increased in affective illness. If affective illness and schizophrenia are genetically related, the problem of persistence is moved back but not yet solved.

The questions of persistence and possible genetic advantage may be related to the problem of age of onset. As already noted, age of onset of schizophrenia is earlier than that of affective disorder, and of bipolar illness earlier than of unipolar illness. Thus there is an inverse relationship between age of onset and severity of illness along the continuum. However, it is also recognised that typical psychotic illnesses seldom have an onset earlier than pubery. It is as though an evolutionary feedback mechanism were hunting for a time of onset in the period following puberty. Perhaps this is a time of particular cerebral growth.

Asymmetrical brain growth is a recent evolutionary development presumably related to the specifically human capacity for speech and perhaps to other intellectual abilities. Its integration with other aspects of brain growth must be critical for optimal cerebral development. One might suppose that the genetic mechanisms responsible require an intrinsic timing device and are also relatively variable between individuals, such variability applying both to the magnitude of the effect and its timing. Pathological effects could arise from inappropriately great enhancements of growth, and their severity might be determined by the stage of development at which they occur.

The findings of a recent CT scan study (Colter et al., in preparation) illustrate a possible sequence. Asymmetries can be observed on CT scan in the temporo-occipital region in the normal brain, the width of the brain being greater on the left. Overall comparison of schizophrenics with other psychiatric patients reveals no difference in the asymmetries. However, patients with early onset (less than 25 years) have diminished, and those with late onset (over 25 years) increased asymmetries, the difference between the groups being significant at the 1% level. The findings reinforce the concept of the disease as a disorder of cerebral asymmetry development. One interpretation is that early disease expression (perhaps as viral particles) causes arrest of development, while later onset is associated with enhanced growth, which also eventually ends in pathology.

Summary

The concept that schizophrenia is a disease induced in genetically predisposed individuals by an exogenous virus has been tested in pairs of affected siblings. Onset is determined by age and not by common exposure to an environmental pathogen. Contagion appears to be excluded.

An alternative hypothesis is that the disease is due to a pathogen (e.g. a retrovirus or other type of mobile element) integrated in the genome. The element is assumed to be acquired either from an affected or predisposed parent or as a result of an early (and season-dependent) genetic rearrangement which leaves the element in the same pathogenic form. If this "hot spot" of genetic recombination has survival value in relation to cerebral growth (e.g. by promoting the development of lateral asymmetry), this could account for the persistence of the disease in the face of a fertility disadvantage. The association between the "virogene" and the mechanisms of lateralised cerebral development provides a possible explanation for the predilection of the disease for the left hemisphere. It may also be relevant to timing of disease onset.

References

Abe K (1969) The morbidity rate and environmental influence in monozygotic co-twins of schizophrenics. Br J Psychiatry 115:519–531

Callahan R, Chin IM, Wong JFH, Tronick SR, Roe BA, Aaronson SA, Schlom J (1985) A new class of endogenous human retroviral genomes. Science 228:1208–1211

Crow TJ (1978) Viral causes of psychiatric disease. Postgrad 54:763–767

Crow TJ (1983) Is schizophrenia an infectious disease? Lancet 1:173–175

Crow TJ (1984) A re-evaluation of the viral hypothesis: is psychosis the result of retroviral integration at a site close to the cerebral dominance gene? Br J Psychiatry 145:243–253

Crow TJ (1986a) Left brain, retrotransposons and schizophrenia. Br Med J 293:3–4

Crow TJ (1986b) The continuum of psychosis and its implications for the structure of the gene. Br J Psychiatry 149:419–429

Crow TJ, Done DJ (1986) Age of onset of schizophrenia in siblings: a test of the contagion hypothesis. Psychiatry Res 18:107–117

Dalen P (1975) Season of birth: a study of schizophrenia and other mental disorders. North Holland, Amsterdam

Hare EH (1983) Was insanity on the increase? Br J Psychiatry 142:439–455

Hickey WE (1982) Selfish DNA: a sexually-transmitted nuclear parasite. Genetics 101:519–531

Jamison KR (1986) Manic-depressive illness and accomplishment: creativity, leadership and social class. In: Goodwin FK, Jamison KR (eds) Manic depressive illness. Oxford University Press, London

Karlsson JL (1984) Creative intelligence in relatives of mental patients. Hereditas 100:83–86

Mager DL, Henthorn PS (1984) Identification of a retrovirus-like repetitive element in human DNA. Proc Natl Acad Sci USA 81:7510–7514

Noreik K, Ødegaard Ø (1966) Psychoses in Norwegians with a background of higher education. Br J Psychiatry 112:43–55

Paulson KE, Doka N, Schmid GW, Misra R, Schindler CW, Rush MG, Kadyk L, Leinwand L (1985) A transposon like element in human DNA. Nature 316:359–361

Steele PE, Rabson AB, Bryan T, Martin MA (1984) Distinctive termini characterise two families of human endogenous retroviral sequences. Science 225:943–947

Torrey EF (1980) Schizophrenia and civilisation . Aronson, New York

Torrey EF, Peterson MR (1976) The viral hypothesis of schizophrenia. Schizophr Bull 2:136–146

Biological Hypotheses of Schizophrenia: Discussion

S. HIRSCH

The five contributions to this session were extremely interesting and will, for most of us, symbolise new developments in our understanding of the biological basis of schizophrenia. There is an interesting overlap between the various papers, both in their finding of laterality differences and in the reports of some of the authors of a tendency for considerable variation between patients in the nature and location of the abnormality. There is an emphasis on left-sided limbic function and an increasing emphasis on developmental abnormalities in the limbic and temporal areas which, it is argued, could be compatible with a virogenic etiology. However, because the results tend to converge, there is a danger that they will be accepted as such when in fact an alternative interpretation is also possible. That is, there is a tendency for each of the studies to quote the same references to support their theories, and in forming the interpretation of their findings, so that the papers may be amplifying the error inherent in each other's work. Each of the papers represent a different technical approach and methodology with its own inherent questions. I will, therefore, briefly discuss each paper in turn before making some general concluding remarks.

Professor Carlsson's paper on dopamine receptors represents a qualitative step forward in our concept of the dopamine receptor. It may be useful if I summarise some of the highlights. He describes substances which were partly active on some dopamine receptors, but not others. $(-)$-3-PPP antagonises the lactotroph receptor 100% but the dopamine autoreceptor by 50%–70%. Moreover, the action of $(-)$-3-PPP varies depending upon the state of the receptor – it has agonist activities on denervated supersensitive receptors but antagonist activities on normoreceptors.

D1 and D2 receptors may act together (coupled) or, under different conditions, independently. Taken together, these findings lead to a concept of a dopamine complex capable of adaptive changes in its confirmation which depends on prevailing pharmacological conditions. The model of neuroleptics simply blocking the dopamine receptor has therefore become more sophisticated. This has implications for the next generation of neuroleptics, because $(-)$-3-PPP does not cause catalepsy, hence it is not likely to affect extrapyramidal functions. This could explain the finding reported by van Kammen (van Kammen et al. 1982) [1] that, contrary to expectation, only 25% of patients showed an increase in symptoms when given a single injection of 20 mg amphetamine, and 29% of patients actually improved; 46% remained unchanged. This suggests that in man, respon-

Charing Cross & Westminster Medical School, London, United Kingdom

siveness to dopamine may change over time. I would like to invite comment from
Dr. Crow and Dr. Reynolds as to how they think this concept of an adaptive dopamine complex fits with their ideas that positive schizophrenic symptoms are related to increased mesolimbic dopaminergic activity. I would also like to ask Professor Beckmann and Dr. Gattaz, who are responsible for the cerebrospinal fluid
(CSF) findings reported above, whether they can fit this more subtle concept of
a dopamine receptor into their model, which, as I understand it, depends on putting each of the neurotransmitters on its own linear scale of high or low activity
and envisages an overall single multiple-neurotransmitter effect.

Dr. Reynold's paper demonstrates an apparently specific finding of a lateralised increase in dopamine in the amygdala (left greater than right) and an increase
in homovanillic acid in amygdala and possibly forebrain. This is consistent with
a considerable body of evidence which implicates dopamine mechanisms in the
pathophysiology of schizophrenic (or should we say psychotic) symptomatology.
The finding is capable of two contrasting interpretations, one being that left-sided
temporal functioning is a likely candidate for pathophysiological changes in psychosis – and this is supported by electrophysiological and brain imaging changes
reported by others. However, the alternative interpretation, which perhaps Dr.
Reynolds favours, is based on the observation reported by others that there is
normally a lateralised difference in the responseiveness of rat brains such that rats
exposed to dopamine infusion show an asymmetric turning response which is
partly dependent on their previously demonstrated turning preference. This suggests that the differences observed in dopamine levels in schizophrenic brain may
be due to inherent left-right differences not related to the illness, which then become evident after the brain has been exposed to neuroleptics. Thus more dopamine neurones in the left amygdala would be reflected in greater presynaptic dopamine release when the postsynaptic neurones are blocked. The interpretation
that the differences in the mean dopamine level are due to pathophysiology which
may be based on structural differences in the brain would be consistent with Professor Beckmann's findings in the CSF and Dr. Crow's virogenic theory. I wonder
if Dr. Reynolds can tell us how he plans to determine whether the asymmetric biochemistry is due to previous exposure to medication and inherent brain differences or due to primary pathology. The failure of depressives to show the same
laterality differences could, of course, be due to a deficiency in the depressives
rather than an excess in the schizophrenics.

Professor Beckmann reports two studies. In the first the CSF of 28 schizophrenics, 13 of whom had been off medication for more than 4 weeks and 14 of
whom were on drugs at the time, is compared with 16 neurological controls. By
use of multidimensional scaling techniques he was able to separate the schizophrenics from controls with almost no overlap, using either 17 CSF biochemical
parameters or the four preselected most relevant ones – dopamine, noradrenaline,
glutamate and cyclic guanosine monophosphate. While there was a wider scatter
with patients on drugs than with those off medication for 4 weeks, the two groups
could not be distinguished. Could the controls be the abnormal group, rather
than the schizophrenics? Could the changes be secondary to the schizophrenic's
response to his environment, rather than a direct expression of the primary lesion?
And how do we interpret the meaning of these differences in multidimensional

scaling, except to conclude that schizophrenics are different from non-schizophrenics?

In the second study Professor Beckmann found that one-third of 64 retrospectively diagnosed DSM-III brains of schizophrenics had histopathological abnormalities in the rostral entorhinal region and that 16 had abnormalities of the ventral insular cortex – another third (22) had equivocal changes. Interestingly in relation to Dr. Reynolds' and Dr. Crow's findings, the abnormalities were asymmetric but apparently in random directions, i.e. not consistently so. There was no reference in their paper to a consistent laterality effect. RDC-diagnosed hebephrenics as opposed to paranoid patients, based on first-admission diagnosis, were more often in the group which showed pathological changes.

Consistent with Dr. Crow, Professor Beckmann hypothesised a genetically induced developmental abnormality based on what can be deduced from the knowledge of the embryological development of the brain. It is interesting that there was a tendency for a consistent localised lesion in this area. Unfortunately oligophrenics were used as controls, which leaves some doubt as to what was normal and what was abnormal. Oligophrenics can be regarded as controls for institutionalisation, and perhaps for diet, if, as I understand it, they come from the same institution at the same period in time, but they do not control for exposure to previous medication, previous treatment with ECT, length of hospitalisation, etc. Underactivity and understimulation persisting over a long period of time could, theoretically, lead to cell atrophy and cell loss. Could this be a possible explanation for the results? Finally, can the reported changes be reconciled with the overlapping but different results reported by Nasrallah – glyosis of the corpus callosum – or Stevens – glyosis of the limbic system? Professor Beckmann's paper does not report glyosis. However, Weinberg has reported atrophy of the cerebral vermis. This was not found in the present study.

Dr. Gattaz participated in the work reported by Dr. Beckmann, but here reports studies of the brain by computerised axial tomography (CAT). In his paper he drew our attention to the variation in the extent of ventricular enlargement reported by previous centres – 6%–60% – and to the fact that the majority of schizophrenics are not affected in this way. Previous findings have not, in a consistent way, been directly related to clinical abnormalities. The possible exception is Professor Huber's studies over a 20-year period which found an association of enlarged ventricles with pure residual symptoms, as well as poor premorbid personality, prominent negative symptoms and a poor response to treatment.

With the use of multidimensional scaling Dr. Gattaz has given us the very interesting finding that two groups of chronic patients could be identified – one fell outside and the other fell within the area of statistical association defined by normal controls. The distinguishing clinical feature of schizophrenics outside the normative area as compared with those inside is that they showed significantly less response to 3 weeks' haloperidol treatment on the BPRS-rated negative symptoms of "anergy" and "anxiety/depression." This is an interesting and persuasive finding, but I don't know how to interpret the apparently inconsistent finding I noted in his Table 2. This is that the "activation" measure also showed significant change – does this conflict with the failure to show response on "anergy"? Were the patients whose mean duration of illness was 5 ± 7 years institutionalised? We would like to know more about the selection of patients in order to generalise back from these findings to other groups of schizophrenics and know whether they apply to the whole of the population of chronic schizophrenics or only to a particular subgroup.

Dr. Gattaz has acknowledged the limitated value of the BPRS, but I think it is time that this instrument be abandoned entirely in such research. Much more precise results might be obtained with other scales such as the Montgomery and Asberg CPRS or the Present State Examination of Wing and others. The BPRS lacks clear definitions and allows for bias, particularly the expectation of change over time. There is a lack of reliability between centres and a poor correspondence between the ratings on the instrument and specific elements of psychopathology.

There is a danger in both Dr. Beckmann's studies and Dr. Gattaz' study which can arise any time patients are not selected using a formal sampling frame. Do the patients represent a special subset who are not generalisable to the entire diagnostic group or subgroup? Patients may get into small samples selectively because they have odd or interesting features or are more severe, less responsive, more neurological, more interesting, or more easily available when one wants to do the study. Thus the results may relate to factors which are not related to the schizophrenic process per se, but may account for poor response to treatment, failure to be discharged from hospital, or whatever. The other aspect of this fallacy is the difficulty of extrapolating from the findings to the diagnostic group as a whole. The remedy is to select patients in a predetermined sampling frame which avoids selection bias.

Moving on to Dr. Crow's paper, I must complement him on his manner of proceeding in the spirit of a true scientist. On the basis of limited observations, he forms a theory from which he deduces a testable hypothesis. He has told us how he then rejected the hypothesis on the basis of the evidence and, again in the scientific spirit, put it forward a second time in a modified form!

Dr. Crow developed the argument for a viral etiology, but in the process of deducing and testing hypotheses disconfirmed his prediction of a contagious element which would support the viral theory. The hypothesis is then nevertheless resurrected on the basis that the virus may be a mobile element integrated into the genetic apparatus that can move within the gamete and therefore not be reflected in a mendelian pattern of genetic transmission. This may be acquired from a parent or occur as a result of genetic rearrangement under environmental influence. This phenomenon has been dscribed in mice. This "hot spot" can survive in the population because, he theorises, it is closely linked to a characteristic which has survival advantage, i.e. to a cerebral dominance gene. I believe this to be a most creative, novel and original contribution. How the virogene then effects the development of schizophrenia and influences the development of cerebral dominance is not stated. I did not understand whether the virogene is meant to explain the evolution of cerebral dominance in man, in which case it must be quite remote from the etiology of schizophrenia in individuals, or whether Dr. Crow is suggesting that cerebral dominance depends in each individual on the presence of the virogene, which in turn may or may not become pathogenic and lead to schizophrenia. I would find this theory implausible.

The theory gives rise to several other questions too: Is the constancy of the schizophrenic inception rate across geographical, cultural and racial groups, as reported earlier in this meeting by Dr. Sartorius, consistent with this hypothesis? Is the WHO finding of a seasonality effect appearing in similar form in schizophrenia, manic-depressive illness and neurosis, but not seen in normal controls, troublesome for this theory? Is the appeal of the virogene hypothesis mainly one of exclusion, i.e. the exhaustion of other theories, as Dr. Crow intimates? I wonder too whether we can be sure he has ruled out contagion, because the age of onset in his data is probably based on date of hospitalisation, in which case it may be subject to many interveneing variables and may not be an adequate test of his hypothesis. One wonders how one would test for horizontal transmission within the gamete, and one would like, of course, to know more about how horizontal transmission could take place.

In general, Drs. Gattaz, Beckmann and Crow all offer us an interesting developmental theory which is the common link between their papers. The concept of a maturational defect is very interesting and could fit with the genetic evidence and explain, as well, the early onset of adult schizophrenia. Dr. Crow referred to the forthcoming paper from his group which suggests that schizophrenia can be separated into an early-onset group with diminished asymmetry and a late-onset group with increased asymmetry. Dr. Graham Shephard, previously in our group, reported a few years ago our study of I believe nine acute first onset unmedicated schizophrenics who underwent positive emission tomography [2]. The main finding in that study was a failure to find laterality in brain metabolism in schizophrenics as compared to normals, who showed the laterality effect. One wonders whether the suggestion of a developmental defect depends on observations which are too small in number for inferences to be drawn and extrapolated to schizophrenics in general. There are many negative studies, not quoted, which do not support these concepts.

To the extent that the findings we have heard in this session are based on a relatively small number of selected patients, be they CAT scan, CSF or histopathological findings, we must ask, as Seymour Kety did in the early 1960s, whether the findings are primary and represent basically etiological differences between schizophrenics and normals, or whether they are secondary to medication, diet, selection of sample etc. Are these findings specific for schizophrenics, or would other chronic institutionalised patients, such as oligophrenics and chronic manic-depressives, show the same changes? Are they secondary to the disease process? CSF and CAT scan findings may reflect changes which are the result of arousal mechanisms, deficient diet, local epidemics etc. It is therefore particularly important that they be replicated in other cohorts in other places.

In the future we will want to know more of the pathophysiology; not only how such lesions and abnormalities develop in schizophrenics, – we have had some suggestions – but also how such diffuse and non-specific changes, which seem to vary from study to study, give rise to the very constant and repeatable pattern of symptoms we see in schizophrenia.

Notwithstanding, we do seem to be moving towards greater specificity of knowledge of the nature of the biological abnormalities which could be found in association with schizophrenia. Although the overlap of different findings and theoretical concepts may be due to an amplification of the error which results from a large number of centres quoting a small number of results, they nevertheless do lead to testable hypotheses, new questions and new technical advances. I think the authors should be congratulated for their careful and creative work and their contribution to the science of our subject.

References

1. van Kammen DP, Docherty JP, Marder SR, Schulz SC, Dalton L, Bunney WE (1982) Antipsychotic effects of pimozide in schizophrenia: treatment response prediction with acute dextroamphetamine response. Arch Gen Psychiatry 39:261–266
2. Shepherd G, Gruzelier J, Manchanda R, Hirsch SR, Wise R, Frackowiack R, Jones T (1983) O positron emission tromographic scanning in predominantly never-treated acute schizophrenic patients. Lance ii:1448–50

Part VI
Vulnerability and Trigger Models/Rehabilitation

Social and Psychological Risk Factors for Episodes of Schizophrenia *

B. P. Dohrenwend, P. E. Shrout, B. G. Link, and A. E. Skodol

Schizophrenia is a disorder or group of disorders that has consistently been found in epidemiological studies to show the highest rate in the lowest social class (see Dohrenwend BP 1983; Eaton and Boyd 1985). This suggests that socioenvironmental factors may be important in etiology (see Faris and Dunham 1939; Mischler and Scotch 1967; Kohn 1972). However, the finding is open to plausible alternative explanations in which low social class is seen as a consequence rather than a cause of disorder (e.g., Dunham 1965; Mechanic 1972), and studies of social mobility focused on this question have provided inconclusive results (see Dohrenwend BP and Dohrenwend BS 1969).

To date, the most direct evidence on the role of socioenvironmental factors has come from a handful of retrospective case-control studies of the relation of recent stressful life events to episodes of schizophrenic or schizophrenia-like disorder (e.g., especially, Brown and Birley 1968; Jacobs and Myers 1976). On the basis of these studies, a consensus has developed over the past 15 years that recent life events have only a trivial impact on the onset of schizophrenia (e.g., Brown et al. 1973a; Hudgens 1974; Gottesman and Shields 1976; Brown and Harris 1978; Rabkin 1980; Day 1981; Lukoff et al. 1984). As Brown and Harris (1978) put it: "For schizophrenia a wide range of events can bring about a sudden onset of florid symptoms. The arousal of any strong emotion, positive or negative, appears to be enough. Events probably bring about a disorder that would have occurred before long in any case" (p. 277).

There have, however, been some differing views. Paykel includes schizophrenia among the disorders for which findings on relative risk attached to recent life events "... indicate effects which are of some importance, particularly in the short term" (Paykel 1978, p. 251), and Dohrenwend BP and Egri (1981) have suggested that the consensus that life events play only a trivial role is premature. Moreover, there is equivocation on both sides of the controversy, with Brown and Harris suggesting that life events may play a larger role, at least in some subgroups of schizophrenia (1978, p. 129), and most reviewers (e.g., Day 1981; Lukoff et al. 1984) calling for further research. Even the best of these studies have been limited to what Lukoff et al. refer to as "a two variable design" in which "life events are recorded ... and subjects are rated on the presence or absence of the onset of the

* This work has been supported by the US National Institute of Mental Health Research Grant MH36208, Clinical Research Center Grant MH30906, and Research Scientist Award 05-MH14663
Social Psychiatry Research Unit, Columbia University, 100 Haven Avenue, New York, NY 10032, USA

illness" (1984, p. 285). If there is unanimity in the reviews, is it that more variables that can affect the impact of the events and/or be compared with such impact need to be studied if the relative importance of recent life events is to be accurately assessed and the process involved understood.

Before turning to our own research, which greatly broadens the range of variables to be studied along with recent life events, let us briefly describe the most important previous studies so that the points of later comparison will be clearer. We will consider for the most part only those investigations that come reasonably near to meeting four criteria for adequate retrospective case/control studies of relations between recent life events and schizophrenia (Dohrenwend BP and Egri 1981). The four constitute the irreducible minimum for providing useful results bearing on the role of recent life events: adequate controls, replicable diagnostic criteria, attention to assessing which events occur independently of the subjects' prior mental state, and careful attention to dating of the occurrence of events in relation to the occurrence of the episodes of psychopathology. Failure to attend to these problems makes much of the published research difficult to interpret. Methodological problems, especially those related to the question of independence, have been particularly serious (see Dohrenwend BS et al. 1984).

A variety of definitions of schizophrenia have been used in case-control studies to date. We will discuss the occurrence of acute psychotic episodes rather than of schizophrenia as defined, for example, by DSM-III, since operationally this is more nearly what was investigated in these studies.

The case-control studies have shown that the number of life events reported by schizophrenics before onset of an episode was significantly greater than the number reported by controls for a comparable period. One of these, by Jacobs and Myers (1976) in New Haven, focused on a survey of 62 first admissions; the other, by Brown and Birley (1968) in London, was concerned with 50 patients admitted for acute episodes of schizophrenia. Although the consistent finding of these two studies was that there was a significantly higher rate of life events in their reporting periods, 1 year in the former and 3 months in the latter study, for patients than for community controls, this excess was due mainly to events that could be dependent on the patient's mental condition.

It is of considerable interest, therefore, that Brown and Birley, who dated the occurrence of events within 1-week periods, also found that events that were judged by the investigators to be independent of any prior psychiatric disorder or possible insidious onset of present episode occurred more frequently in the 3-week period preceding episodes of schizophrenia than in a comparable period in the lives of their controls. Forty-six percent of the patients but only 12% of the controls experienced a build up of at least one independent event in this 3-week period. This difference was not found in earlier 3-week periods. Moreover, this finding is not an isolated one, since Leff and colleagues (1973) found a relatively high frequency of events in the period just prior to relapse in a sample of schizophrenics being treated in a randomized trial of phenothiazine in the community by contrast with the larger number of nondrug controls who relapsed. In addition, Brown and Birley (1968) showed that their results held regardless of first admission vs readmission status of the patient, and also for first episodes vs relapses.

How severe were the events that preceded the onset of schizophrenic episodes? It is possible to envision a set of events that, when they occur close together in a brief period of time, could approximate the conditions of extreme situations, such as combat (Dohrenwend BP 1979). These consist of fateful loss events, such as death of loved ones occurring outside the person's actual or potential control; events that exhaust the individual physically, especially those involving physical illness or injury that is life-threatening; and, finally, events not previously classified in these two categories that are likely to disrupt social supports, events such as a move from one community to another, a change of job, or a marital separation. When events of each of these three types co-occur in a brief period of time, we have the presence of what we hypothesize to be a pathogenic triad approximating the stress conditions of extreme situations such as prolonged exposure to combat during wartime. Fortunately, Brown and Birley (1968) provide information on the actual events experienced in the 13-week period prior to onset or relapse. It is clear from this material that not one of the cases experienced events from all three elements of our hypothesized pathogenic triad. Moreover, when Brown et al. (1973 b) reanalyzed the data after rating the threatening implications of the events, they found that events with little or no threatening implications were prominent in the build-up of events in the 3-week period prior to onset that differentiated the schizophrenic cases from the well controls. Thus 32% of the cases as against only 13% of the controls had a relatively trivial event in the 3-week period prior to onset (Brown et al. 1973 b, pp. 84–85). On the other hand, these investigators reported that about 16% of the cases experienced events that the investigators judged to be markedly severe over the 13-week period, three times the rate of such events among the controls (Brown et al. 1973 b, p. 84). Both sets of differences were said to hold when checks were run for independent events only. The first result of this reanalysis is one of the main reasons for Brown and colleagues' conclusion that recent events play only a trivial role in onset. The latter result may be one of the reasons they are somewhat tentative about their general conclusion, at least so far as a subgroup of schizophrenics is concerned (Brown et al. 1973 a).

Rogler and Hollingshead (1965) have provided additional relevant data from a study of 20 couples, at least one of whom was diagnosed as schizophrenic following their first contact with a mental health agency. They are compared to very carefully selected matched controls from a slum section of San Juan, Puerto Rico. The particular result of interest is that death of a child was a frequent antecedent to the onset of disorder. Of 12 child deaths in the 40 San Juan families, 11 were concentrated in seven of the families containing one or more schizophrenic parents. Questions can be raised about the role of negligence on the part of the parents, due, perhaps, to personality problems that occurred prior to onset of psychotic episodes. However, there is little evidence of such negligence in the descriptive material provided by Rogler and Hollingshead. There is also evidence in this study of histories of far more serious physical illness and injury in the schizophrenics than in the controls, but the dating of these illnesses with reference to the onset of the disorders is not clear.

In the present retrospective case-control study, we have been investigating a variety of stress-related variables as possible risk factors for episodes of schizophrenic disorder by contrast with episodes of major depression. As a theoretical guide for selecting and organizing these variables, we conceive of life stress processes as having three main structural components (Dohrenwend BS and Dohrenwend BP 1981). The first is *recent events* that occur within a relatively brief time interval (usually a few months to a year). These events can range from extreme situations, such as combat and natural disasters, to the more usual life events that most of us experience at one time or another, such as birth of a child, marriage, death of a loved one, getting a new job, losing a job, and so on. For some purposes, especially when it is possible to take multiple measurements at brief intervals over time, smaller events may be included such as some of those that Lazarus and his colleagues associate with daily "hassles" (Kanner et al. 1981).

In the second major component, the *ongoing social situation*, we include the kinds of circumstances that Brown and Harris (1978) refer to as "ongoing difficulties" and some of the things that Pearlin and Lieberman (1979) refer to as "role strains." Here, the origins of the various elements of the situation antedate the observation period for recent events, but have an impact within the period – a current impact. We pay particular attention to the presence or absence of what we call supportive social networks.

The third component, *personal dispositions*, we conceive of as including genetic or other vulnerabilities related to family history of disorders in first-degree relatives and the residues of remote events, such as early childhood bereavement. With regard to the latter, although we do not know what the current dispositional residue of a remote event such as childhood bereavement might be, we measure whether there was bereavement and we assume that, if it has a current impact, it is via personal dispositions since its effects would long since have been internalized. We also include the presence of prior disorder. And, of central importance, we consider a set of normal personality variables that range from attitudes of mastery to helplessness and include locus of control, Type A behavior pattern, masculinity-femininity (especially with regard to depression), and denial.

The Problem

The questions we address in this paper can be summarized as follows: Are recent stressful life events risk factors in the development of schizophrenic disorders? Are other factors in the ongoing situation risk factors as well? If recent life events and/or variables in the ongoing situation are risk factors, is this evidence that stress from the social environment is an important cause of schizophrenia? In trying to answer the last of these questions, it is necessary to assess the extent to which the events and factors in the ongoing situation are independent not only of prior disorder or insidious onset of disorder, but also of the individual's prior personal dispositions, characteristics, and behavior in general, since we want to evaluate the role of environmentally induced stress. To the extent that the events and situations are themselves functions of personal dispositions, they are by definition of secondary importance compared to the dispositional variables – including, but not limited to, prior disorder or manifestations of the insidious onset of disorder.

Method

The respondents consist of 65 persons with recent schizophrenic episodes, 122 with recent episodes of major depression, and 197 well controls sampled from the general population. The research setting is the Washington Heights section of New York City surrounding the Columbia Presbyterian Medical Center.

The majority of the 65 cases of "schizohrenic disorder" (including mainly DSM-III schizophrenia, but also schizophreniform disorder, brief reactive psychosis, schizoaffective disorders, and atypical psychosis) and of the 122 cases of DSM-III major depression to whom they are being compared were recruited from psychiatric facilities at New York State Psychiatric Institute and the Columbia Presbyterian Medical Center. A small subsample, 24, of the cases of major depression were located in a general population sample from which 197 well controls were also selected. Details of the sampling procedures have been reported elsewhere (Dohrenwend BP et al. 1986).

The psychiatric status of the patients was assessed independently in the form of DSM-III diagnoses. These were either made or supervised by members of the Biometrics Department at New York State Psychiatric Institute under the direction of Robert Spitzer, using clinical records and unstructured clinical interviews (Spitzer et al. 1982; Skodol et al. 1984). Of the schizophrenic disorder cases, 21 were in their first episode, as were 50 of the cases of major depression. The majority (25 of 44) of the repeat episode cases in the schizophrenic disorder group met DSM-III criteria for schizophrenia. Probably because of the 6-month duration of symptoms criterion, the majority (15 of 21) of the first-episode cases were diagnosed as having one of the other nonaffective psychoses mentioned above, rather than DSM-III schizophrenia itself.

To identify the 197 well controls we examined the scores of respondents in the community sample on a set of screening scales that we developed (Dohrenwend BP et al. 1980; Shrout et al. 1986). The Diagnostic Interview Schedule (DIS, Robins et al. 1981), modified to encourage more probing, was also administered by Master's-level mental health professionals to all persons in the community sample who reported high levels of nonspecific distress on one of the screening measures (Dohrenwend BP et al. 1980). More information about the operational definitions of the various case and control groups can be found in Dohrenwend BP et al. (1986).

While it has weaknesses, especially in the representativeness of the case samples, which, except for the small sample of community major depressives, are composed largely of patients, our case-control study has strong points that are missing from previous investigations of this kind. For example, previous case-control studies have compared one type of case with controls or two types of cases without controls. In the present study, the two different types of cases together with a community control group are compared in the same design. Only with such a design can questions be answered about the specificity of potential risk factors, as well as their relative magnitude in comparison to norms in the general population.

In a separate risk factor interview, information was obtained from the cases and controls about their current social circumstances, social network, recent life events, remote landmark events, family history of illness, and personality characteristics by a trained, experienced interviewer. Most questions were asked verbally, although some paper and pencil measures were filled out by the respondent in the presence of the interviewer. Events were probed for date of occurrence and qualitative descriptive information was obtained about what actually happened and the circumstances under which the event occurred (Dohrenwend BP et al. 1987a).

The onsets of disorder for which the cases were selected were established using available clinical data and respondent self-reports. We found that slightly over three-quarters (16/21) of the first-episode cases of schizophrenic disorder involved an acute onset with clear-cut psychotic symptomatology. Sixty-one percent (27/44) of the repeat episodes also showed acute onsets. Among the minority of cases where the development of the disorder was insidious, the date of onset was defined by the earliest significant change from the respondent's usual self that could be attributed to the disorder. Symptoms such as social withdrawal or impairment in personal hygiene were taken to indicate the onset of an episode in these cases.

Our analyses to date have involved comparisons of the schizophrenic disorder case group with the depressed cases and well controls on several of the possible risk factors from each of the three components of the life stress process: recent events, the ongoing situation, and personal dispositions.

Table 1. Demographic characteristics of case and control groups

	Schizophrenic disorder ($n=65$)	Major depression ($n=122$)	Well controls ($n=197$)
Sex			
Male	32 (49%)	30 (25%)	98 (50%)
Female	33 (51%)	92 (75%)	99 (50%)
Ethnicity			
Hispanic	12 (19%)	35 (29%)	44 (22%)
Black	28 (43%)	38 (31%)	56 (28%)
Other	25 (38%)	49 (40%)	97 (49%)
Marital status			
Married	6 (9%)	37 (30%)	113 (57%)
Separated or divorced	25 (39%)	45 (37%)	36 (18%)
Single or widowed	34 (52%)	40 (33%)	48 (24%)
Education			
Not high school graduate	25 (39%)	35 (29%)	38 (19%)
High school graduate	32 (49%)	59 (48%)	92 (47%)
College graduate	8 (12%)	28 (23%)	67 (34%)
Family income			
Less than $ 7000	39 (60%)	48 (39%)	23 (12%)
$ 7000–$ 15000	18 (28%)	35 (29%)	50 (25%)
$ 15000–$ 25000	5 (8%)	27 (22%)	76 (39%)
Over $ 25000	3 (4%)	12 (10%)	48 (24%)
Mean age (standard deviation)	34.2 (12.7)	36.8 (11.9)	40.8 (12.2)
Mean father's occupational prestige (standard deviation) (Treiman 1977)	37.4 (11.6)	42.7 (14.8)	43.0 (13.6)

The life events section of PERI was used to elicit life events (Dohrenwend BS et al. 1978). This is what Katschnig (1980) would describe as "level 3" measurement, in which events are differentiated as to type but not as to detail within type. We are currently working on refining these measures with descriptive data obtained about the nature and details of the events and the changes that occurred following them (Dohrenwend BP et al. 1987 a) and will use some of this information in this paper. In most of the present analyses, however, the life event variables involve level 3 measurement and are simple counts of self-reported events of various theoretically meaningful types that occurred in the year prior to the episode of disorder for which the cases were selected, and the year prior to the interview for controls. The network variables are adapted from the work of Claude Fischer and colleagues (1977). The personality variables are self-report measures developed and/or tested in the course of this project and include such well-known scales as Rotter's (1966) measure of locus of control and the Jenkins activity checklist (Jenkins et al. 1967). More information about and references to published sources on the measures are provided in the summary of results below and elsewhere (Dohrenwend BP et al. 1986).

Our procedure in these analyses has involved testing differences among the case and control groups on the potential risk factors after statistically controlling with analyses of covariance for demographic factors that may have resulted in spurious associations.

The need for the controls is evident from the results in Table 1, which shows that the case groups differ demographically from each other and from the well controls. Note especially the differences on variables indicating present social class status and class background, where the schizophrenic cases are at a pronounced disadvantage to the well controls and, to a lesser extent, the major depressives.

On the basis of these results and a series of further analyses, we decided to control in every comparison the variables of sex, ethnicity (black, Hispanic, other), education (less than high school, high school graduate, college graduate), marital status (never married, divorced or separated, married), age (as a continuous variable), income (in four categories), father's occupational prestige (also continuous), and interaction between ethnicity and father's occupational prestige.

Results

Recent Life Events

The respondents in the risk factor interview were asked about 76 categories of events on the PERI life events list (Dohrenwend BS et al. 1978, 1984). These event categories were combined on a priori grounds into a variety of life event indices that we considered important on theoretical (Dohrenwend BP 1979) and empirical (Dohrenwend BS et al. 1984) grounds. The most important of these a priori groupings are summarized in Table 2.

For purposes of our first set of analyses, an individual's score on each of the indices shown in Table 2 is simply the number of events reported as present in the

Table 2. A priori classifications used to define event variables

---

Event categories in pathogenic triad

A. Fateful loss event occuring to respondent. Examples: child died, laid off,   (12 events)
   physically assaulted or attacked
B. Nonfateful disruptions of supports to respondent Examples: divorced,   (10 events)
   fired, went to jail
C. Illnesses and injuries to respondent. Example: serious illness started or   (2 events)
   got worse

Other event classes mutually exclusive with those above

D. Positive events reflecting respondent's roles or performance. Examples: (13 events)
   graduated from school or training program, promoted, relations with
   spouse changed for better
E. Negative events reflecting respondent's roles or performance. Examples: (17 events)
   relations with spouse changed for worse, demoted, went on welfare

---

year prior to the episode for the cases and the year prior to the interview for controls.

Table 3 compares schizophrenic disorder cases, major depressives, and well controls on each of these indices. Unadjusted means are presented in the left half of the table. Differences adjusted on the basis of controls on demographic variables and tests of significance of these differences are shown on the right.

The first thing to note is that total events did not differentiate cases of either type from controls. This was true whether we considered all events in which the individual was the central figure or all events that happened to another person who was significant to the individual (e.g., spouse or child). Rather, it is the various indices that we constructed on prior theoretical and empirical grounds that show differences; all of those used in the present analysis involve the individual as central figure. The major depressives score higher than the well controls on all four of these indices that are composed of negative life events and the schizophrenic disorder group respondents are higher than the well controls on two out of the four. The well controls score higher than either case group on the index of positive life events.

Fateful loss events (other than physical illness or injury) are negative events that occur outside the actual or potential control of the individual. They are thus independent of his or her personality characteristics and behaviors, including, but not limited to, characteristics and behaviors indicating prior disorder or insidious onset of present disorder. Of the various life event indices shown in Table 3, therefore, fateful loss events have the strongest claim to causal status as a measure of environmentally induced stress. Note that only the major depressives show an elevated rate on this measure, differing significantly from both the schizophrenic disorder group and the controls.

We checked to see if there was a build-up of fateful loss events for the schizophrenics in the month or two prior to the episode, since Brown and Birley (1968) found such a build-up for what they termed "independent events." We find no such build up for fateful loss events. This may be because our definition of fateful loss differs markedly, as we mentioned earlier, from Brown and Birley's more in-

Table 3. Means on life event indices across schizophrenic disorder group, major depressives, and well controls

Life event index	Unadjusted means (n)			Significance of overall	Adjusted differences between groups		
	A Schizophrenic	B Depressed	C Well	F	A vs C	B vs C	A vs B
Total events	4.77	5.98	5.21	0.29	−0.45	0.83	−1.28
Triad events:							
Fateful loss to respondent	0.38	0.80	0.46	0.02	0.02	0.38[b]	−0.36[a]
Physical illness or injury to respondent	0.25	0.30	0.11	0.001	0.14[b]	0.21[d]	−0.07
Events likely to induce losses in network support	0.77	0.69	0.25	0.001	0.39[d]	0.36[d]	0.03
Events indicating negative role performance	0.62	0.70	0.36	0.014	0.13	0.38[c]	−0.25
Events indicating positive role performance	0.69	0.64	1.28	0.027	−0.54[a]	−0.58[c]	0.04

[a] $p < 0.1$; [b] $p < 0.05$; [c] $p < 0.01$; [d] $p < 0.001$.

clusive definition of "independence," which turns on whether the event could be influenced by prior disorder or the insidious onset of the present disorder but not on other kinds of personal dispositions; thus, Brown and colleagues included under "independence" not only what we call fateful loss events but also, for example, positive events related to the respondent's performance. Moreover, in the index of fateful loss used here, the respondent is always the central figure in the event, while Brown and colleagues included positive and negative events occurring to significant others in their measure of independent events.

Next to the fateful loss events, serious physical illnesses and injuries appear most likely to have causal status as sources of environmentally induced stress, since many occur outside the actual or potential control of the individual. Like the depressives, the schizophrenic disorder cases show a significantly elevated rate of such events. However, we used the qualitative descriptions by the respondent of what actually happened in each event to check on whether these illnesses and injuries introduced a substantial change in the lives of the respondents. When illness and injury events rated by us as showing "no change lasting a week or more" were removed from the analysis, the difference between the schizophrenic cases and the controls disappeared. Only the depressives continued to show an elevated rate. This was the only major modification that resulted when this check was extended to all of the measures reported in Table 3.

The one type of event from our pathogenic triad (fateful loss, physical illness and injury, and nonfateful events likely to disrupt social supports) in which the schizophrenic disorder respondents show a higher rate than controls even when trivial (no change) events are excluded is nonfateful events that are likely to disrupt their social supports. The schizophrenic disorder cases also have fewer events related to positive role performance than controls and show a tendency, which becomes significant when "no change" events are removed, to score higher on events indicating negative role performance. In these respects, they tend to resemble the major depressives.

With one exception, the results just described appear to hold for both first-episode and repeat-episode cases of schizophrenic disorder. The exception is for events indicating positive role performance. These are reported almost as frequently by first-episode cases, 0.905, as by well controls, 1.025, by contrast with only 0.312 in repeat-episode cases. The difference may well be evidence of a deficit in social functioning consequent upon factors associated with the occurrence of prior disorder in the repeat episode cases.

Social Networks

As mentioned earlier, we followed the procedure developed by Claude Fischer and colleagues (1977) for eliciting the members of the social networks of our cases and controls. Briefly, this involved asking each person in the study to name those individuals with whom he or she had or could have had supportive exchanges in areas of activity such as care of children, watching the house while he or she was away, discussion of decisions at work, discussion of personal problems, borrowing money, and social recreational activities. From this information we constructed such network variables as size and extensiveness (the number and density of coverage of the areas of activity).

The networks of the schizophrenic disorder cases in the year prior to their episodes were particularly weak compared to those of both the depressives and the controls. As Table 4 shows, the networks of the schizophrenic disorder cases are the smallest, least extensive, have the fewest instrumental supporters, and tend to have the fewest social companions and confidants. By and large, these differences hold for both first-episode and repeat-episode cases of schizophrenic disorder, although the networks of the first-episode cases appear somewhat larger, 6.38 vs 5.57.

Personality Variables

Under the general heading of personal dispositions, we are investigating a set of variations in normal personality ranging from attitudes of mastery at one pole to helplessness at the other. This basic dimension can be seen to have interesting variants at each extreme, some of them likely to lead to poor coping in certain stress situations. At the mastery end, for example, one can put extreme Type A personality reactions that may well lead to problems in coping (Matthews and Glass 1983). And it is interesting to consider how closely attitudes of mastery appear to coincide with masculine personality characteristics and helplessness with feminine ones, as measured, for example, by the Spence-Helmreich scales (1978). This particular variant of the mastery-helplessness dimension may have implications for the development of depression, a disorder that is far more prevalent in women than in men.

With this introduction, our choice of some of the personality measures should come as no surprise. They include the measures of locus of control developed by Rotter (1966) and Levenson (1973), Jenkins' measure of Type A behavior (Jenkins et al. 1967), and a set of items that we are calling "mastery orientation" from Spence and Helmreich (1978). They also include a scale of denial that we constructed from various sources such as Crowne and Marlowe (1960) and Epstein and Fenz (1967).

Table 5 summarizes the comparisons on these personality variables. Note that by contrast with the controls, the respondents in the schizophrenic disorder group tend to be high on external locus of control, high on denial, and low on mastery orientation. They share these characteristics with the major depressives, differing from them only in showing less Type A behavior and less tendency to endorse negative femininity items. There are no differences between first- and repeat-episode cases of schizophrenic disorder on these personality variables.

Remote Events and Situations

We have inquired into a number of past events and situations in the lives of our respondents and have been able to analyze some of them. The results are presented in Table 6.

Table 4. Means on network variables across schizophrenic disorder group, major depressives, and well controls

Risk factor variable	Unadjusted means (n)			Significance of overall	Adjusted differences between groups		
	A Schizophrenic	B Depressed	C Well	F	A vs C	B vs C	A vs B
Size of social network	5.83 (65)	8.25 (122)	10.24 (197)	0.01	-2.3^c	-0.93^a	-1.41^a
Extensiveness of network	8.06 (65)	9.32 (122)	10.04 (197)	0.001	-1.19^d	-0.42^a	-0.77^c
Multiplexity of network	45.79 (65)	54.87 (122)	43.56 (197)	0.004	-5.54	5.36^b	-10.90^d
Density of network	0.47 (53)	0.38 (109)	0.46 (191)	0.004	-0.02	-0.12^c	0.10^b
Number of instrumental supporters	3.43 (65)	5.09 (122)	6.01 (197)	0.013	-1.41^c	-0.26	-1.16^c
Number of social companions	2.74 (65)	4.03 (122)	5.19 (197)	0.002	-2.13^c	-1.27^c	0.86
Number of confidants	2.37 (65)	3.42 (122)	3.21 (197)	0.17	-0.34	0.32	-0.66^a

[a] $p<0.1$; [b] $p<0.05$; [c] $p<0.01$; [d] $p<0.001$.

Table 5. Means on personality variables across schizophrenic disorder group, major depressives, and well controls

Risk factor variable	Unadjusted means (n)			Significance of overall	Adjusted differences between groups		
	A Schizophrenic	B Depressed	C Well	F	A vs C	B vs C	A vs B
Levenson internal-external locus of control	3.38 (63)	3.16 (121)	2.69 (197)	0.001	0.56^d	0.41^d	0.15
Rotter internal-external locus of control	1.46 (64)	1.48 (120)	1.37 (192)	0.001	0.05^a	0.08^d	-0.03
Jenkins speed and impatience factors type A behavior pattern	0.35 (58)	0.42 (120)	0.34 (196)	0.001	0.05^a	0.11^d	-0.06^b
Spence-Helmreich selected positive masculinity items – mastery	3.28 (62)	3.15 (121)	3.74 (197)	0.001	-0.48^d	-0.55^d	0.07
Negative keyed negative items selected from Crowne-Marlowe, Epstein-Fenz – denial	1.42 (62)	1.46 (122)	1.35 (197)	0.001	0.06^b	0.11^d	-0.05^a
Spench-Helmreich selected negative femininity items	3.45 (61)	3.74 (122)	3.18 (197)	0.001	0.13	0.44^d	-0.31^b

[a] $p<0.1$; [b] $p<0.05$; [c] $p<0.01$; [d] $p<0.001$.

Table 6. Rates of selected remote events and situations experienced by schizophrenic disorder group, major depressives, and well controls

Remote event or situation	Unadjusted percentages			Significance of overall F	Adjusted differences in log odd ratios between groups		
	A Schizophrenic (n=65)	B Depressed (n=122)	C Well (n=197)		A vs C	B vs C	A vs B
Death of mother before respondent reached age 11	3.1	3.3	2.1	ns	0.13	0.50	−0.37
Separation from parents for a year or more before age 18 (parents still alive when respondent reached age 18)	27.1 (n=48)	42.5 (n=87)	33.1 (n=145)	<0.10	−0.61	0.37	−0.97[a]
Mother household head	52.3	41.0	36.1	ns	0.17	0.03	0.14
Raised mainly by mother (no knowledge of father)	9.2	10.7	1.5	<0.03	1.84[b]	1.83[b]	0.01
Raised mainly by institution (no knowledge of father)	6.2	3.3	3.0	ns	−0.11	−0.54	0.43
Friends in trouble with authorities before age 18 (available for subsample only)	47.1 (n=34)	34.4 (n=61)	19.4 (n=98)	<0.02	1.31[b]	1.08[b]	−0.23
Trouble with law enforcement authorities before age 18 (available for subsample only)	20.6 (n=34)	14.8 (n=61)	7.1 (n=98)	ns	1.51[a]	0.52	−0.99
Noisome first occupation	32.2	13.1	10.2	<0.005	1.46[c]	0.46	1.0[b]
Death of one or more children (among those with children)	19.0 (n=21)	18.6 (n=70)	13.7 (n=117)	ns	−0.16	0.14	−0.31
Past life-threatening illness or injury to respondent	41.5	44.3	28.4	<0.001	1.05[c]	0.96[d]	0.09

[a] $p<0.1$; [b] $p<0.05$; [c] $p<0.01$; [d] $p<0.001$.

Two of the variables that we included because of findings from previous research do not appear to differentiate our groups of cases from controls. One of these is death of mother before age 11, which we thought might show a higher rate in the depressive cases. We did not find an elevated rate, even in community cases where Brown and Harris' (1978) results would lead us to expect one. The other remote event we thought might be important is death of one or more children, which differentiated schizophrenic cases from controls in the study by Rogler and Hollingshead (1965). These variables excepted, Table 6 shows a pattern of past adversity and past problems for both case groups, but especially for the schizophrenic disorder group, by contrast with the controls.

Respondents in both case groups were more likely to be raised mainly by their mothers with no knowledge of their fathers, to have had friends who got into trouble with authorities before they were age 18, and to have suffered one or more life-threatening physical illnesses or injuries. In addition, the schizophrenic disorder cases tended to get in trouble with authorities themselves before age 18, to have blue-collar first jobs that were characterized by noisome features such as danger, physical arduousness, noise, or dirt. We have analyzed this last factor in considerable detail and concluded that it cannot be explained away by selective factors, since, for example, these first jobs proved to be no lower in prestige than the first jobs of controls from similar backgrounds and actually paid somewhat higher than blue-collar jobs that were not characterized by noisome characteristics of this kind (Link et al. 1986). These differences appear to hold for both first-episode and repeat-episode cases, but the difference on noisome occupations is sharper for the first-episode cases (Link et al. 1986). This suggests that exposure to noisome occupational characteristics may sometimes, at least, act as a factor in the ongoing situation or even as a recent event rather than as a remote situation or event. We will conduct further analyses on this question.

Family History of Psychiatric Disorders

Our measure of family history is primitive. We use reports by the respondents about the psychiatric problems of their first-degree relatives rather than the more satisfactory procedure of conducting direct interviews with the relatives themselves (Orvaschel et al. 1982), and we did not question in detail about symptomatology. Each respondent was asked whether each of his or her first-degree relatives had ever had "serious mental or emotional problems such as problems with depression, suicide attempts, odd or violent behavior, or difficulties with drugs or alcohol." If the answer was affirmative, the respondent was further asked to name "the specific mental or emotional problem(s) that the relative(s) had" and whether the relative was "ever in a hospital" for the specific problem. If outpatient treatment was mentioned, this was also recorded. Two psychiatrists independently rated the replies, with quite satisfactory reliability (Dohrenwend BP et al. 1986). Matthias Angermeyer took the lead in developing this measure.

Table 7 shows that family history provides one of the sharpest contrasts of any of the possible risk factors so far tested between the case groups and the well controls. Majorities of the two case groups have at least one first-degree relative

Table 7. Comparisons of percentages of individuals with positive family history for psychiatric disorder in general and of four specific types across schizophrenic disorder group, major depressives, and well controls

Family history type	Unadjusted percentages			Significance of overall	Adjusted differences in log odd ratios between groups		
	A Schizophrenic (n=65)	B Depressed (n=122)	C Well (n=197)	F	A vs C	B vs C	A vs B
One or more first-degree relatives with probable mental disorder of any type	52.3	62.3	25.9	0.000	1.16[c]	1.63[e]	−0.47
One or more first-degree relatives with each of the following subtypes:							
Affective	16.9	31.1	11.2	0.000	1.16[b]	1.77[e]	−0.61
Psychotic	12.3	4.1	0.5	0.000	3.90[c]	2.66[b]	1.24[a]
Alcoholism	27.7	27.0	11.7	0.025	0.89[b]	0.96[c]	−0.08
Antisocial	9.2	9.8	2.0	0.05	1.34[a]	1.51[b]	−0.17

[a] $p<0.1$; [b] $p<0.05$; [c] $p<0.01$; [d] $p<0.001$; [e] $p<0.0001$.

with a probable mental disorder, by contrast with only a quarter of the controls. Note that the cases have more alcoholism and more antisocial behavior among their first-degree relatives. Finally, note that the schizophrenic disorder cases describe the highest rate of psychotic disorder in their first-degree relatives while the depressives describe the highest rate of affective disorder, although the latter difference is not statistically significant between the two case groups. These differences hold for both first- and repeat-episode cases.

DSM-III Schizophrenia

In the preceding analyses, we checked on whether differences in the various possible risk factors held for first- and repeat-episode cases. This provided an indication of whether they might be important for both onset and course of disorder.

Two-thirds of the repeat-episode cases met criteria for DSM-III schizophrenia, by contrast with slightly less than 30% of the first-episode cases. While number of episodes and diagnostic type within the schizophrenic disorder group are highly correlated, the question can still be raised as to whether, given the diagnostic heterogeneity of the group, the results would hold for the more homogeneous diagnostic subgroup of DSM-III schizophrenics. We have, therefore, repeated the above analyses excluding all but the DSM-III schizophrenics from the schizophrenic disorder group. Although we did not attempt statistical tests due to the decrease of power, the differences with the controls and depressives seem even sharper. There is, however, one unaccountable anomaly – a tendency for the DSM-III schizophrenics to have a lower proportion of first-degree relatives with psychotic disorders and a higher proportion of relatives showing antisocial behavior than other members of the schizophrenic disorder group.

Discussion

Let us return to the questions with which we began: How important are recent life events and factors in the ongoing situation in episodes of schizophrenic disorder? Do they indicate that environmentally induced stress is an important cause of schizophrenia?

The most important set of findings with regard to our question about the role of environmentally induced stress from recent events and the ongoing situation has to do with fateful loss events. Fateful loss events are the type of recent event most likely to be independent of personal dispositions and hence the clearest source of environmentally induced stress. This type of event showed an elevated rate prior to the episodes of depressed cases but not prior to the episodes of the schizophrenic disorder cases. Nor was there a build-up of such events in the 3-week period prior to onset of schizophrenic episodes such as Brown and Birley (1968) found for events they defined as "independent." This difference between our results and theirs is important for our questions. As we noted earlier, our definition of fateful loss overlaps but differs from that of Brown and his colleagues.

The nature of the difference and its implications can be understood in the context of Rutter's recent discussion of the notion of independence:

One of the important methodological advances in life events research was the recognition that it is necessary to separate events that might have been brought about by the mental disorder from those that were independent (e.g. Brown et al. 1973 b). For obvious reasons, the causal hypothesis could be tested adequately only through the use of independent events. However, that leaves several crucial matters unaddressed. To begin with, the notion of independence from the illness is by no means the same as independence from the person. Some investigators (Brown and Harris 1978) have largely restricted the concept to the illness, but this allows all sorts of events to be classified as "independent" when in fact the person's own behavior may have played a role in bringing the event about (Rutter 1986, p. 1084).

The fact that "all sorts of events" (not only what we define as fateful loss events, but also positive events and events that occurred to significant others) were defined as "independent" was the basis for the finding, in the Brown and Birley study, not only that an excess of independent events built up in the 3 weeks prior to onset but also that these events tended to embody little or no threat. We must agree with Brown and colleagues that this finding indicates that life events play only a trivial role in causing schizophrenic disorder. Given their definition of "independence" we cannot tell, moreover, whether the build-up of events indicated any direct role for environmentally induced stress. Again, Rutter's discussion will help clarify the issue:

The issue of what causes life stressors is not just a methodological quibble over the criteria for independence; the question is central to the study of life events. If acute stressors and chronic adversities play a role in the causation of psychiatric disorder, we must ask why it is that some people have more adverse experiences than do others. Is it chance or ill luck? Or, rather, are the negative experiences explicable in terms of individual characteristics or past adversities? Insofar as they are due to individual features, are these ones that are linked genetically with hereditary influences that predispose to ... (disorder)? It is now appreciated that to an important extent, genetically determined qualities can serve to create environments. Equally, it is evident, however, that adult functioning is shaped in part by chains of indirect environmental linkages deriving from adversities in childhood (Rutter 1986, p. 1084).

Physical illness and injury events are the types of events that, next to fateful loss events, are most likely to be sources of environmentally induced stress. When we removed trivial physical illness and injury events, there was no difference between the schizophrenic disorder cases and controls. As with fateful loss events, this is again in contrast with the depressives who show elevations on both types of events even when trivial events are removed. Other types of recent events (e.g., nonfateful events likely to disrupt social supports) and aspects of the ongoing social situation (e.g., weak social networks) that are less likely than fateful loss events or physical illness and injury events to be independent of the personal dispositions of the individual did differentiate between schizohrenic disorder cases and well controls. Moreover, the networks of the schizophrenic cases were weaker than those not only of the controls but also of the depressives.

Present personality characteristics together with family history of mental disorders, remote events, and other past adverse circumstances that might be expected to have shaped current personal dispositions differentiated schizophrenic disorder cases from well controls. More past adverse circumstances differentiated the schizophrenic disorder group than differentiated the depressives from the controls.

Taking these findings at face value, what are their implications for our questions? There is a clear contrast with the major depressive cases. For the major depressives, recent environmentally induced stress appears to be an important risk factor. For the schizophrenic disorder cases, although recent events and weak networks play a role among the factors leading to a schizophrenic episode, the events themselves and the weak networks are likely to have occurred in considerable part, at least, because of sets of more important factors, the personal dispositions of the individual that are indicated by measured personality characteristics, remote events and circumstances, and family histories of mental disorder. We are investigating ways to examine relationships among these sets of variables directly in further analyses.

Does the prominence of personal dispositions in our results mean that socioenvironmental factors are not important risk factors for schizophrenic episodes? We think that it would be incorrect to draw this conclusion at this point. Schizophrenia is a disorder that is inversely related to social class and this relationship is probably stronger for schizophrenia than for major depression (Dohrenwend BP 1983). While the results of previous research are not consistent on whether parental social class is also lower (Turner and Wagenfeld 1967) or no different from what would be expected (Goldberg and Morrison 1963), it is certainly lower in this sample. We think that it will prove lower in general if a clear distinction is made between white collar and blue collar occupations in defining the class difference. For the present sample of schizophrenic disorder cases there is a sharp difference in own and parental class between the schizophrenic disorder cases and both the depressives and the controls (see Table 1). It seems likely, therefore, that at least some of the differences we have found on indicators of personal dispositions stem from the adverse social environments associated with lower-class backgrounds. Perhaps this is most evident in the results on noisome first occupations which are almost invariably blue collar (Link et al. 1986).

Although we controlled on class background, we did not control on the multitude of factors that are associated with such backgrounds. Some of these early adverse circumstances appear to apply to both major depressives and schizophrenic disorder cases: a family history of mental disorder in first-degree relatives, having friends in trouble with authorities, being raised by mother alone with no knowledge of father, and having past life-threatening illnesses. Others, however, appear specific to the schizophrenic disorder cases: having one or more first-degree relatives with psychotic disorders, getting in early trouble with authorities, having a first occupation with noisome characteristics. Thus, while personal dispositions appear to be more important than recent events and/or network characteristics that are environmentally induced, another issue must be raised if we are to answer the larger question of the role of socioenvironmental factors of remote as well as recent origin. To what extent are the dispositions themselves a function of socialization in adverse environments, and to what extent are they a function of genetic inheritance? And if, as is highly likely, both are involved, what are the relations between the two sets of factors?

We must raise the question, however, of whether these results should be taken at face value. Consider two weaknesses in our study that could be the basis for calling the results into question. The first has to do with the possibility that the differences on the personality variables may turn out to be state-dependent (see Hirschfeld et al. 1983 a, b). Unlike the life event and network variables, the personality items were meant to measure enduring traits of the respondents. We did not ask the respondents in the two case groups, therefore, to refer their responses to our personality questions to a particular time period prior to the episodes of disorder for which we recruited them. It is possible, nevertheless, that their responses to the items are affected by the episode of disorder. If the responses are in fact state-dependent consequences of the episode, the personality differences would of course lose their status as risk factors in the development of the disorders. We shall try to investigate this possibility by following the cases into episode-free periods, readministering the personality measures, and checking to see if the earlier differences from the controls tend to disappear.

The second problem has to do with the possibility of biases in our sample of cases. One basis for Dohrenwend BP and Egri's (1981) earlier conclusion that environmentally induced stress related to recent life events might be more important in schizophrenia than was generally assumed was the lack of representativeness of case samples in previous studies. Like the earlier London (Brown and Birley 1968) and New Haven (Jacobs and Myers 1976) studies, however, the present study has also focused on cases of schizophrenic disorder recruited largely from psychiatric inpatients. Zubin and Spring (1977) have suggested that as a result of relying on such samples, "Our information is biased by the fact that many episodes in highly competent individuals are not recorded in our statistics and by the fact that those who fill our hospitals and clinics are largely poor premorbid, relapsing patients" (1977, p. 123). Following Zubin and Spring, and drawing as well on the military literature and the WHO cross-cultural studies (Sartorius et al. 1978), Dohrenwend BP and Egri (1981) argued that possible sampling biases may have led to results that underestimate the role of recent life events. By extension, such a bias could have also affected the results of the present study (see Cohen and Cohen 1984).

We will get help on these questions about the effects of possible sampling biases from data that we are now collecting in Israel from more representative samples of persons with these and other types of psychiatric disorder (Dohrenwend BP et al. 1987 b). Meanwhile, probably our best evidence that the findings will replicate is the fact that the present results hold, by and large, for the more acute first-episode cases as well as the more chronic repeat-episode cases, and for those schizophrenic disorder cases who meet DSM-III criteria for schizophrenia as well as those who meet criteria for other nonaffective, nonorganic psychoses.

Conclusion

If they hold up with tests of state dependence and more representative samples of cases, the results we have reported suggest that one of us will have to modify his earlier conclusion. Recent environmentally induced stress from life events does not appear to be of primary importance as a risk factor for episodes of schizophrenia. Accepted at face value, the results suggest that in the search for environmental causes we give greater emphasis to class-related socialization experiences in adverse family and other early social environments. Relative to such factors, recent stressful life events and networks appear to be of secondary and derivative, though not necessarily negligible, importance.

References

Brown GW, Birley JLT (1968) Crises and life changes and the onset of schizophrenia. J Health Soc Behav 9:203–214

Brown GW, Harris TO (1978) Social origins of depression. Free Press, New York

Brown GW, Harris TO, Peto J (1973a) Life events and psychiatric disorders, part 2: nature of the causal link. Psychol Med 3:159–176

Brown GW, Sklair F, Harris TO, Birley JLT (1973b) Life events and psychiatric disorders, part 1: some methodological issues. Psychol Med 3:74–87

Cohen P, Cohen J (1984) The clinician's illusion. Arch Gen Psychiatry 41:1178–1182

Crowne DP, Marlowe D (1960) The approval motive: studies in evaluative dependence. Wiley, New York

Day R (1981) Life events and schizophrenia: the "triggering" hypothesis. Acta Psychiatr Scand 64:97–122

Dohrenwend BP (1979) Stressful life events and psychopathology: some issues of theory and method. In: Barrett JF, Rose RM, Klerman GL (eds) Stress and mental disorder. Raven, New York, pp 1–15

Dohrenwend BP (1983) The epidemiology of mental disorders. In: Mechanic D (ed) Handbook of health, health care, and the health professions. Free Press, New York, pp 157–194

Dohrenwend BP, Dohrenwend, BS (1969) Social status and psychological disorder: a causal inquiry. Wiley, New York

Dohrenwend BP, Egri G (1981) Recent stressful life events and episodes of schizophrenia. Schizophr Bull 7:12–23

Dohrenwend BP, Dohrenwend BS, Gould MS, Link B, Neugebauer R, Wunsch-Hitzig R (1980) Mental illness in the United States: epidemiologic estimates. Praeger, New York

Dohrenwend BP, Shrout PE, Link B, Martin J, Skodol A (1986) Overview of initial results from a risk factor study of depression and schizophrenia. In: Barrett JE (ed) Mental disorders in the community: progress and challenge. Guilford Press, New York, pp 184–215

Dohrenwend BP, Link BG, Kern R, Shrout PE, Markowitz J (1987a) Measuring life events: the problem of variability within event categories. In: Cooper B (ed) Psychiatric epidemiology: progress and prospects. Croom Helm, London

Dohrenwend BP, Levav I, Shrout PE, Link BG, Skodol AE (1987b) Life stress and psychopathology. Am J Community Psychol (to be published)

Dohrenwend BS, Dohrenwend BP (1981) Life stress and psychopathology. In: Regier DA, Allen G (eds) Risk factor research in the major mental disorders. National Institute of Mental Health DHHS Publ No (ADM) 81–1068. Superintendent of Documents, US Government Printing Office, Washington, DC 20402, pp 131–141

Dohrenwend BS, Krasnoff L, Askenasy AR, Dohrenwend BP (1978) Exemplification of a method for scaling life events: the PERI life events scale. J Health Soc Behav 19:205–229

Dohrenwend BS, Dohrenwend BP, Dodson M, Shrout PE (1984) Symptoms, hassles, social supports and life events: the problem of confounded measures. J Abnorm Psychol 93:222–230

Dunham WH (1965) Community and schizophrenia: an epidemiological analysis. Wayne State University Press, Detroit

Eaton WW, Boyd JH (1985) Epidemiology of schizophrenia. Epidemiol Rev 7:105–126

Epstein S, Fenz WD (1967) The detection of areas of emotional stress through variations in perceptual threshold and psychological arousal. J Exp Res Personality 2:191–199

Faris R, Dunham WH (1939) Mental disorders in urban areas. University of Chicago Press, Chicago

Fischer CS, Jackson RM, Stueve CA, Gerson K, Jones LM, Baldassare M (1977) Networks and places: social relations in the urban setting. Free Press, New York

Goldberg EM, Morrison SL (1963) Schizophrenia and social class. Br J Psychiatry 109:785–802

Gottesman II, Shields J (1976) A critical review of recent adoption, twin, and family studies of schizophrenia: behavioral genetics perspectives. Schizophr Bull 2:360–401

Hirschfeld R, Klerman G, Clayton P, Keller M (1983a) Personality and depression. Arch Gen Psychiatry 40:993–998

Hirschfeld R, Klerman GL, Clayton PJ, Keller MB, McDonald S, Larkin BH (1983b) Assessing personality: effects of the depressive state on trait measurement. Am J Psychiatry 140:695–699

Hudgens RW (1974) Personal catastrophe and depression: a consideration of the subject with respect to medically ill adolescents, and a requiem for retrospective life event studies. In: Dohrenwend BS, Dohrenwend BP (eds) Stressful life events: their nature and effects. Wiley, New York, pp 110–134

Jacobs SC, Myers JK (1976) Recent life events and acute schizophrenic psychosis: a controlled study. J Nerv Ment Dis 162:75–87

Jenkins CD, Roseman RH, Friedman M (1967) Development of an objective psychological test for the determination of the coronary-prone behavior pattern. J Chronic Dis 20:371–379

Kanner AD, Coyne JC, Schaefer C, Lazarus RS (1981) Comparison of two modes of stress measurement: daily hassles and uplifts versus major life events. J Behav Med 4:1–39

Katschnig H (1980) A critique of the global approach in life event research. In: Katschnig H (ed) Sozialer Streß und psychische Krankheit. Urban and Schwarzenberg, Wien

Kohn M (1972) Class family and schizophrenia: a reformulation. Soc Forces 50:295–304

Leff JP, Hirsch S, Gaind R, Rohde PD, Stevens BS (1973) Life events and maintenance therapy in schizophrenic relapse. Br J Psychiatry 123:659–660

Levenson H (1973) Multidimensional locus of control in psychiatric patients. J Consult Clin Psychol 41:397–404

Link BG, Dohrenwend BP, Skodol AE (1986) Socioeconomic status and schizophrenia: noisome occupational characteristics as a risk factor. Am Sociol Rev 51:242–258

Lukoff D, Snyder K, Ventura J, Nuechterlein KH (1984) Life events, familial stress, and coping in the developmental course of schizophrenia. Schizophr Bull 10:258–292

Matthews KA, Glass DC (1983) Type A behavior, stressful life events, and coronary heart disease. In: Dohrenwend BS, Dohrenwend BP (eds) Stressful life events and their contexts. Rutgers University Press, New Brunswick, pp 167–177

Mechanic D (1972) Social class and schizophrenia: some requirements for a plausible theory of social influence. Soc Forces 50:305–309

Mischler EG, Scotch NA (1965) Sociocultural factors in the epidemiology of schizophrenia: a review. Int J Psychiatry 1:258–293

Orvaschel HO, Thompson WD, Belanger A, Prusoff BA, Kidd KK (1982) Comparison of the family history method to direct interview: factors affecting the diagnosis of depression. J Affective Disord 4:49–59

Paykel ES (1978) Contribution of life events to causation of psychiatric illness. Psychol Med 8:245–253

Pearlin LI, Lieberman MA (1979) Social sources of emotional distress. In: Simmon RG (ed) Research in community and mental health, vol 1. JAI Press, Greenwich CT, pp 217–247

Rabkin JG (1980) Stressful life events and schizophrenia: a review of the research literature, Psychol Bull 87:408–425

Robins L, Helzer JE; Crougham R, Ratcliff KS (1981) National Institute of Mental Health Diagnostic Interview Schedule: its history, characteristics and validity. Arch Gen Psychiatry 38:381–389

Rogler LH, Hollingshead AB (1965) Trapped. Families and schizophrenia. Wiley, New York

Rotter JB (1966) Generalized expectancies of internal versus external control of reinforcement. Psychol Monogr 80:609

Rutter M (1986) Meyerian psychobiology, personality development, and the role of life experiences. Am J Psychiatry 143(9):1077–1087

Sartorius N, Jablensky A, Shapiro R (1978) Cross-cultural differences in the short-term prognosis of schizophrenic psychoses. Schizophr Bull 4:102–113

Shrout PE, Dohrenwend BP, Levav I (1986) A discriminant rule for screening cases of diverse diagnostic types: preliminary results. J Consult Clin Psychol (54)3:314–319

Skodol AE, Williams JBW, Spitzer RL, Gibbon M, Kass F (1984) Identifying common errors in the use of DSM-III through diagnostic supervision. Hosp Community Psychiatry 35:251–255

Spence JT, Helmreich R (1978) Masculinity and femininity: their psychological dimensions, correlates and antecedents. University of Texas Press, Austin

Spitzer R, Skodol AE, Williams J et al. (1982) Supervising intake diagnosis: a psychiatric Rashomon. Arch Psychiatry 39:1299–1305

Treiman (1977) Occupational prestige in comparative perspective. Academic, New York

Turner RJ, Wagenfeld MO (1967) Occupational mobility and schizophrenia: an assessment of the social causation and social selection hypotheses. Am Sociol Rev 32:104–113

Zubin J, Spring B (1977) Vulnerability: a new view of schizophrenia. J Abnorm Psychol 86:103–126

Vulnerability Models for Schizophrenia: State of the Art

K. H. NUECHTERLEIN

Rationale for Vulnerability Models

Vulnerability models for schizophrenic disorders have been developed to take into account several basic observations regarding the nature of these illnesses. First, the evidence for genetic factors in schizophrenic disorders is strong, yet the occurrence of schizophrenia among biological relatives does not seem to follow any simple, single-gene, Mendelian pattern (Matthysse and Kidd 1976; Gottesman and Shields 1982). Furthermore, although monozygotic twins have a concordance rate for schizophrenia that is clearly higher than that of dizygotic twins, the probandwise concordance rate is far from 100%, typically being 40%–50% in recent studies (Gottesman and Shields 1982). Thus, clinical schizophrenia per se is not directly inherited, but rather genes are viewed as influencing vulnerability to schizophrenic disorders.

A second observation about the nature of schizophrenia that favors a vulnerability conception is the increasing recognition that a substantial proportion of patients with schizophrenic disorders, at least under current treatment conditions, are characterized by periods of active psychosis interspersed with periods of substantial improvement or recovery rather than by continuous psychosis (Zubin and Spring 1977; Bleuler 1978; Ciompi 1980; Zubin et al. 1983). The connecting link in repetition of schizophrenic episodes in such individuals can be conceptualized as a continued level of personal vulnerability to schizophrenic psychotic episodes, which causes certain individuals to be more likely than others to have such episodes even after improvement or recovery occurs.

A final observation that favors a vulnerability conception is that environmental potentiators or stressors appear to play a role in the return of schizophrenic psychotic episodes in some patients (Brown and Birley 1968; Brown et al. 1972; Vaughn and Leff 1976; Vaughn et al. 1984; Nuechterlein et al. 1986b). Other patients, however, show an onset or return of episodes that is very gradual and not related to environmental stressors in any obvious way (reviewed by Lukoff et al. 1984). Postulating a continuum of vulnerability for schizophrenic psychosis accommodates this observation by suggesting that substantial environmental stress is necessary to precipitate episodes of schizophrenic psychosis in persons with only moderate vulnerability levels, whereas little or no particular environmental stress is needed to generate schizophrenic psychotic symptoms in those with very high levels of personal vulnerability.

Department of Psychiatry and Biobehavioral Sciences, University of California, Los Angeles, 760 Westwood Plaza, Los Angeles, CA 90024, USA

Of course, the view that the onset and course of illness are influenced by personal vulnerability factors or predispositions and by environmental potentiators and stressors is not unique to schizophrenia but is shared with a wide variety of psychiatric and medical disorders (Elliott and Eisdorfer 1982; Lazarus and Folkman 1984). However, the nature of the vulnerability factors and of the mechanisms by which they affect symptom formation would be expected to differ across disorders, such that some vulnerability factors and mechanisms would be relatively specific to schizophrenic disorders, whereas others would have more general relevance to a variety of illnesses.

Strategies for Isolation of Vulnerability Factors

Several different strategies for identification of potential factors in vulnerability to schizophrenia can be distinguished. One set focusses on groups at "high risk" for schizophrenic psychosis, because studies that contrast patients who have already developed schizophrenia with matched, nonschizophrenic groups can offer clues to possible vulnerability factors but have great difficulty separating vulnerability factors for schizophrenic disorders from the consequences of such disorders (Garmezy and Streitman 1974; Mednick and McNeil 1968).

The study of groups at heightened risk for schizophrenic disorders allows observations to be gathered before the onset of major psychotic symptoms and associated treatment, thereby eliminating retrospective bias in reporting and confusion of precursors with consequences. The most popular means of selecting subjects at heightened risk is to study children born to a schizophrenic parent, who have a 10%–15% risk of developing adult schizophrenia as compared to a general population risk of 1% or less (Rosenthal 1970; Gottesman and Shields 1982). A variant of this is to study siblings of schizophrenic patients. Studying first-degree relatives has the advantages of well-documented risk figures and the availability of genetic models to quantify expected frequencies of a vulnerability factor under different modes of transmission.

A second high-risk strategy is to study people who present with hypothesized schizotypal personality characteristics to determine whether they have nonsymptomatic characteristics that might be vulnerability factors for psychosis (Chapman et al. 1978; Steronko and Woods 1978; Nuechterlein 1985). A third high-risk strategy has been the longitudinal study of families of adolescents with nonpsychotic disturbances to determine those characteristics that discriminate the families of adolescents who later develop a schizophrenia spectrum disorder from those with more benign outcomes (Goldstein et al. 1978; Rodnick et al. 1984). Finally, a recently developed high-risk strategy that reverses the usual dependent and independent variables has been to select subjects on the basis of the presence of potential vulnerability factors and then examine associated personality or symptomatic features that are believed to indicate increased risk for schizophrenia (Buchsbaum et al. 1978; Venables et al. 1978; Asarnow et al. 1983; Nuechterlein 1985).

Although these strategies differ substantially in the extent to which the heightened risk for later schizophrenia for their targeted group is documented, the use of multiple strategies for selection of high-risk samples has the advantage of allowing the generalization of findings to be assessed. This process should help to suggest the possible effects of sampling biases that may be involved in any single strategy (Lewine et al. 1984; Nuechterlein 1985).

Another important type of approach to identification of possible vulnerability factors for schizophrenic disorders involves demonstrating that similar deficits occur across premorbid, psychotic, and postpsychotic periods in schizophrenic individuals, in order to show that a potential vulnerability indicator has an enduring nature in this population and is more than a component of the acute psychotic period (Asarnow and MacCrimmon 1978, 1982; Nuechterlein and Dawson 1984a). Zubin and Spring (1977) and Zubin and Steinhauer (1981) have emphasized the distinction between vulnerability markers, which show stable abnormalities across clinical states, and episode markers, which are abnormal during episodes but return to normal during recovery periods. We have recently (Nuechterlein and Dawson 1984a) suggested an elaboration into a tripartite distinction, which is shown in Fig. 1.

Whereas we maintain the designation "episode indicator" for measures of internal processes of the individual that show abnormalities only during the psychotic episode and are at normal levels before and after psychotic periods, we make a distinction between "stable vulnerability indicators" and "mediating vulnerability factors." Stable vulnerability indicators are measures that index stable,

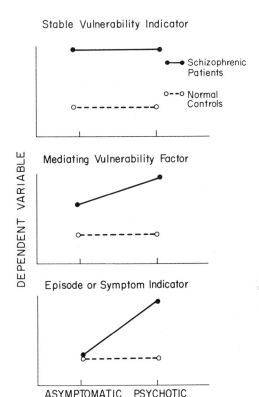

Fig. 1. Characteristic patterns across clinical states for stable vulnerability indicator, mediating vulnerability factor, and episode or symptom indicator (from Nuechterlein and Dawson 1984a)

traitlike abnormalities of schizophrenic patients which are independent of symptomatic state. These measures might be very helpful in identifying schizophrenia-prone individuals but are likely to be rather distant from processes that trigger schizophrenic psychotic episodes. Mediating vulnerability factors, on the other hand, are distinguished by showing deviance from normal levels during both psychotic and asymptomatic states but also covarying with the level of symptomatology. Careful longitudinal and experimental analyses would be expected to show that some of these mediating vulnerability factors become more deviant before specific groups of schizophrenic symptoms appear or intensify, due to proximal roles in the causal chain leading to these symptoms.

Evidence for Particular Vulnerability Factors

Although the data regarding potential vulnerability factors in schizophrenic disorders drawn from studies of high-risk populations and of relatively remitted schizophrenic patients are still in a fairly early stage of analysis, some results are noteworthy at this time. It should be mentioned that many of the available findings are cross-sectional, so clear, longitudinal, predictive relationships between these abnormalities and subsequent schizophrenic psychosis have often not yet been established. An additional consequence of the cross-sectional nature of most of the data is that the distinction between stable vulnerability indicators and mediating vulnerability factors cannot usually be made yet. Finally, the extent to which the potential vulnerability characteristics are specific to schizophrenia and related disorders has also not been fully examined. After a review of domains that currently show promise, some tentative heuristic schemas for their synthesis will be described.

Abnormalities in Information Processing and Attentional Functioning

The concern with schizophrenic deficits in attentional functioning can be traced to Emil Kraepelin, a very influential early figure in psychiatry at the University of Heidelberg who critically shaped our current conception of schizophrenia through his classic descriptions of dementia praecox: "It is quite common for (dementia praecox patients) to lose both inclination and ability on their own initiative to keep their attention fixed for any length of time ... In psychological experiments the patients cannot stick to the appointed exercise" (1919/1971, p. 6). Furthermore, Kraepelin noted that this deficit appeared to be connected to aspects of formal thought disorder: "With this loss of capacity to follow a lead is connected *a certain unsteadiness of attention*; the patients digress, do not stick to the point, let their thoughts wander without voluntary control in the most varied directions" (1919/1971, p. 6).

Recent studies have suggested that similar, but more subtle, deficits may serve as indicators of vulnerability to schizophrenic disorder. Certain laboratory measures of information processing and attentional processes have revealed subtle deficits in 7- to 16-year-old children of schizophrenic parents, in the absence of evidence of psychosis. These deficits have often been evident in mean differences relative to comparison samples, but possibly more importantly, deficient performance has been found in a disproportionately large subgroup among children born to schizophrenic parents compared to normal children. An excess of low-performance outliers is congruent with the genetic expectation that only some children of a schizophrenic parent will be at a truly high risk for schizophrenia.

We have suggested that the performance measures detecting a deficit in the processing of information by children of schizophrenic parents have the common property of a high momentary processing load (Nuechterlein and Dawson 1984 b). Demanding versions of a visual vigilance task, the continuous performance test (CPT), have produced some of the most robust results thus far. In three different samples of children of schizophrenic patients (Rutschmann et al. 1977; Nuechterlein 1983; Rutschmann et al. 1986), identification of very briefly presented, randomly placed target stimuli within a continuous series of similar nontarget stimuli has been found to be impaired under conditions that involve perceptually degraded images or substantial short-term memory burden. Furthermore, the two studies that included children of nonschizophrenic psychiatric patients as a comparison group found that these children did not show this discrimination deficit (Nuechterlein 1983; Rutschmann et al. 1986). Using an alternative high-risk strategy, a study from our laboratory examined young adults without a history of psychiatric disorder. It showed that those with a poor level of this signal/noise discrimination in a demanding degraded-stimulus version of the CPT had significantly higher scores than the remaining subjects on personality inventory scales believed to reflect schizotypal characteristics, such as the Physical Anhedonia Scale (Chapman et al. 1976) and the Minnesota Multiphasic Personality Inventory (MMPI) schizophrenia scale (Nuechterlein 1985; Nuechterlein et al., in preparation).

Other research indicates the potential predictive utility of CPT deficits for later disturbance among high-risk children and the persistence of such deficits in schizophrenic patients. In the New York State Psychiatric Institute high-risk project, children of a schizophrenic parent who developed clinical levels of deviance (including but not limited to schizophrenia) during late adolescence had earlier shown lower signal/noise discrimination during a demanding CPT at age 7–12 years than the nondeviant children of schizophrenic parents (Erlenmeyer-Kimling et al. 1984). Furthermore, many actively symptomatic schizophrenic patients (Asarnow and MacCrimmon 1978; Orzack and Kornetsky 1966; Walker 1981) and also relatively remitted schizophrenic outpatients (Asarnow and MacCrimmon 1978; Wohlberg and Kornetsky 1973) show a similar target detection deficit in the CPT. Finally, longitudinal evidence indicates that the signal/noise discrimination level in the demanding degraded-stimulus CPT is relatively stable over time among chronic schizophrenic patients, which is congruent with the view that it may index an enduring vulnerability factor (Nuechterlein 1985).

Another information-processing deficit that may be related to vulnerability to schizophrenic disorder is disruption of effortful rehearsal processes by distraction. When strings of items are presented for memory under distraction conditions, short-term recall is impaired among children of schizophrenic parents for items presented in early serial positions, which must be actively rehearsed to allow successful later recall (Harvey et al. 1981). No deficit is found for recall of the most recently presented items, which can be stored through more passive processes. This pattern does not characterize children of a parent with bipolar or unipolar affective disorder (Harvey et al. 1981). Furthermore, this deficit among children at risk for schizophrenia parallels impaired recall for early-serial-position items that has been demonstrated among actively psychotic schizophrenic patients (Oltmanns 1978) and among partially recovered schizophrenic patients (Frame and Oltmanns 1982).

In addition to deficits in tasks that demand voluntary attention, dysfunctions in smooth-pursuit eye movements are a very promising vulnerability indicator for schizophrenia that may show a deficit in an involuntary form of attention. Evidence for the status of this dysfunction as a vulnerability indicator has come from studies of parents, siblings, and twins rather than children of schizophrenic patients (Holzman et al. 1974, 1978, 1980, 1984). Twin data support genetic transmission of this dysfunction. Smooth-pursuit eye movement dysfunctions are found in 50%–85% of schizophrenic patients (e.g., Holzman et al. 1974) and in relatively remitted schizophrenic patients (Iacono et al. 1981). Recent evidence supports the relative specificity of this dysfunction to families of schizophrenic patients as compared to families of affective disorder patients (Holzman et al. 1984). Readers should see Holzman (1985) for an excellent recent review of this research.

Additional research that follows high-risk subjects to their eventual diagnostic outcome is needed to determine the extent to which specific antecedents of schizophrenia can be found in particular aspects of information processing or, alternatively, in the degree of generalization of deficit across perceptual and cognitive tasks that involve high momentary processing loads. The interrelationship among the deficits in this domain still requires clarification. Finally, the study of correlations between various types of information-processing deficits and specific types of schizophrenic symptoms is currently of great interest.

Autonomic Nervous System Anomalies

The early findings of Mednick and Schulsinger (1968) from the first large-scale longitudinal study emphasized autonomic hyperresponsivity and abnormally fast recovery among children of schizophrenic parents, particularly as evident in electrodermal responses to loud, irritating noise stimuli. An early-breakdown subgroup of the high-risk children was also characterized by these autonomic abnormalities (Mednick and Schulsinger 1968). Subsequent follow-up revealed that a composite index of these adolescent electrodermal characteristics was predictive of later schizophrenic symptomatology among male but not among female offspring of schizophrenic mothers (Mednick et al. 1978).

Later attempts by other investigators to replicate the cross-sectional electrodermal findings in other samples of children born to a schizophrenic parent have led to inconsistent results. Two studies found some evidence that agrees with hyperresponsivity (Van Dyke et al. 1974; Prentky et al. 1981), although they did not replicate many of the original findings for particular measures of hyperresponsivity and fast recovery. Two other, more recent reports (Erlenmeyer-Kimling et al. 1984; Kugelmass et al. 1985) have found that children of a schizophrenic parent in general showed no abnormalities in electrodermal activity, except for some evidence of hyporesponsivity, a tendency which is the reverse of the initial Mednick and Schulsinger (1968) result. Possible reasons for these varying results include differences in family intactness, associated severity and chronicity of parental disorder, children's age, and genetic contribution of the nonschizophrenic parent. It remains plausible that a mixture of underlying subgroups with differing autonomic abnormalities might contribute to differences across samples (as suggested by Dawson and Nuechterlein 1984) or that instability of autonomic responsivity rather than either stable hyperresponsivity or stable hyporesponsivity is present. In any case, any abnormalities in electrodermal activity among high-risk subjects are likely to be more complex than originally suggested.

For schizophrenic patients, the electrodermal results are quite consistent in showing that 40%–50% of symptomatic patients fail to have any skin conductance orienting responses (SCR-ORs) to innocuous, novel stimuli, compared to only 5%–10% of normal subjects (reviewed by Dawson and Nuechterlein 1984). The remaining schizophrenic patients often show tonic sympathetic hyperarousal when unmedicated. Clinically, the SCR-OR nonresponder schizophrenic patients are viewed as more withdrawn and conceptually disorganized, whereas the SCR-OR responders are described as more excited and active (Gruzelier 1976; Straube 1979; Bernstein et al. 1981).

Electrodermal abnormalities have also been predictive of short-term prognosis. In acute schizophrenic patients, hyperarousal as compared to relatively normal autonomic arousal has been found to be predictive of poor prognosis (Frith et al. 1979; Zahn et al. 1981). In older, chronic schizophrenic patients on the other hand, poor prognosis has been associated with hypoarousal (Schneider 1982). My colleague Dr. Dawson and I have suggested that these results can best be interpreted as indicating that either deviation from normal levels of autonomic arousal may predict a poorer outcome (Dawson and Nuechterlein 1984). Additional research is needed to examine the possibility that each type of deviation predicts and may contribute to a certain pattern of schizophrenic symptoms. For example, present evidence could be interpreted as suggesting that autonomic hypoarousal in schizophrenic patients foretells a continuation or return of schizophrenic negative symptoms, whereas hyperarousal predicts the return of blatant psychotic symptoms. Given the consistent findings of autonomic abnormalities in schizophrenic patients and the inconsistent findings in children of schizophrenic parents, it would appear that a role for autonomic abnormalities in the return or continuation of schizophrenic symptoms is more likely than a role in the initial onset of a schizophrenic disorder, unless the initial autonomic abnormality is very heterogeneous across schizophrenia-prone individuals or does not manifest itself until fairly shortly before the initial episode.

Neurointegrative Defect and Neurological Soft Signs

Several investigators have reported various neurological signs in children born to schizophrenic parents. In one early study, Dr. Barbara Fish found "neurointegrative" deficits, such as uneven neurological maturation, physical growth, and cognitive functioning that she has termed pandysmaturation (e.g., Fish 1957, 1984). In the Israeli Kibbutz-City High-Risk Study, Marcus (1974) and Marcus, Hans, Lewow, Wilkinson, and Burack (1985a) observed that school-age children of a schizophrenic parent had a greater number of neurological soft signs than children of normal parents. These signs included deficient sensory-perceptual functioning and motor coordination. Marcus et al. (1985a) found that these deficits showed moderate stability over 5 years.

Soft signs of neurological or motor deficit in childhood and early adolescence have also been found in other studies of children born to schizophrenic parents (Hanson et al. 1976; Rieder and Nichols 1979; Erlenmeyer-Kimling et al. 1982; Marcus et al. 1985b). Substantial variation across studies appears to be present for the types of soft neurological signs that are more prevalent among children of schizophrenic parents. However, one area of relatively consistent deficit is impaired fine motor coordination. A recent analysis of siblings and parents of schizophrenic patients found that these first-degree relatives also had more neurological signs than matched normal subjects, this time including more motor system abnormalities of localizing significance (Kinney et al. 1986).

Early evidence suggests that neurological soft signs, if combined with attentional performance, might help to predict later psychiatric disorder in children born to a schizophrenic parent. Using late adolescent ratings of overall level of psychiatric disturbance as the criterion, Erlenmeyer-Kimling et al. (1982) found that childhood neuromotor functioning had little direct predictive role but did have a strong concurrent relationship to attentional functioning, which in turn did presage the late adolescence disturbance ratings. A similar pattern is evident in the Israeli data of Marcus, Hans, Nagler, Auerbach, Mirsky, and Aubrey (1987), who report that all of their early cases of schizophrenic psychotic breakdowns among offspring of schizophrenic patients had shown a combination of attentional and motor abnormalities at 8–14 years of age.

As the motor and sensory-perceptual deficits in the children of schizophrenic mothers appear at a gross level to be similar to those in certain other psychiatric conditions (such as childhood attention deficit disorder), the specificity of these dysfunctions to vulnerability for schizophrenia needs to be examined carefully. However, as noted by Nuechterlein (1983) and Marcus (1986), children with attention deficit disorder apparently have no particular risk for later schizophrenia. This suggests that more detailed analyses of the types of motor and sensory-perceptual anomalies characterizing attention deficit disorder and risk for schizophrenia may reveal separate underlying abnormalities associated with each condition. Hyperactive children, for example, appear to be characterized by a lower level of response caution during at least some versions of the CPT than children of a schizophrenic parent (Nuechterlein 1983).

Schizotypal Personality Characteristics and Social Deficits

A number of anomalies in the social behavior of offspring of schizophrenic patients have been found, particularly in the areas of emotional instability, aggressiveness, and social isolation. The most frequently observed social characteristics of children of a schizophrenic parent are: being highly reactive to stress, unhappy, moody, excitable, anxious, and easily frustrated, a combination that has been summarized as emotional instability. Components of this pattern have been found in at least five different samples of children born to a schizophrenic parent (Rolf 1972 – females only; Weintraub et al. 1978; John et al. 1982; Watt et al. 1982; Janes et al. 1984).

Abnormalities in adolescent social behavior have shown some predictive value for later schizophrenia, although it is not clear whether any truly distinctive pattern predicts schizophrenia specifically. In the Danish high-risk study, teacher ratings indicating that an adolescent was nervous, anxious, and excitable presaged an increased likelihood of later schizophrenic outcome in offspring of schizophrenic mothers (John et al. 1982). A retrospective study of the school records of adolescents who later developed schizophrenia also found that such children showed more emotional instability than their peers (Watt et al. 1979).

In addition to evidence of emotional instability, children born to a schizophrenic parent have been found to have higher levels of withdrawal and social isolation (Mednick and Schulsinger 1968; Weintraub et al. 1978; MacCrimmon et al. 1980; Sohlberg and Yaniv 1985) and also aggressive, disruptive behavior (Rolf 1972; Weintraub et al. 1978; Watt et al. 1982; Weintraub and Neale 1984) than their peers. These characteristics may also have some predictive value within samples of children of schizophrenic mothers. In the Danish high-risk project, the adolescent female offspring of schizophrenic mothers who did eventually develop schizophrenia were more likely to be characterized as lonely, withdrawn, and anhedonic than other adolescent females in the high-risk group (John et al. 1982). The adolescent male offspring of schizphrenic mothers who later developed schizophrenia were more likely than the remaining high-risk males to be seen as disruptive, emotional, and disciplinary problems as well as lonely and rejected (John et al. 1982).

The uncertainty whether a certain pattern of social behavior precedes schizophrenia as opposed to other disorders derives from evidence that similar abnormalities in social behavior have been found among children of a depressed parent (e.g., Weintraub et al. 1978; Weintraub and Neale 1984). Furthermore, many of these social characterisitics seem to have too high a population base rate to be specific vulnerability indicators for schizophrenia. At the present time, combinations of social anomalies with vulnerability indicators from other areas seem more likely to detect distinctive preschizophrenic patterns.

It is perhaps noteworthy that the range of social behavior abnormalities found in children of schizophrenic patients seems to overlap partially with the criteria for schizotypal personality disorder in the *Diagnostic and Statistical Manual of Mental Disorders*, 3rd Edn (DSM-III; American Psychiatric Association 1980). The DSM-III criteria, which were developed to operationalize a personality disorder that was found to be genetically associated with schizophrenia in the Danish adoption studies (Kety et al. 1978; Kendler et al. 1981), include (1) social isolation, (2) inadequate face-to-face rapport, and (3) undue social anxiety or hypersensitivity to real or imagined criticism. These symptoms seem to be in the general domain of the social isolation, withdrawal, and emotional instability findings in the children of schizophrenic patients. Rather than social deficits, most of the remaining DSM-III criteria refer to oddities of perception, thought, and speech that are likely to be more strongly related to the subtle deficits in information processing that were reviewed in an earlier section. Thus, the combination of cognitive and social symptoms in the DSM-III schizotypal personality disorder criteria is consistent with the present suggestion that social deficits among children of schizophrenic parents might be best combined with vulnerability indicators from other domains for optimal description of preschizophrenic patterns.

Vulnerability/Stress Models of Schizophrenic Disorder

A vulnerability/stress or diathesis/stress framework for understanding the possible contributors to schizophrenia continues to be a popular and productive way to summarize the view that predispositional factors, some of which are strongly influenced by genetic factors, combine with environmental stressors to precipitate episodes of schizophrenic psychosis (Rosenthal 1970; Garmezy 1974; Zubin and Spring 1977; Gottesman and Shields 1982). Some recent conceptual frameworks or working models for schizophrenia (e.g., Mednick et al. 1978; Erlenmeyer-Kimling et al. 1982) or for schizophrenic episodes (e.g., Zubin and Spring 1977; Nuechterlein and Dawson 1984a) have been formulated to reflect current evidence regarding vulnerability factors.

As Strauss, Hafez, Lieberman, and Harding (1985) have suggested, early vulnerability/stress models did not recognize sufficiently the role of active coping efforts on the part of the individual. Some vulnerability/stress formulations also placed too little emphasis on possible protective influences in the environment. However, as discussed by Liberman (1986), these deficiencies are not intrinsic to a vulnerability/stress framework and have been corrected in the overall framework for schizophrenic episodes that I and my colleagues Drs. Robert Liberman and Michael Dawson have developed at the UCLA Clinical Research Center for the Study of Schizophrenia.

Figure 2 presents this overall heuristic schema of schizophrenic psychotic episodes, which should be viewed as a guiding summary of available evidence or a working framework rather than as a formal hypothetico-deductive model. It includes four classes of variables that may contribute to schizophrenic psychotic episodes: personal vulnerability factors, personal protective factors, environmental protective factors, and environmental potentiators and stressors. Personal vulnerability factors are enduring individual predispositional characteristics which, when combined with sufficient environmental potentiators and stressors, are hypothesized to lead to transient intermediate states that precede schizophrenic symptom formation. On the other hand, personal and environmental protective factors serve to reduce the likelihood of schizophrenic symptom development for an individual with a given level of vulnerability under a given level of stress. Figure 2 suggests some of the vulnerability factors, potentiators, stressors, and protective factors that are postulated at the present time to be related to schizophrenic episodes, although this figure is not intended to include all possible factors. Evidence for some of these factors has been reviewed in this chapter.

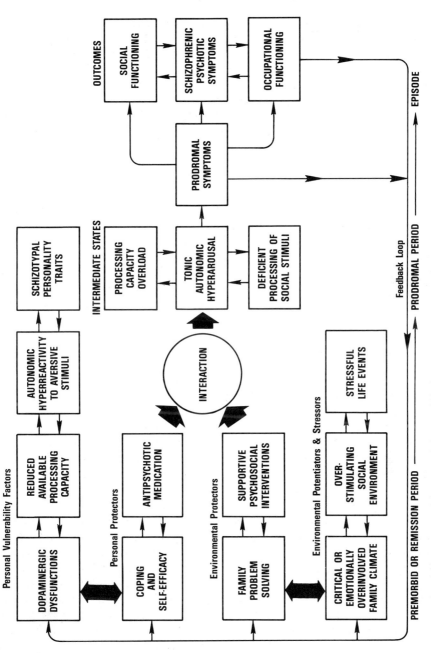

Fig. 2. A heuristic conceptual framework for possible factors in the development of schizophrenic episodes

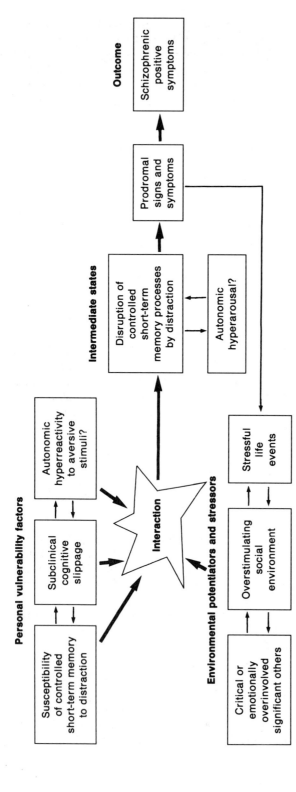

Fig. 3. A tentative conceptual framework for possible vulnerability and stress factors in the development of schizophrenic positive symptoms

A further differentiation between possible vulnerability factors for development of positive vs negative symptoms of schizophrenia (Crow 1985; Andreasen 1985) in information processing, psychophysiological, and social behavior domains may be heuristic, although the following suggestions are quite speculative at this juncture. Neurotransmitter and brain structural anomalies are not represented in the figures that follow, but such factors are viewed as likely underlying contributors to the level of analysis represented here. A tentative conceptual framework for possible vulnerability and stress factors (omitting protective factors for simplicity of presentation) related to development of positive symptoms is presented in Fig. 3.

The personal vulnerability factors from studies of high-risk populations that appear potentially relevant to development of the blatant positive symptoms of schizophrenia (i.e., hallucinations, delusions, and positive forms of formal thought disorder) include susceptibility of controlled short-term memory processes to distraction, subclinical cognitive slippage, and possibly autonomic hyperreactivity to aversive stimuli. Although direct evidence of a link between premorbid distraction effects on short-term memory and later positive symptoms of schizophrenia is not available from studies of high-risk populations, possible cross-sectional interrelationships among schizophrenic patients have been reported recently. Oltmanns, Ohayon, and Neale (1978) reported that short-term recall deficits due to auditory distraction were strongly correlated with formal thought disorder within a schizophrenic sample. Green and Walker (1986b) found that schizophrenic patients with predominantly positive symptoms, compared to those with predominantly negative symptoms, showed greater auditory distractibility on the task used by Oltmanns et al. (1978), while Cornblatt, Lenzenweger, Dworkin, and Erlenmeyer-Kimling (1985) described a parallel correlation between a positive symptom index and a distractibility index on another task.

Subclinical cognitive slippage is another potential vulnerability index among children of schizophrenic parents that would be expected to show a relationship to later development of positive symptoms of schizophrenia. Arboleda and Holzman (1985) have recently reported that the Rorschach-based Thought Disorder Index reveals elevated levels of cognitive slippage in children who have a psychotic parent (although the specificity to children at risk for schizophrenia is not yet clear). Interview ratings from the Danish high-risk study indicate that adolescent evidence of "incoherence" and "pathology of associations" before diagnosable schizophrenia is predictive of a later diagnosis of schizophrenia or borderline schizophrenia (Parnas et al. 1982).

Finally, the initial findings of Mednick and Schulsinger (1968) and the follow-up data of Mednick et al. (1978) suggest the possibility that autonomic hyperreactivity to aversive stimuli might be a vulnerability factor for development of blatant positive symptoms of schizophrenia. However, the failure of other groups to replicate clearly the cross-sectional findings make the status of this factor ambiguous at this time.

Figure 3 also suggests possible environmental potentiators and stressors that predict relapse of schizophrenic positive symptoms and that might have relevance as precipitants of the initial episode as well, at least for cases in which the vulnera-

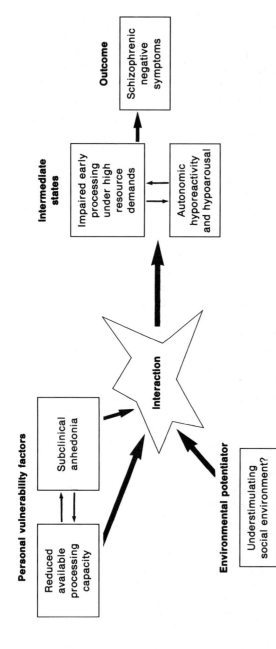

Fig. 4. A tentative conceptual framework for possible personal vulnerability and environmental potentiator factors in the development of schizophrenic negative symptoms

bility factors do not alone lead to a critical liability level for schizophrenia. These factors include discrete life event stressors and the critical or emotionally overinvolved attitudes of significant others (high "expressed emotion"). We hypothesize that these potentiators and stressors interact with the personal vulnerability factors to influence development of intermediate states and prodromal symptoms, a process that continues on to florid psychotic symptoms if the vicious circle of feedback between prodromal symptoms and environmental stressors is not broken.

In a parallel fashion, Fig. 4 illustrates some potential vulnerability factors for negative symptoms of schizophrenia (e.g., flat affect, poverty of speech, avolition) that might be drawn from a similar level of analysis. The phrase "reduced available processing capacity" is used to summarize a personal vulnerability factor that may influence performance on information-processing tasks with high momentary processing demands (Nuechterlein and Dawson 1984 b), such as versions of the CPT with high perceptual discrimination or short-term memory loads or the forced-choice span of apprehension task. More circumscribed factors underlying deficits measured by these tasks may be clarified in the future, but emphasis on the lack of sufficient allocation of processing capacity (Kahneman 1973; Posner 1982) in such situations describes one important deficit which would lead to the observed pattern of characteristics in high-risk populations. Among recent-onset schizophrenic patients, Nuechterlein, Edell, Norris, and Dawson (1986 a) have shown that poor signal discrimination under high-processing-load CPT and span of apprehension conditions is associated with higher levels of negative symptoms, both cross-sectionally during an inpatient period and longitudinally between an inpatient psychopathology assessment and an outpatient performance assessment. Green and Walker (1984, 1986 a) have demonstrated that visual backward masking deficits are associated cross-sectionally with negative symptoms in schizophrenics. Given the linkage of backward masking and forced-choice span of apprehension deficits to early components of visual information processing, the overall pattern of findings in high-risk and schizophrenic populations suggests that impaired early visual information processing under high processing resource demands is a possible intermediate state associated with the development of negative symptoms.

Subclinical anhedonia is shown in Fig. 4 as a potential additional personal vulnerability factor for negative symptoms due to its conceptual relationship to clinical levels of flattened affect and avolitional symptoms. The related phenomena of withdrawal and social isolation, as noted previously, have been found among the children of schizophrenic patients. In addition, we have noted a relationship between anhedonia and signal discrimination deficits on a high-processing-load, degraded-stimulus version of the CPT in young adults with other schizotypal features but without major psychopathology (Nuechterlein, Asarnow, and Marder, in preparation), which suggests that these factors may form a meaningful complex.

Other potential factors in the development of negative symptoms in schizophrenia are autonomic hyporeactivity, as has been proposed by Venables (1984), and an understimulating social environment, as proposed by Wing (1978). Although the status of these factors as potential components in the development of negative symptoms does not derive primarily from studies of first-degree relatives of schizphrenic patients, these factors are included in Fig. 4 to stimulate thinking about the possible interplay of these variables with the suggested personal vulnerability factors for negative symptoms. In addition, it should be noted that the possible relationship of negative symptoms to underlying brain structural changes, such as abnormal cell loss as has been posited by Crow (1980, 1985), appears compatible with the personal vulnerability factors of reduced available processing capacity and subclinical anhedonia (Fig. 4).

Beyond the possible heuristic value of the particular combination of factors included in Fig. 3 and 4, these figures are intended to indicate the probability that certain clusters of schizophrenic symptoms, or alternatively, different forms of schizophrenic disorder, may be found to be associated with particular sets of personal vulnerability factors and environmental potentiators and stressors. Recognition of the need for several separate vulnerability/stress models to address subforms of schizophrenia that have at least partially separable etiologies can be expected in the years to come.

Acknowledgements. The preparation of this chapter was aided by support from NIMH research grant MH37705, by NIMH research grant MH30911, which supports the UCLA Clinical Research Center for the Study of Schizophrenia, and by MacArthur Foundation support to the UCLA node of the Network on Risk and Protective Factors in Major Mental Disorders. The conceptual frameworks presented at the end of this chapter were developed through discussions with Michael Dawson, Michael Green, and Robert Liberman.

References

American Psychiatric Association (1980) Diagnostic and statistical manual of mental disorders, 3rd edn. American Psychiatric Association Press, Washington

Andreasen NC (1985) Positive vs. negative schizophrenia: a critical evaluation. Schizophr Bull 11:380–389

Arboleda C, Holzman PS (1985) Thought disorder in children at risk for psychosis. Arch Gen Psychiatry 42:1004–1013

Asarnow RF, MacCrimmon DJ (1978) Residual performance deficit in clinically remitted schizophrenics: a marker of schizophrenia? J Abnorm Psychol 87:597–608

Asarnow RF, MacCrimmon DJ (1982) Attention/information processing, neuropsychological functioning and thought disorder during the acute and partial recovery phases of schizophrenia: a longitudinal study. Psychiatry Res 7:309–319

Asarnow RF, Nuechterlein KH, Marder SR (1983) Span of apprehension performance, neuropsychological functioning, and indices of psychosis-proneness. J Nerv Ment Dis 171:662–669

Bernstein AS, Taylor KW, Starkey P, Juni S, Lubowsky J, Paley H (1981) Bilateral skin conductance, finger pulse volume, and EEG orienting response to tones of differing intensities in chronic schizophrenics and controls. J Nerv Ment Dis 169:513–528

Bleuler M (1978) The schizophrenic disorders: long-term patient and family studies (Clemens S, trans). Yale University Press, New Haven (Original work published 1972)

Brown GW, Birley JL (1968) Crises and life changes and the onset of schizophrenia. J Health Soc Behav 9:203–214

Brown GW, Birley JL, Wing JK (1972) Influence of family life on the course of schizophrenic disorders: a replication. Br J Psychiatry 121:241–258

Buchsbaum MS, Murphy DL, Coursey RD, Lake CR, Ziegler MG (1978) Platelet monoamine oxidase, plasma dopamine-beta-hydroxylase, and attention in a "biochemical high risk" sample. J Psychiatr Res 14:215–224

Chapman LJ, Chapman JP, Raulin ML (1976) Scales for physical and social anhedonia. J Abnorm Psychol 85:374–382

Chapman LJ, Chapman JP, Raulin ML, Edell WS (1978) Schizotypy and thought disorder as a high risk approach to schizophrenia. In: Serban G (ed) Cognitive defects in the development of mental illness. Brunner/Mazel, New York, pp 351–360

Ciompi L (1980) The natural history of schizophrenia in the long term. Br J Psychiatry 136:413–420

Cornblatt BA, Lenzenweger MF, Dworkin RH, Erlenmeyer-Kimling L (1985) Positive and negative schizophrenic symptoms, attention, and information processing. Schizophr Bull 11:397–408

Crow TJ (1980) Molecular pathology of schizophrenia: More than one disease process? Br Med J 280:66–68

Crow TJ (1985) The two-syndrome concept: origins and current status. Schizophr Bull 11:471–486

Dawson ME, Nuechterlein KH (1984) Psychophysiological dysfunctions in the developmental course of schizophrenic disorders. Schizophr Bull 10:204–232

Elliott GR, Eisdorfer C (1982) Stress and human health. Springer, Berlin Heidelberg New York

Erlenmeyer-Kimling L, Cornblatt B, Friedman D, Marcuse Y, Rutschmann J, Simmens S, Devi S (1982) Neurological, electrophysiological, and attentional deviations in children at risk for schizophrenia. In: Henn FA, Nasrallah HA (eds) Schizophrenia as a brain disease. Oxford University Press, New York, pp 61–98

Erlenmeyer-Kimling L, Marcuse Y, Cornblatt B, Friedman D, Rainer JD, Rutschmann J (1984). The New York high-risk project. In: Watt NF, Anthony EJ, Wynne LC, Rolf JE (eds) Children at risk for schizophrenia: a longitudinal perspective. Cambridge University Press, New York, pp 169–189

Fish B (1957) The detection of schizophrenia in infancy. J Nerv Ment Dis 125:1–24

Fish B (1984) Characteristics and sequelae of the neurointegrative disorder in infants at risk for schizophrenia: 1952–1982. In: Watt NF, Anthony EJ, Wynne LC, Rolf JE (eds) Children at risk for schizophrenia: a longitudinal perspective. Cambridge University Press, New York, pp 423–439

Frame CL, Oltmanns TF (1982) Serial recall by schizophrenic and affective patients during and after psychotic episodes. J Abnorm Psychol 91:311–318

Frith CD, Stevens M, Johnstone EC, Crow TJ (1979) Skin conductance responsivity during acute episodes of schizophrenia as a predictor of symptomatic improvement. Psychol Med 9:101–106

Garmezy N (1974) Children at risk: the search for the antecedents of schizophrenia: part 2. Ongoing research programs, issues and intervention. Schizophr Bull 1(9):55–125

Garmezy N, Streitman S (1974) Children at risk: the search for the antecedents of schizophrenia: part I. Conceptual models and research methods. Schizophr Bull 1(8):14–90

Goldstein MJ, Rodnick EH, Jones JE, McPherson SR, West KL (1978) Familial precursors of schizophrenia spectrum disorders. In: Wynne LC, Cromwell RL, Matthysse S (eds) The nature of schizophrenia: new approaches to research and treatment. Wiley, New York, pp 487–498

Gottesman II, Shields J (1982) Schizophrenia: the epigenetic puzzle. Cambridge University Press, New York

Green M, Walker E (1984) Susceptibility to backward masking in schizophrenic patients with positive or negative symptoms. Am J Psychiatry 141:1273–1275

Green M, Walker E (1986a) Symptom correlates of vulnerability to backward masking in schizophrenia. Am J Psychiatry 143:181–186

Green M, Walker E (1986b) Attentional performance in positive and negative symptom schizophrenia. J Nerv Ment Dis 174:208–213

Gruzelier JH (1976) Clinical attributes of schizophrenic skin conductance responders and nonresponders. Psychol Med 6:245–249

Hanson DR, Gottesman II, Heston LL (1976) Some possible childhood indicators of adult schizophrenia inferred from children of schizophrenics. Br J Psychiatry 129:142–154

Harvey P, Winters K, Weintraub S, Neale JM (1981) Distractibility in children vulnerable to psychopathology. J Abnorm Psychol 90:298–304

Holzman PS (1985) Eye movement dysfunctions and psychosis. Int Rev Neurobiol 27:179–205

Holzman PS, Proctor LR, Levy DL, Yasillo N, Meltzer HY, Hurt SW (1974) Eye tracking dysfunctions in schizophrenic patients and their relatives. Arch Gen Psychiatry 31:143–151

Holzman PS, Kringlen E, Levy DL, Proctor LR, Haberman S (1978) Smooth pursuit eye movements in twins discordant for schizophrenia. J Psychiatr Res 14:111–122

Holzman PS, Kringlen E, Levy DL, Haberman SJ (1980) Deviant eye tracking in twins discordant for psychosis: a replication. Arch Gen Psychiatry 37:627–631

Holzman PS, Solomon CM, Levin S, Waternaux CS (1984) Pursuit eye movement dysfunctions in schizophrenia: family evidence for specificity. Arch Gen Psychiatry 41:136–139

Iacono WG, Tuason VB, Johnson RA (1981) Dissociation of smooth pursuit and saccadic eye tracking in remitted schizophrenics. Arch Gen Psychiatry 38:991–996

Janes CL, Worland J, Weeks DG, Konen PM (1984) Interrelationships among possible predictors of schizophrenia. In: Watt NF, Anthony EJ, Wynne LC, Rolf JE (eds) Children at risk for schizophrenia: a longitudinal perspective. Cambridge University Press, New York, pp 160–166

John RS, Mednick SA, Schulsinger F (1982) Teacher reports as a predictor of schizophrenia and borderline schizophrenia: a Bayesian decision analysis. J Abnorm Psychol 91:399–413

Kahneman D (1973) Attention and effort. Prentice-Hall, Englewood Cliffs

Kendler KS, Gruenberg AM, Strauss JS (1981) An independent analysis of the Copenhagen sample of the Danish Adoption Study of Schizophrenia: I. The relationship between schizotypal personality disorder and schizophrenia. Arch Gen Psychiatry 38:982–984

Kety SS, Rosenthal D, Wender PH, Schulsinger F, Jacobsen B (1978) The biologic and adoptive families of adoptive individuals who became schizophrenic: prevalence of mental illness and other characteristics. In: Wynne LC, Cromwell RL, Matthysse S (eds) The nature of schizophrenia: new approaches to research and treatment. Wiley, New York

Kinney DK, Woods BT, Yurgelun-Todd D (1986) Neurologic abnormalities in schizophrenic patients and their families: II. Neurologic and psychiatric findings in relatives. Arch Gen Psychiatry 43:665–668

Kraepelin E (1919) Dementia praecox and paraphrenia (Barclay RM, trans). Krieger, Huntington, New York (1971 reprint of original translation)

Kugelmass S, Marcus J, Schmueli J (1985) Psychophysiological reactivity in high-risk children. Schizophr Bull 11:66–73

Lazarus RS, Folkman S (1984) Stress, appraisal, and coping. Springer, Berlin Heidelberg New York

Lewine RRJ, Watt NF, Grub TW (1984) High-risk-for-schizophrenia research: sampling bias and its implications. In: Watt NF, Anthony EJ, Wynne LC, Rolf JE (eds) Children at risk for schizophrenia: a longitudinal perspective. Cambridge University Press, New York, pp 557–564

Liberman RP (1986) Coping and competence as protective factors in the vulnerability-stress model of schizophrenia. In: Goldstein MJ, Hand I, Hahlweg K (eds) Treatment of schizophrenia: family assessment and intervention. Springer, Berlin Heidelberg New York, pp 201–215

Lukoff D, Snyder K, Ventura J, Nuechterlein KH (1984) Life events, familial stress, and coping in the developmental course of schizophrenia. Schizophr Bull 10:258–292

MacCrimmon DJ, Cleghorn JM, Asarnow RF, Steffy RA (1980) Children at risk for schizophrenia: clinical and attentional characteristics. Arch Gen Psychiatry 37:671–674

Marcus J (1974) Cerebral functioning in offspring of schizophrenics: a possible genetic factor. Int J Ment Health 3:57–73

Marcus J (1986) Schizophrenia and attentional deficit disorder (ADD): reply to Kaffman. Schizophr Bull 12:337–339

Marcus J, Hans SL, Lewow E, Wilkinson L, Burack CM (1985a) Neurological findings in high-risk children: childhood assessment and 5-year follow-up. Schizophr Bull 11:85–100

Marcus J, Hans SL, Mednick SA, Schulsinger F, Michelsen J (1985b) Neurological dysfunctioning in offspring of schizophrenics in Israel and Denmark. Arch Gen Psychiatry 42:753–761

Marcus J, Hans SL, Nagler S, Auerbach JG, Mirsky AF, Aubrey A (1987) A review of the NIMH Israeli High-Risk Study and the Jersualem Infant Development Study. Schizophr Bull (to be published)

Matthysse S, Kidd KK (1976) Estimating the genetic contribution to schizophrenia. Am J Psychiatry 133:185–191

Mednick SA, McNeil TF (1968) Current methodology in research on the etiology of schizophrenia: serious difficulties which suggest the use of the high-risk group method. Psychol Bull 70:681–693

Mednick SA, Schulsinger F (1968) Some premorbid characteristics related to breakdown in children with schizophrenic mothers. In: Rosenthal D, Kety SS (eds) Transmission of schizophrenia. Pergamon Press, New York, pp 267–291

Mednick SA, Schulsinger F, Teasdale TW, Schulsinger H, Venables PH, Rock DR (1978) Schizophrenia in high-risk children: sex differences in predisposing factors. In: Serban G (ed) Cognitive defects in the development of mental illness. Brunner/Mazel, New York, pp 169–197

Nuechterlein KH (1983) Signal detection in vigilance tasks and behavioral attributes among offspring of schizophrenic mothers and among hyperactive children. J Abnorm Psychol 92:4–28

Nuechterlein KH (1985) Converging evidence for vigilance deficit as a vulnerability indicator for schizophrenic disorders. In: Alpert M (ed) Controversies in schizophrenia: changes and constancies. Guilford, New York, pp 175–198

Nuechterlein KH, Dawson ME (1984a) A heuristic vulnerability/stress model of schizophrenic episodes. Schizophr Bull 10:300–312

Nuechterlein KH, Dawson ME (1984b) Information processing and attentional functioning in the developmental course of schizophrenic disorders. Schizophr Bull 10:160–203

Nuechterlein KH, Edell WS, Norris M, Dawson ME (1986a) Attentional vulnerability indicators, thought disorder, and negative symptoms. Schizophr Bull 12:408–426

Nuechterlein KH, Snyder KS, Dawson ME, Rappe S, Gitlin M, Fogelson D (1986b) Expressed emotion, fixed-dose fluphenazine decanoate maintenance, and relapse in recent-onset schizophrenia. Psychopharmacol Bull 22:633–639

Nuechterlein KH, Asarnow RF, Marder SR (in preparation) Perceptual sensitivity during vigilance as an indicator of psychosis proneness

Oltmanns TF (1978) Selective attention in schizophrenic and manic psychosis: the effect of distraction on information processing. J Abnorm Psych 87:212–225

Oltmanns TF, Ohayon J, Neale JM (1978) The effect of antipsychotic medication and diagnostic criteria on distractibility in schizophrenia. J Psychiatr Res 14:81–91

Orzack MH, Kornetsky C (1966) Attention dysfunction in chronic schizophrenia. Arch Gen Psychiatry 14:323–326

Parnas J, Schulsinger F, Schulsinger H, Mednick SA, Teasdale TW (1982) Behavioral precursors of schizophrenia spectrum. Arch Gen Psychiatry 39:658–664

Posner MI (1982) Cumulative development of attentional theory. Am Psychol 37:168–179

Prentky RA, Salzman LF, Klein RH (1981) Habituation and conditioning of skin conductance responses in children at risk. Schizophr Bull 7:281–291

Rieder RO, Nichols PL (1979) The offspring of schizophrenics: 3. Hyperactivity and neurological soft signs. Arch Gen Psychiatry 36:789–799

Rodnick EH, Goldstein MJ, Lewis JM, Doane JA (1984) Parental communication style, affect, and role as precursors of offspring schizophrenia-spectrum disorders. In: Watt NF, Anthony EJ, Wynne LC, Rolf JE (eds) Children at risk for schizophrenia: a longitudinal perspective. Cambridge University Press, New York, pp 81–92

Rolf JE (1972) The social and academic competence of children vulnerable to schizophrenia and other behavior pathologies. J Abnorm Psychol 80:225–243

Rosenthal D (1970) Genetic theory and abnormal behavior. McGraw-Hill, New York

Rutschmann J, Cornblatt B, Erlenmeyer-Kimling L (1977) Sustained attention in children at risk for schizophrenia: report on a continuous performance test. Arch Gen Psychiatry 34:571–575

Rutschmann J, Cornblatt B, Erlenmeyer-Kimling L (1986) Sustained attention in children at risk for schizophrenia: findings with two visual continuous performance tests in a new sample. J Abnorm Child Psychol 14:365–385

Schneider SJ (1982) Electrodermal activity and therapeutic response to neuroleptic treatment in chronic schizophrenic inpatients. Psychol Med 12:607–613

Sohlberg SC, Yaniv S (1985) Social adjustment and cognitive performance of high-risk children. Schizophr Bull 11:61–65

Steronko RJ, Woods DJ (1978) Impairment in early stages of visual information processing in nonspsychotic schizotypal individuals. J Abnorm Psychol 87:481–490

Straube ER (1979) On the meaning of electrodermal nonresponding in schizophrenia. J Nerv Ment Dis 167:601–611

Strauss JS, Hafez H, Lieberman P, Harding CM (1985) The course of psychiatric disorder: III. Longitudinal principles. Am J Psychiatry 142:289–296

Van Dyke JL, Rosenthal D, Rasmussen PV (1974) Electrodermal functioning in adopted-away offspring of schizophrenics. J Psychiatr Res 10:199–215

Vaughn C, Leff JP (1976) The influence of family and social factors on the course of psychiatric illness. Br J Psychiatry 129:125–137

Vaughn C, Snyder KS, Jones S, Freeman WB, Falloon IRH (1984) Family factors in schizophrenic relapse: a California replication of the British research on expressed emotion. Arch Gen Psychiatry 41:1169–1177

Venables PH (1984) Cerebral mechanisms, autonomic responsiveness, and attention in schizophrenia. In: Spaulding WD, Cole JK (eds) Nebraska Symposium on Motivation 1983, vol 31: Theories of schizophrenia and psychosis. University of Nebraska Press, Lincoln, pp 47–91

Venables PH, Mednick SA, Schulsinger F, Raman AC, Bell B, Dalais JC, Fletcher RP (1978) Screening for risk of mental illness. In: Serban G (ed) Cognitive defects in the development of mental illness. Brunner/Mazel, New York, pp 273–303

Walker E (1981) Attentional and neuromotor functions of schizophrenics, schizoaffectives, and patients with other affective disorders. Arch Gen Psychiatry 38:1355–1358

Watt NF, Fryer JH, Lewine RRJ, Prentky RA (1979) Toward longitudinal conceptions of psychiatric disorder. Prog Exp Pers Res 9:199–283

Watt NF, Grubb TW, Erlenmeyer-Kimling L (1982) Social, emotional, and intellectual behavior at school among children at high risk for schizophrenia. J Consult Clin Psychol 50:171–181

Weintraub S, Neale JM (1984) Social behavior of children at risk for schizophrenia. In: Watt NF, Anthony EJ, Wynne LC, Rolf JE (eds) Children at risk for schizophrenia: a longitudinal perspective. Cambridge University Press, New York, pp 279–285

Weintraub S, Prinz RJ, Neale JM (1978) Peer evaluations of the competence of children vulnerable to psychopathology. J Abnorm Child Psychol 6:461–473

Wing JK (1978) Clinical concepts of schizophrenia. In: Wing JK (ed) Schizophrenia: toward a new synthesis. Academic, London, pp 1–30

Wohlberg GW, Kornetsky C (1973) Sustained attention in remitted schizophrenics. Arch Gen Psychiatry 28:533–537

Zahn TP, Carpenter WT, McGlashan TH (1981) Autonomic nervous system activity in acute schizophrenia: II. Relationships to short-term prognosis and clinical state. Arch Gen Psychiatry 38:260–266

Zubin J, Spring B (1977) Vulnerability – a new view of schizophrenia. J Abnorm Psychol 86:103–126

Zubin J, Steinhauer S (1981) How to break the logjam in schizophrenia: a look beyond genetics. J Nerv Ment Dis 169:477–492

Zubin J, Magaziner J, Steinhauer S (1983) The metamorphosis of schizophrenia: from chronicity to vulnerability. Psychol Med 13:551–571

A Model of Schizophrenic Vulnerability to Environmental Factors

J. Leff

Introduction

It is no longer possible to view schizophrenia as a purely endogenous psychosis, the product of some biological process that is impervious to environmental influences. The most striking recent evidence for the responsiveness of schizophrenia to social factors has come from the WHO international studies of incidence and outcome. These have shown that even when schizophrenia is diagnosed in a standardised way, there are major differences in outcome across cultures (WHO 1979). This builds on the earlier work demonstrating that the hospital environment influences the clinical picture shown by schizophrenic patients, including both positive and negative symptoms (Wing and Brown 1970; Wing and Freudenberg 1961). These studies have addressed the issue of social influences on the *course* of the established illness. Theories about the role of social factors in the *causation* of schizophrenia can only be tested by long-term prospective studies of the kind that have been mounted in the United States (Garmezy 1974). Until these come to fruition, we are constrained to study patients who have already developed the illness, with all the limitations on identifying aetiological factors that entails. However, within these limits it has been possible to establish some links between environmental stressors and biological features of schizophrenia.

That environmental factors play a role in precipitating episodes of schizophrenia is suggested by the relapse rate on maintenance neurolepetic drugs. There is no doubt that such treatment improves the outlook for schizophrenic patients (Leff and Wing 1971; Hogarty and Goldberg 1973; Hogarty et al. 1979; Crow et al. 1986). However, even when compliance is assured by intramuscular depot preparations, the relapse rate is still as high as one-third over 1–2 years. A relapse rate of this magnitude could be due to the nature of the biological defect in schizophrenia, relapsing patients having a more severe abnormality than non-relapsers. Studies of environmental factors that we will review in this paper make this an unlikely explanation.

Life Events and Episodes of Schizophrenia

The bulk of work on life events has involved patients with depression and with non-psychotic conditions. Only a small number of studies have been conducted

MRC Social Psychiatry Unit, Outstation: Friern Hospital, Friern Barnet Road, London N11 3BP, United Kingdom on patients with schizophrenia. The area of life events research is fraught with the dangers of circular reasoning unless certain technical precautions are taken. These include conservative dating of the onset of episodes of illness and the exclusion of events which may have resulted from changes in the patient's behavior through prodromal symptoms. Observing these precautions, Brown and Birley (1968) found a significant concentration of independent events in the 3 weeks preceding onset or relapse of schizophrenia, compared with a control group of healthy adults. This finding has now been replicated in a WHO study in six of the seven centres participating (Day et al., in press).

As the centres are located in places as diverse as Prague, Ibadan and Nagasaki, the results suggest that the susceptibility of schizophrenic patients to the stress of life events is likely to be universal. However, since life events have been linked with the onset of numerous psychiatric and non-psychiatric conditions, they must represent a *non-specific* form of stress in schizophrenia.

In Brown and Birley's original study, there was a suggestion from the data that more patients relapsing while on regular phenothiazine medication might have experienced life events prior to relapse than those off regular drugs. The numbers in their study were too small to test this observation, but it was subsequently investigated by Leff et al. (1973) in the context of two controlled trials of maintenance neuroleptics, and confirmed. The interpretation of the second group of researchers was that patients unprotected by drugs relapsed as a result of the disturbing effect of everyday social interactions, while those on drugs were unlikely to relapse unless exposed to some additional stress in the form of a life event. This formulation, though plausible, failed to take into account another stress factor influencing the course of schizophrenia, the expressed emotion (EE) of other members of the patient's household.

Expressed Emotion and the Course of Schizophrenia

Relatives' EE is an empirically constructed measure of the relatives' emotional attitudes towards the schizophrenic patient. The method of assessment was devised by Brown and Rutter (1966) and modified by Vaughn and Leff (1976a) to make it more practical. The ratings are made from audiotapes of a semistructured interview (the Camberwell Family Interview) with a relative. The relative's emotional attitudes as expressed to the interviewer are assumed to reflect behaviour towards the patient over long periods of time. Studies comparing relatives' EE with ratings made from direct relative-patient interaction have provided evidence for this assumption (Miklowitz et al. 1984; Szmuckler et al., in press; Strachan et al., 1986).

EE is rated on five separate scales, four of which have proved to be linked with the outcome of schizophrenia. High levels of criticism or overinvolvement, or the presence of hostility are associated with a poor outcome over 9 months (Brown et al. 1972; Vaughn and Leff 1976b) and 2 years (Leff and Vaughn 1981; MacMillan et al. 1986). High levels of warmth, in the absence of the adverse components, are linked with a good outcome. Hostility is almost always found together with high criticism, so that it is a redundant measure. Consequently, families are cat-

Table 1. Relapse rates (%) of schizophrenia over 9 months in various studies

	City				
	London		Los Angeles		Chandigarh
Ethnic group					
	British	British	Anglo-Americans	Mexican Americans	Indians
Study	Brown et al. (1972)	Vaughn and Leff (1976)	Vaughn et al. (1984)	Jenkins et al. (1986)	Leff et al. (in press)
High EE	58	50	56	58	31
Low EE	16	12	17	26	9

Table 2. Percentage of high-EE households in different cultural groups

City					
Los Angeles	London	Aarhus	Los Angeles	Chandigarh	
Ethnic group					
Anglo-Americans	British	Danish	Mexican Americans	Indians	
				Urban	Rural
67	48	54	41	30	8

egorised as high EE on the basis of high criticism (six or more critical comments) and/or high overinvolvement (score of 3 or more on the 0–5 scale). Over the course of 9 months post discharge, the relapse rate in high-EE homes has been found to be three or more times that in low-EE households in a number of studies conducted in a wide variety of cultures (see Table 1).

The low rates in Chandigarh are partly explained by the fact that unlike any of the other samples, the Chandigarh patients were all making their first contact with the services. One of the surprising features of this group of studies is that the same cut-off points for high criticism and overinvolvement predicted relapse across the populations included, despite major cultural differences in the distribution of the EE components.

These are illustrated in Table 2, from which it can be seen that there appears to be a gradient in the proportion of high-EE households, with highly industrialised and westernised cultures at the high end and a rural, traditional community at the low end. Some of the cultural influences that may shape relatives' EE are discussed by Jenkins et al. (1986) in relation to a Mexican American population.

Protective Factors in High-EE Homes

In the first British EE study by Brown et al. (1972) two factors were identified, each of which appeared to confer some degree of protection from relapse on patients in high-EE households. One was regular maintenance with neuroleptic drugs, while the other was low social contact with high-EE relatives. Social contact was estimated by constructing a time budget of a typical week and adding up the number of hours the relative and patient spent together in the same room. This measure was termed face-to-face contact and was arbitrarily divided at 35 h per week into high and low contact. In a replication study, Vaughn and Leff (1976 b) confirmed the protective nature of each factor, and showed by an analysis of pooled data that the two factors together exerted an additive effect. In the California replication conducted by Vaughn et al. (1984), each factor on its own did *not* appear to be protective, but in conjunction they seemed to give complete protection against the pathogenic effect of a high-EE environment. Thus while the two factors appeared to be *additive* in the London studies, their effect was *interactive* in the California study.

The amount of social contact made no difference to outcome in the Mexican American study (Jenkins et al. 1986), while information on this factor was incomplete in the Chandigarh study, so that the relevant analysis could not be performed. It appears that cultural factors influence the role of social contact in protecting patients in high-EE homes, in contrast to the association between high EE and relapse, which is stable across cultures.

Experimental Intervention in High-EE Families

The technique of separating independent life events from other types of life event avoids the problem of circularity and allows us to interpret the association between life events and the onset of episodes of schizophrenia as being causal in nature. Of course, it has no bearing on the issue of whether life events are a sufficient or necessary cause of schizophrenia. As we shall argue, neither adjective can be applied to independent life events in relation to schizophrenia.

The association between high-EE and the outcome of schizophrenic episodes cannot be clarified in the same way. Whatever statistical manipulations are carried out on data from naturalistic studies, the direction of cause and effect remains contentious. For example, both Vaughn and Leff (1976 b) and MacMillan et al. (1986) found an association between acuteness of onset and EE status of relatives. The duration of illness was significantly longer in high-EE than in low-EE households. Furthermore, in both studies, long duration of illness was associated with poor outcome. When Vaughn and Leff conducted a log linear analysis to investigate the relationship between these factors, they found that when the link between duration of illness and outcome was taken into account, the association between EE and outcome remained significant. By contrast, when MacMillan's group performed a similar analysis, the link between EE and outcome was no longer significant.

More definite conclusions are likely to emerge from an experimental approach, in which the family environment is altered in the desired direction and a consequent reduction in relapse rate is looked for. This strategy was employed in a recent controlled trial of social treatments for high-EE families of schizophrenic patients (Leff et al. 1982, 1985). Patients in high contact with high-EE relatives were maintained on regular neuroleptic drugs and the families were randomly assigned to routine care or a package of social interventions. The package comprised an educational programme, a relatives' group and family therapy in the home. The intervention was aimed at reducing EE and/or social contact, and achieved one or both of these aims in nine of the 12 experimental families. In these families the relapse rate of patients who remained on prophylactic medication was nil at 9 months compared with 50% in the control group ($p=0.022$). At 2 years the relapse rates were 14% and 78% respectively ($p=0.020$). These findings strongly support the view that relatives' EE exerts a causal influence on the outcome of schizophrenia over a 2-year period following discharge from hospital. They further suggest that reducing EE and/or social contact is genuinely protective as long as patients remain on prophylactic neuroleptics.

The Non-Specificity of EE

In replicating the study of Brown et al. (1972), Vaughn and Leff (1976 b) also extended the work to include a group of neurotic depressive patients in order to determine whether the link between EE and outcome was specific to schizophrenia or not. In fact, relatives' EE also proved to be predictive of the outcome for depressive neurosis, although in a slightly different way. Whereas a cut-off point of six critical comments best predicted relapse of schizophrenia, for depressive neurosis the cut-off point had to be adjusted to two critical comments to achieve prediction. This finding has recently been replicated by Hooley et al. (1986).

A study of obese women in California (Havstad 1979) showed that their ability to maintain weight loss through dieting was significantly related to their husband's level of critical comments, the same threshold predicting a poor outcome as with depression. Other studies still to be completed have identified high-EE attitudes in the relatives of patients with anorexia, children with uncontrolled epilepsy, and diabetics. It is clear from this diversity that criticism and overinvolvement can develop in relatives in families containing patients with a wide range of psychiatric and non-psychiatric disorders. We would speculate that such attitudes will be found wherever there are chronic or relapsing conditions in family members. It is clear that the association between relatives' EE and the outcome of schizophrenia is non-specific, and cannot account for the particular form of the disorder.

The Relationship Between Life Events, Relatives' EE and Drug Treatment

At the time that Vaughn and Leff were planning their replication of the earlier study of EE, the association between life events and the onset of episodes of

Table 3. Independent life events in the 3 weeks before onset in patients not on regular medication

	Number	Number with life event	%
High-EE homes	15	1	6.7
Low-EE homes	16	9	56.3

Exact $p = 0.004$.

schizophrenia had already been established by Brown and Birley (1968) and Leff et al. (1973). It was therefore considered advisable to include the life events history in the study of EE, and this was done. The use of this technique made it possible to examine the relationship between these two forms of environmental stress in the precipitation of episodes of schizophrenia. Of the 37 patients included in the study, only six were on regular maintenance neuroleptics at the time of the key admission, when the environmental factors were measured. This group is too small for statistical analysis and has thus been excluded from the data under consideration. Of the remaining 31 patients, 15 were living with high-EE relatives and 16 with low-EE relatives. The occurrence of independent life events in these groups in the 3 weeks before onset of an episode of schizophrenia is shown in Table 3.

The proportion of patients in high-EE homes experiencing an independent life event in the 3 weeks before onset is no higher than one would find in the general population (12%). By contrast, more than half the patients in low-EE homes experienced an event during the same period. This finding has recently been replicated in the WHO study in Chandigarh, India (Leff et al., in press), where the comparable proportions were 14% in high-EE homes and 57% in low-EE homes.

These results were interpreted as indicating that patients unprotected by maintenance drugs and exposed to the chronic stress of a high-EE household do not require any additional event to precipitate relapse. Patients living with low-EE relatives are not subjected to continual stress in their everyday lives, so that the majority of them require the occurrence of a life event to provoke an episode of illness.

A group of patients in high-EE homes who relapsed while receiving maintenance neuroleptics was accumulated during the trial of social intervention. A history of independent life events was taken either at the time of relapse or at the 9-month follow-up if the patient remained well. At follow-up 14 patients were still living with high-EE relatives and had been regularly maintained on prophylactic medication, in almost every case a depot preparation. Of these, six had relapsed while the other eight remained well. Five of the six relapses had experienced an independent life event in the 3 weeks prior to relapse, compared with three of the eight who remained well. This is not a significant difference, because of the surprisingly high rate of life events in the well patients. One would ordinarily have expected a rate similar to that in the general population (one in eight), unless the hospital admission within the previous year had itself led to an increased likelihood of life events. However, when the rate of life events in high-EE patients on drugs (83%) is compared with the rate in high-EE patients off drugs (7%), a highly significant difference emerges (exact $p = 0.001$).

These data suggest that the great majority of high-EE patients on maintenance drugs require the occurrence of an independent life event to precipate relapse. There is one category of patient not considered so far, namely low-EE patients taking regular maintenance drugs. We have now followed 15 such patients for 2 years without recording a single relapse.

A Model for the Interaction of Life Events, Relatives' EE and Prophylactic Medication

The factors just considered appear to explain a considerable proportion of the variance of episodes of schizophrenia in patients living with relatives. It should be emphasized that we have not included patients living alone. Among those living with family, one group is not accounted for by these factors, namely the unmedicated patients in low-EE homes who have not experienced a recent life event; about 44% of low-EE patients off drugs. It is possible that in these patients biological factors play a more salient role in the aetiology of schizophrenic episodes.

The interrelationship between the three factors can be represented by a model, as depicted in Fig. 1. The basic assumption of this model is that there is an underlying biological fault, either inherited or acquired, which confers on the individual a vulnerability to develop schizophrenic symptoms in response to particular environmental stresses. It is evident from the preceding discussion that the specific nature of schizophrenia must lie in the biological fault and does not stem

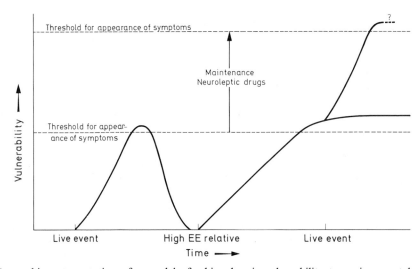

Fig. 1. A graphic representation of a model of schizophrenic vulnerability to environmental stressors

from the characteristics of the stressors. The model postulates that an individual prone to develop schizophrenia has a baseline level of vulnerability which is above that of the general population. This level rises and falls in response to environmental stress. When a certain threshold is exceeded, characteristic symptoms appear. As vulnerability falls with the lapse of time after the experience of stress it descends below the threshold again, and the symptoms resolve.

The response of vulnerability to the abrupt stress of a life event would be a rapid rise and rapid fall, producing a schizophrenic episode with an onset shortly after the event (the crucial period seems to be 3 weeks or less). Assuming that the psychological impact of the event would diminish quite rapidly, the episode of illness would be relatively short-lived. There is a correspondence between this formulation and Kasanin's (1933) description of schizoaffective psychoses. By contrast, patients living in high-EE homes are exposed to long-term stress, which would provoke a slow rise in vulnerability to above threshold levels, and then a slow fall, resulting in a longer episode of florid symptoms. This aspect of the model is readily testable, utilising measures of life events, relatives' EE and course of schizophrenic symptoms in a clinical setting. It is postulated that prophylactic neuroleptic drugs raise the threshold for development of schizophrenic symptoms. For patients in low-EE homes protected by medication, the new elevated threshold is above the peak level of vulnerability reached in response to a life event, so that this group of patients rarely relapses. Patients in high-EE homes on regular drugs are subject to a slow rise in vulnerability, which would not ordinarily exceed the new elevated threshold for the appearance of symptoms. However, the additional stress occasioned by a life event would increase the patient's vulnerability above the new threshold, resulting in a florid episode of illness. It is uncertain from the model whether the patient's vulnerability would then fall sharply, as after a life event in a low-EE patient, or would remain elevated for some time.

One advantage of this model is that it subsumes well-established findings; namely, that low-EE patients on drugs rarely relapse, and that high-EE patients off drugs do not require a life event to precipitate a relapse, whereas high-EE patients on drugs do. Furthermore, it generates predictions that can be tested. We have already spelled out the difference in the clinical course of an episode to be expected following a life event, and in unmedicated high-EE patients. In no way does it indicate the nature of the vulnerability, but assuming that some biological measure is employed, it does predict the manner in which the measure should vary over time in response to different environmental stresses.

Some studies of psychophysiological measures have been carried out with schizophrenic patients which are of relevance to certain aspects of the model. Most of them were completed before the model was constructed, but nevertheless can be used to test some predictions that follow from the model.

Psychophysiological Studies of Schizophrenia

In planning psychophysiological studies we were concerned to examine possible links between psychophysiological measures and the environmental stresses that had been identified as influencing the course of schizophrenia. Hence measures of life events and relatives' EE were included in addition to psychophysiological parameters.

Studies of Patients in Remission

The first study was conducted on a sample of patients who had already taken part in Vaughn and Leff's (1976b) replication of the EE work. The patients were contacted on average 2 years after their last admission, when the majority were in remission. A variety of psychophysiological measures were made, including heart rate, blood pressure, skin conductance level and spontaneous fluctuations of skin conductance (SF). The recordings were carried out in the patient's own homes using portable equipment.

Since face-to-face contact with relatives had been found to influence the relapse rate of schizophrenia, it was our intention to expose the patients to a key relative and look for changes in the psychophysiological measures. Hence the recordings were initially made for 15 min while the patient was alone with the experimenter, and then the relative entered the room and a further 15 min of recordings took place. The EE rating of the relative had been made 2 years previously in Vaughn and Leff's study, but was unknown to the experimenter. He repeated the procedure three times at 3-monthly intervals and on each occasion took a history of life events. In doing so he covered a period of 3 weeks preceding the testing occasion, since this was known to be the crucial period of sensitivity for schizophrenic patients.

Of the 37 patients included in Vaughn and Leff's study, 21 were available and asked to take part. Twenty-one age- and sex-matched normal subjects with no history of psychiatric illness were recruited as a control group and underwent identical procedures (Tarrier et al. 1979).

The most significant findings concerned the rate of SFs per minute. Over the whole 30-min period of recording, the two groups of patients, high and low EE, had higher mean SF rates than the controls (high EE = 5.9, low EE = 5.6, controls = 2.8: $p < 0.001$). If the SF rate in some way represented a vulnerability to development of schizophrenia, this finding would be predicted by the model.

For the first 15 min, the SF rates of high-EE and low-EE patients were indistinguishable. However, after the entry of the relative, the high-EE patients showed no change in SF rate, while the SF rate of low-EE patients fell rapidly over 5 min and reached the low level of the control subjects. This resulted in a significantly lower rate than the high-EE patients while in the presence of the relative ($p < 0.01$). This unexpected finding was interpreted as indicating that low-EE relatives have a calming effect on patients, enabling them to habituate, whereas high-EE relatives sustain a high level of arousal in the patients. We have already encountered the problem of determining the direction of cause and effect, and it confounds the interpretation of these findings, too. It is conceivable that some characteristic of the patients causes them to react differently in terms of arousal and also determines the nature of the relatives' emotional response to them.

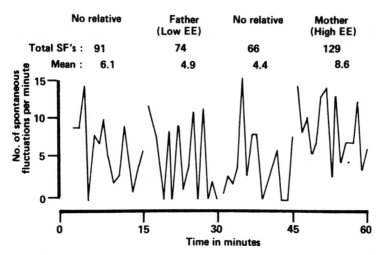

Fig. 2. Spontaneous fluctuations of skin conductance (*SFs*) in a patient exposed successively to a low-EE and a high-EE relative. (Reproduced from Tarrier and Barrowclough 1984, with permission of the authors and the British Journal of Psychiatry)

Tarrier and Barrowclough (1984) subsequently produced some striking evidence which makes this explanation most unlikely. They carried out the recording procedure in families with one high-EE and one low-EE relative, and exposed the patient to them alternately, with the results shown in Fig. 2.

In this case, the mean SF rate was significantly higher in the presence of the high-EE relative (8.6) than when the patient was alone (4.4) or with the low-EE relative (4.9). This finding has now been replicated with other pairs of relatives disparate for EE level and strongly supports the view that the patients' psycho-physiological responses are environmentally determined.

The other relevant finding to emerge from this study related to life events. Of the 21 patients taking part, seven had experienced an independent life event in the 3 weeks prior to one of the recording sessions. These patients acted as their own controls, a comparison being made between sessions preceded by a life event and sessions without a prior life event. The two sets of recordings did not differ for the first 15 min when the patient was alone with the experimenter. After the entry of the relative, however, there was a steep rise in the SF rate, but only on occasions preceded by a life event. This resulted in a significantly higher rate during the second half of the recording for event-preceded occasions than for event-free occasions ($p < 0.05$). It is evident from this finding that independent life events do produce an increase in arousal, but this is only apparent in the presence of the relative. It seems to be the combination of a recent life event and the relative's presence that elevates the SF rate. According to the model, this should only occur in high-EE households. Unfortunately the number of patients experiencing a life event (seven) was too small to perform a meaningful analysis comparing high-EE and low-EE homes. Nevertheless, it is worth noting that the only group that showed a mean *increase* in SFs over the second 15 min of the session was that of patients in high-EE homes who had experienced a recent life event.

As far as we are aware, no patient who had experienced a recent independent event relapsed shortly afterwards. Therefore, if the SF rate does bear some relationship to the vulnerability to develop symptoms, it must be assumed that the rises recorded did not exceed the threshold for the appearance of symptoms, and that they were transient. These assumptions can only be adequately tested by serial measurements at short intervals over long periods of time.

Studies in Acutely Ill Patients

Subsequent to the studies of patients in remission, similar work has been undertaken with patients during an acute episode of schizophrenia. The subjects were part of the sample included in the trial of social intervention (Leff et al. 1982, 1985) and were tested in hospital on average 6 weeks after admission. The procedures used in the earlier study were repeated, including a 15-min period of recording while the patient was alone with the experimenter followed by a further 15 min in the presence of a relative. It took about 6 weeks to obtain a recording because of the need to identify suitable patients, interview and rate relatives and arrange a convenient time for the session. The difference between patients from high- and low-EE homes in the presence of the relative which had emerged from the study of patients in remission was not replicated (Sturgeon et al. 1984). Instead, patients from both kinds of household showed a significant reduction in SF rate in the presence of their relative.

However, another major difference between the two types of patient was found: the mean SF rate for the whole 30 min of recording for the high EE patients (11.5) was more than double that for the low-EE patients (5.4, $p = 0.006$). The patients in the two groups did not differ in terms of the severity of their clinical state on admission as assessed by the Present State Examination (Wing et al. 1974). The SF rate for high-EE patients, then, was markedly elevated 6 weeks after admission for an episode of schizophrenia compared with the rate during a period of remission (11.5 vs 5.9). This is predicted by the model if the SF rate represents an index of vulnerability. By contrast, the SF rate recording during admission for low-EE patients was the same as that when they were in remission (5.4 vs 5.6). Either the SF rate is *not* an index of vulnerability for low-EE patients, or they had experienced a transient rise in SF rate, which had already returned to a baseline level by the time the recording was made 6 weeks after admission. Since the majority of low-EE patients relapse following a recent life event, this explanation would fit with the model. To test its validity it would be necessary to record the SF rate as close to admission as possible. This has now been carried out on a series of unmedicated patients, although the data have not yet been published.

Patients were tested within 48 h of admission to a research ward, before any psychotropic medication was instituted. Unfortunately, the demands of this design make it impossible to arrange for relatives to be present at the recording session, hence we were unable to employ the method used in the previous studies. Instead the standard paradigm for recording the orienting response was utilised, and the number of SFs occurring during the session was measured. As it happened, no patient admitted during the period of the study was living in a low-EE home.

However, it was possible to compare patients from high-EE homes with those living alone who had experienced an independent life event in the 3 weeks before admission. The mean number of SFs for these two groups was 16.3 and 26.4 respectively. This is a non-significant difference, and indicates that patients admitted following the acute stress of a life event are at least as highly aroused (in terms of SFs) on admission as patients admitted from the long-term stress of a high-EE home.

According to the model, the vulnerability of patients experiencing a life event should fall more rapidly during an episode of illness than that of patients in high-EE homes. A second recording session was arranged 4 weeks after the first, but unfortunately too few patients in the two groups of interest completed both sessions to enable meaningful statistical analysis. Nevertheless, the means for the two groups are worth presenting as they are suggestive. For those experiencing a life event, the mean number of SFs fell between the first and second recording sessions from 39.8–9.5. For those admitted from high-EE homes, the mean *rose* from 14.0–31.0.

The data are clearly incomplete and it is not easy to compare across the three studies, since the method in the last study differed from that in the other two. However, the data assembled so far do not contradict the model, and indeed suggest that it is worth conducting a longitudinal study of psychophysiological measures, environmental stressors and change in clinical symptoms to test the predictions of the model more adequately.

Psychophysiological Measures and Psychological Symptoms

One of the links that remains to be forged in the chain of causality is that between a biological measure of vulnerability and the characteristic symptoms of schizophrenia. With this in mind, we designed a study of the association between SFs and a symptom that fluctuates rapidly over time, auditory hallucinations (Cooklin et al. 1983). As patients cannot be relied on to report accurately on their experiences of auditory hallucinations, a group was selected who showed clear nonverbal evidence of these phenomena. In nearly all the ten patients studied, the onset of auditory hallucinations was reliably signalled by an abrupt lateral deviation of the eyes. Judgements of the onset of periods of auditory hallucinations were made from video tapes, while SFs were rated independently from continuous skin conductance recordings.

Recordings were made under two randomly alternated conditions; a maximum of 15 min sitting alone, and 15 min in conversation with an interviewer when only neutral, non-arousing topics were discussed. The aim of this design was to induce changes in SF rate and to determine whether they were followed by changes in the frequency of observable auditory hallucinations.

In fact, a significant association ($p < 0.01$) was established between the onset of hallucinatory periods and a rise in the SF rate. However, while the proportion of time spent hallucinating when alone (55%) was significantly greater ($p < 0.001$) than that with the interviewer (9%), no such differences were observed in the SF rate. Thus it was not possible to clarify the direction of cause and effect. It is equally plausible to maintain that the experience of auditory hallucinations produces a rise in SF rate, as that a rise in SF rate triggers the pathological experience.

Conclusions

Psychophysiological studies that included measures of social stress have identified the rate of spontaneous fluctuations of skin conductance as a possible index of the vulnerability of schizophrenic patients to develop episodes of illness. The evidence is patchy and in certain respects equivocal. Nevertheless, it seems worth pursuing the hypotheses generated by the model, and in particular mounting prospective studies that include psychophysiological parameters, measures of relatives' EE and independent life events and careful charting of the onset and course of the symptoms characteristic of schizophrenia. This type of multidimensional research offers hope of advancing our understanding of the complex problems posed by schizophrenia.

References

Brown GW, Birley JLT (1968) Crises and life changes and the onset of schizophrenia. J Health Soc Behav 9:203

Brown GW, Rutter M (1966) The measurement of family activities and relationships: a methodological study. Human Relations 19:241–263

Brown GW, Birley JLT, Wing JK (1972) Influence of family life on the course of schizophrenic disorders: a replication. Br J Psychiatry 121:241–258

Cooklin R, Sturgeon D, Leff J (1983) The relationship between auditory hallucinations and spontaneous fluctuations of skin conductance in schizophrenia. Br J Psychiatry 142:47–52

Crow TJ, MacMillan JF, Johnson AL, Johnstone EC (1986) A randomised controlled trial of prophylactic neuroleptic treatment. Br J Psychiatry 148:120–128

Day R et al. (in press) Stressful life events preceding the acute onset of schizophrenia: a cross national study from the World Health Organisation. Cult Med Psychiatry

Garmezy N (1974) Children at risk: the search for the antecedents of schizophrenia. Part II: ongoing research programs, issues, and intentions. Schizophr Bull 1 (9):55–125

Havstad LF (1979) Weight loss and weight loss maintenance as aspects of family emotional processes. PhD thesis, University of California, Los Angeles

Hogarty GE, Goldberg SC, Collaborative Study Group (1973) Drug and sociotherapy in the aftercare of schizophrenic patients: one-year relapse rates. Arch Gen Psychiatry 28:54–64

Hogarty GE, Schooler NR, Ulrich RF, Mussare F, Ferro P, Herron E (1979) Fluphenazine and social therapy in the aftercare of schizophrenic patients. Arch Gen Psychiatry 36:1283–1294

Hooley JM, Orley J, Teasdale JT (1986) Levels of Expressed Emotion and relapse in depressed patients. Br J Psychiatry 148:632–641

Jenkins JH, Karno M, De La Selva A, Santana F (1986) Expressed Emotion in cross-cultural context: familial responses to schizophrenic illness among Mexican Americans. In Goldstein MS, Hand I, Hahlweg K (eds) Treatment of schizophrenia: family assessment and intervention. Springer, Berlin Heidelberg New York Tokyo

Kasanin (1933) The acute schizoaffective psychoses. Am J Psychiatry 13:97–126

Leff JP, Vaughn C (1981) The role of maintenance therapy and relative expressed emotion in relapse of schizophrenia: a two-year follow-up. Br J Psychiatry 139:102–104

Leff JP, Wing JK (1971) Trial of maintenance therapy in schizophrenia. Br Med J 3:599–604

Leff JP, Hirsch SR, Gaind R, Rohde PD, Stevens BC (1973) Life events and maintenance therapy in schizophrenic relapse. Br J Psychiatry 123:659–660

Leff JP, Kuipers L, Berkowitz R, Eberlein-Vreis R, Sturgeon D (1982) A controlled trial of social intervention in the families of schizophrenic patients. Br J Psychiatry 141:121–134

Leff J, Kuipers L, Berkowitz R, Sturgeon D (1985) A controlled trial of social intervention in the families of schizophrenic patients: two year follow-up. Br J Psychiatry 146:594–600

Leff J, Wing N, Ghosh A, Bedi H, Menon DK, Kuipers L, Korten A, Ernberg G, Day R, Sartorius N, Jablensky A (in press) Influence of relatives' Expressed Emotion on the course of schizophrenia in Chandigarh. Br J Psychiatry

MacMillan JF, Gold A, Crow TJ, Johnson AL, Johnstone EC (1986) Expressed emotion and relapse. Br J Psychiatry 148:133–144

Miklowitz DJ, Goldstein MJ, Falloon IRH, Doane JA (1984) Interactional correlates of expressed emotion in the families of schizophrenics. Br J Psychiatry 144:482–487

Strachan AM, Leff JP, Goldstein MJ, Doane JA, Burtt C (1986) Emotional attitudes and direct communication in the families of schizophrenics: a cross-national replication. Br J Psychiatry 149:279–287

Sturgeon D, Turpin G, Kuipers L, Berkowitz R, Leff J (1984) Psychophysiological responses of schizophrenic patients to high and low expressed emotion relatives: a follow-up study. Br J Psychiatry 145:62–69

Szmuckler G, Berkowitz R, Eisler I, Leff J, Dare C (in press) Expressed Emotion in independent and family settings: a comparative study. Br J Psychiatry

Tarrier N, Barrowclough C (1984) Psychophysiological assessment of Expressed Emotion in schizophrenia – a case example. Br J Psychiatry 145:197–200

Tarrier N, Vaughn C, Lader MH, Leff JP (1979) Bodily reactions to people and events in schizophrenia. Arch Gen Psychiatry 36:311–315

Vaughn CE, Leff JP (1976a) The measurement of expressed emotion in the families of psychiatric patients. Br J Soc Clin Psychol 15:157–165

Vaughn CE, Leff JP (1976b) The influence of family and social factors on the course of psychiatric illness: a comparison of schizophrenic and depressed neurotic patients. Br J Psychiatry 129:125–137

Vaughn CE, Snyder KS, Freeman W, Jones S, Falloon IRH, Liberman RP (1984) Family factors in schizophrenic relapse. Arch Gen Psychiatry 41:1169–1177

Wing JK, Brown GW (1970) Institutionalism and schizophrenia. Cambridge University Press, London

Wing JK, Freudenberg RK (1961) The response of severely ill chronic schizophrenic patients to social stimulation. Am J Psychiatry 118:311–322

Wing JK, Cooper JE, Sartorius N (1974) The description and classification of psychiatric symptoms: an instruction manual for the PSE and Catego system. Cambridge University Press, London

World Health Organisation (1979) The International Pilot Study of Schizophrenia, vol 1. WHO, Geneva

Theoretical Implications
of Psychosocial Intervention Studies on Schizophrenia

M. C. ANGERMEYER

Changing Paradigms

During the last decade a new generation of psychosocial interventions has emerged that represents a radical departure from traditional psychotherapeutic approaches to the treatment of schizophrenia. As theoretical framework serves the vulnerability-stress model – or, to be more precise, various versions of it, as there is not only one vulnerability-stress model (Zubin and Spring 1977; Gottesman and Shields 1982; Zubin et al. 1983; Nuechterlein and Dawson 1984; Ciompi 1986; Zubin 1986). It is maintained that an underlying core defect of yet unknown origin – perhaps inherited or due to prenatal or perinatal complications, adverse psychosocial influences during early developmental stages, etc. – is necessary for the appearance of schizophrenic symptomatology. However, this vulnerability in most cases does not suffice to bring about a manifestation of schizophrenic disorder. The second key feature of the model is the concept of stress in terms of socioenvironmental conditions (e.g., life events) which may provoke schizophrenic symptoms. The impact of stress on the individual may be moderated by his/her personal dispositions (e.g., coping capacity) or factors located in his/her social environment (e.g., supportive social network). Interventions to prevent development of psychotic episodes are primarily aimed at the manipulation and/or modification of these moderating factors.

Besides reference to two totally different conceptualizations of the development of schizophrenic disorders, the new and the traditional treatment approach differ in a number of other important aspects. This becomes most evident if modern psychosocial interventions are contrasted with psychoanalytically oriented individual psychotherapy (Table 1).

In this review I shall discuss only controlled outcome studies of psychosocial interventions with explicit reference to the vulnerability-stress model. Two different types of intervention studies can be distinguished: those which aim primarily at the modification of the family environment (family-focused intervention) and those which intend changes of the individual's attitudes and behavior (patient-focused intervention). Tables 2 and 3 contain the most important data on sample composition, form and intensity of treatment, etc. In addition, it should be mentioned that all family-focused interventions were carried out during aftercare immediately following discharge from inpatient treatment. Patient-focused interventions, on the other hand, took place in various treatment settings: outpatient

Department of Psychiatry, University of Hamburg, Martinistr. 52, 2000 Hamburg 20, Federal Republic of Germany

Table 1. Comparison between the most salient features of new psychosocial interventions and psychoanalytic individual psychotherapy of schizophrenia

	Individual psychotherapy	Psychosocial intervention
Theoretical framework	Psychodynamic developmental model	Vulnerability-stress model
Treatment goal	Treatment of "cause" of disorder, "cure," changes in intrapsychic structure	Management of illness, rehabilitation
Focus of therapy	"Inner life," unconscious processes, symbolic meaning of illness, past	"Real life," concrete problems current situation
Empirical basis	Clinical evidence, data collected from psychotherapy	Empirical studies, results of psycho-physiological experiments and research into social stress
Pathogenic role attributed to psychosocial factors	Specific causal processes	Unspecific stressors or moderators
Role of family environment in pathogenic process	Etiological factor	Determinant of course (source of chronic stress, support system)
Attitude toward labeling	Avoidance of labeling	Explicit labeling of symptomatic behavior as symptoms of schizophrenic disease
Attitude toward psycho-pharmacotherapy	Considered as necessary evil	Integrated part of intervention serving to reduce vulnerability

(Buchkremer and Fiedler, in press; Hartwich and Schumacher 1985), day-hospital (Bellack et al. 1984), or inpatient (Liberman et al. 1986a, b; Brenner et al. 1980).

Goals of Psychosocial Interventions

The psychosocial interventions discussed here have differing targets. An overview is given in Fig. 1, which is based on the concept, developed by Dohrenwend and Dohrenwend (1981), of the "life stress process," consisting of the three main structural components "life events," "ongoing social situation," and "personal dispositions." I should emphasize that the interactive version of this concept has been chosen only for illustration purposes, I do not intend to imply that this version is best suited for the depiction of the pathogenic process resulting in schizophrenic relapse. In intervention studies the ongoing situation reduces to family environment, personal dispositions to the vulnerability and coping capacity of the individual.

Family-Focused Interventions

The family environment proved to be highly influential in a series of studies conducted at the MRC Social Psychiatry Unit in London, which established a robust

Table 2. Overview of family-focused intervention studies

Authors	Males (%)	Mean age (years)	First-admission patients (%)	Diagnostic criteria	Assignment to study groups	Intervention			Control group		
						Type	n	Intensity	Description	n	Medication
Goldstein et al. (1978)	55	23.4	69	New Haven schizophrenia index score ≥4	Random	Crisis-oriented family therapy	52	Weekly for 6 weeks	Patients involved in dosage study of neuroleptics	52	Parenteral, continuous control (first 6 weeks)
Leff et al. (1982, 1985)	50	34.5	33	CATEGO S	Random	Education program and relatives' group Family therapy (eclectic)	12	Two sessions Biweekly for 9 months[a] No fixed schedule[b]	Routine out-patient care	12	Parenteral, continuous control
Falloon et al. (1982, 1985)	67	25.8	36	CATEGO S or P, DSM-III	Random	Behavioral family therapy	18	25 sessions for 9 months, monthly sessions thereafter	Individual case management	18	Oral, continuous control
Köttgen et al. (1984)	65	23	69	Nuclear symptoms (based on PSE)	Random	Relatives' group and group therapy (both eclectic-psychodynamic)	15	Weekly or monthly for 9 months[c] Weekly of monthly for 9 months[d]	Routine out-patient care	14	Mostly parenteral, no continuous control
Hogarty et al. (1986)	66	27	23	RDC schizophrenia or schizo-affective disorder	Random	Psychoeducational family therapy	21	First weekly, then biweekly for several months, monthly thereafter, duration 2 years	Patients involved in dosage study of neuroleptics	29	Parenteral continuous control
						Social skills training	20	Weekly in the first year, biweekly or monthly thereafter, duration 2 years			
						Psychoeducational family therapy and social skills training	20				

[a] Six to twenty-one attendances, $\bar{x} = 9.1$.
[b] One to twenty-five sessions, $\bar{x} = 5.6$.
[c] Two-fifths regular attendance.
[d] One-third regular attendance.

Table 3. Overview of patient-focused intervention studies

Authors	Males (%)	Mean age (years)	Mean number of admissions / Duration of illness (years)	Diagnostic criteria	Assignment to study groups	Intervention			Control group		
						Type	n	Intensity	Description	n	Medication
Bellack et al. (1984)	59	37.7	4.9 / 10.5	Feighner criteria	Random	Social skills training	29	Three hours per week for 12 weeks	Unspecific group therapy	14	Oral or parenteral, no continuous control
Liberman et al. (1986) Lukoff et al. (1986)	100	?	?	CATEGO S, DSM-III[a]	Random	Social skills training and multiple family group (behavioral)	14	Five sessions/week for 10 weeks			Oral, continuous control
						Holistic health therapy and multiple family group (dynamic)	14	Seven sessions/week for 10 weeks, weekly sessions during 10 weeks			
Brenner et al. (1980)	55	37.2	– / 5.7	ICD-8	Sequentially as admitted to inpatient treatment	Training of cognitive, communicative and social skills	14	Four to five sessions/ week, maximum duration 2 months	Unspecific group activities Routine out-patient care	15 14	Oral or parenteral, no continuous control
Hartwich and Schumacher (1985)	38	32.7	3.4	ICD-8	Parallelized groups	Group therapy (eclectic)	20	Weekly sessions for 5 years	Routine out-patient care	22	Mostly parenteral, no continuous control
Buchkremer and Fiedler (in press)	60	31.6	3 / 7.9	ICD-8	Parallelized groups	Social skills training and relatives' group (only subsample)	19	Weekly sessions for 10 weeks	Routine out-patient care	24	No specified, no continuous control
						Cognitive therapy and relatives' group (only subsample)	18	Weekly sessions for 10 weeks			

[a] Except two patients.

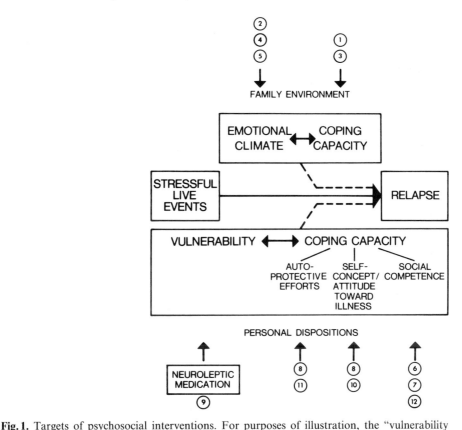

Fig. 1. Targets of psychosocial interventions. For purposes of illustration, the "vulnerability model" (adapted from Dohrenwend and Dohrenwend 1981) has been used.
① "Crisis-oriented family therapy" (Goldstein et al. 1978); ② education program, relatives' group, and family therapy (Leff et al. 1982); ③ "behavioral family therapy" (Falloon et al. 1982); ④ relatives' group and group therapy (Köttgen et al. 1984); ⑤ "psychoeducational family therapy" and/or social skills training (Hogarty et al. 1986); ⑥ social skills training (Bellack et al. 1984); ⑦ social skills training (Liberman et al. 1986); ⑧ holistic health therapy (Lukoff et al. 1986); ⑨ "integrated training of cognitive, communicational and social skills" (Brenner et al. 1980); ⑩ group therapy (eclectic approach) (Hartwich and Schumacher 1985); ⑪ "cognitive therapy" (Buchkremer and Fiedler, in press); ⑫ social skills training (Buchkremer and Fiedler, in press)

link between certain *emotional attitudes of relatives* ("expressed emotion," EE) and the risk of schizophrenic relapse (Brown et al. 1962, 1972; Vaughn and Leff 1976; Leff and Vaughn 1981). Three intervention studies relied directly on the EE concept (Leff et al. 1982, 1985; Köttgen et al. 1984a, b, c; Hogarty et al. 1986).

The main goal of these was to reduce the relatives' criticism and emotional overinvolvement with the patient as measured by EE. Consequently, all three studies selected only patients from homes high on EE. Using a package of psychosocial techniques consisting of an education program, relatives' groups, and family therapy, Leff et al. attempted to work directly on relatives' emotional attitude and modify their high-EE to low-EE. The second goal of their intervention was to reduce exposure of patients to high-EE relatives by cutting back face-to-face contact to the critical limit of 35 h per week. In previous studies reduced contact with high-EE relatives had proved to be associated with significantly lower relapse rates. Köttgen et al. tried to improve the family atmosphere by offering group meetings to the relatives and group therapy to the patients. Hogarty et al. designed a psychoeducational family treatment and/or social skills training with the patient – the latter with the declared intention of indirectly "cooling down" the emotional climate in the family.

Two intervention studies aimed essentially at improving the *family's coping capacity*. In Goldstein et al.'s crisis-oriented family therapy (Goldstein and Ko-peikin 1981), four stress-coping objectives were pursued sequentially: (1) stress identification, (2) stress avoidance and coping, (3) evaluation of the attempts at using stress-management strategies, and (4) anticipatory planning. The behavioral family therapy developed by Falloon et al. (1981, 1984) attempted to enhance coping skills by increasing the efficiency of family problem-solving. The major aim of the therapy was to train the family to employ a structured problem-solving method that involved sitting down together, specifying a problem issue, considering a broad range of possible solutions, and agreeing on a detailed plan to implement the best solution. Where families displayed deficits in their interpersonal communication that precluded effective problem-solving discussions, training in communication skills was implemented.

Patient-Focused Interventions

The goal of most patient-focused interventions was to enhance the *individual's ability to cope*. Main emphasis was put on strengthening *problem-solving and social skills* considered necessary to establish a social network and on reducing stress in interpersonal encounters (Bellack et al. 1984; Liberman and Evans 1985; Liberman et al. 1981, 1986b; Buchkremer and Fiedler, in press). According to Liberman et al., three kinds of social skills can be distinguished: receiving skills necessary to perceive a situation correctly; processing skills which enable the person to evaluate possible responses and choose one that is appropriate; and sending skills allowing the effective presentation of the response selected. In two intervention studies an attempt was made to train patients in the use of so-called *autoprotective techniques* in the sense of efforts on the part of patients at self-stabilization when their psychic equilibrium threatens to collapse as a result of internal or external stress (e.g., Böker 1986). Buchkremer and Fiedler's "cognitive therapy" was meant to enable the patients to recognize crises early on and to take steps written down in a "crisis plan" for each patient to forestall relapses. The holistic health therapy developed by Lukoff et al. (1986) also included autoprotective components: to train the patients in stress-reduction techniques, including meditation and physical exercise. In addition to reducing stress, a key issue in holistic treatment was mobilizing an individual's volition. The goal was to increase positive expectations of recovery from illness and to increase positive *attitudes toward the illness*. Hartwich and Schumacher (1985), on the other hand, aimed at helping patients to accept that they were handicapped by the illness.

Brenner et al. are the only investigators who have attempted specifically to treat illness-related cognitive deficits and in so doing to influence the vulnerability of the patients. They developed an integrated program to train cognitive differentiation, social perception, communicational skills, social skills, and problem-solving behavior. This program was based on a hierarchical model of the development and organization of schizophrenic patients' behavior (Brenner 1986; Stramke and Brenner 1983).

Outcome – And Its Relation to Stated Intervention Goals

Table 4 gives an overview of the effect of psychosocial interventions on relapse rates. The studies of Brenner et al. and Hartwich and Schumacher are not included as no relapse rates are reported. For ease of comparison, rates for the 12-month follow-up were exponentially extrapolated from 6- or 9-month rates if missing in the research reports. One should be aware that relapse was not uniformly defined. Manque de mieux, in studies (Bellack et al.; Brenner et al.) rehospitalization rates had to be used. Since at present too few relevant data have been published I will dispense with a discussion of the effect of psychosocial interventions on negative symptoms and social functioning.

Among *family-focused interventions* those by Leff et al. (1982, 1985), Hogarty et al. (1986), and Falloon et al. (1982, 1985) appeared to be highly successful. In all three studies the relapse rates in the experimental groups did not exceed 10% during the first 9 months post discharge, compared with rates between 28% and 50% in the control groups. Concerning the 24-month follow-up, Leff et al. and Falloon et al. report relapse rates as low as 17% and 20% respectively for the experimental groups; Hogarty et al.'s estimates range between 22% and 35%. By contrast, the corresponding rates for the control groups reached between 75% and 83%. Only in the studies by Goldstein et al. (1978) and Köttgen et al. (1984 a, b, c) could no statistically significant reduction of relapse rates be attained.

Let us now investigate whether these outcomes represented achievement of the intervention goals. Only if it can be shown that the assumed underlying "mechanism of action" could be positively influenced by the intervention does an evaluation of the relevance of postulated pathogenic models seem possible. The most convincing results were produced by Leff et al. (1982, 1985), who were able to show that in all nine of the 12 experimental families where at least one of the two intervention goals was reached (change from high to low EE, reduction of face-to-face contact to below 35 h per week), none of the patients relapsed during the 9-month follow-up. Hogarty et al. (1986) arrived at similar results: there was also no relapse in any household that had changed from high to low EE – regardless of treatment condition. However, it seems necessary to caution against premature causal inferences regarding EE and relapse. It is quite possible that the high-EE status of households with a relapsed patient is a response to the relapse event itself. In the absence of interim EE evaluations, it remains unknown whether some or all of these households had, in fact, already changed from high to low EE – and then returned to high-EE status (Hogarty et al. 1986). As has been shown,

Table 4. Relapse rates (%). For number of cases see Tables 1 and 2

Study	Type of intervention	Six-month relapse rates		Nine-month relapse rates		Twelve-month relapse rates		Two-year relapse rates	
		Experimental	Control	Experimental	Control	Experimental	Control	Experimental	Control
Goldstein et al. (1978)	Crisis-oriented family therapy	0[a], 22[c,g]	17[a,g], 48[c]			39[b,c]	31[a,b], 73[b,c]		
Leff et al. (1982, 1985)	Education program, relatives' group, and family therapy			8	50	12[b]	60[b]	20	78
Falloon et al. (1982, 1985)	Behavioral family therapy			6[d]	44[d]	8[b,d]	54[b,d]	17[d]	83[d]
Köttgen et al. (1984)	Relatives' group and group therapy			33	50	41[b]	60[b]		
Hogarty et al. (1986)	Psychoeducational family treatment			9	28	19	41	25[e]	75[e]
	Social skills training			10		20		35[e]	
	Psychoeducational family treatment and social skills training			0		0		22[e]	
Bellack et al. (1984)	Social skills training					48[f]	50[f]		
Liberman et al. (1969)	Social skills training and multiple family group			21		27[b]		50	
	Holistic health therapy and multiple family group			50		60[b]		79	
Buchkremer and Fiedler (in press)	Social skills training and relatives' group (subsample)	26				53	54	53	54
	Cognitive therapy and relatives' group (subsample)	6				22		33	

[a] High-dose neuroleptic medication.

[b] Exponentially extrapolated rates based on 6-month or 9-month rates (source for data from studies by Leff et al., Falloon et al., and Köttgen et al.: Hogarty et al. 1986, p. 640).

[c] Low-dose neuroleptic medication.

[d] Only major exacerbations of schizophrenia.

[e] Uncontrolled estimates (Hogarty et al. 1986).

[f] Rehospitalization.

criticism may decrease "spontaneously" over time in a remarkable proportion of households (Brown et al. 1972; Dulz and Hand 1986).

Another finding from the Hogarty et al. study also deserves mention. Among households whose EE remained high, relapse rates continued to be elevated and did not differ among controls and those who received either family treatment or social skills training alone; the combination of both treatment modalities, however, produced a significant prophylactic effect (no relapse) in households that remained high in EE. This phenomenon could not be explained by differences in the amount of face-to-face contact between patient and relative, as no significant differences were found among the four study groups in this regard. Thus, other mechanisms apart from those implied by the EE concept must have had some effect.

The most confusing findings as regards the relationship between EE and relapse were reported by Köttgen et al. (1984 a, b, c). In sharp contrast to the other two studies (Leff et al. 1982, 1985; Hogarty et al. 1986), relapse occurred in 44% of families that were seen to change from high to low EE and in only 37.5% of families in which EE remained high. Unfortunately, a number of serious limitations in method makes it difficult to draw conclusions from these results (e.g., no reliabilities on EE ratings on the basis of the original criterion tapes are provided; a majority of patients did not live at home throughout the follow-up period; only 65% of the patients received continuous neuroleptic medication).

Falloon's group did provide evidence for having achieved its intervention goal of enhancing family coping by strengthening the family's problem-solving capacity. After 3 months of treatment the families participated in two audiotaped direct interaction tasks involving the parent(s) and the patient. The comparison with the initial pretreatment assessment revealed a significant increment in constructive problem-solving behavior (Doane et al. 1986). In addition, the effectiveness of families' efforts to cope with everyday minor and major life changes, or to resolve intrafamilial and other sources of ambient stress, was assessed continously throughout the first 12 months of the study. Coping behavior improved steadily in families who received family therapy over the 9 months of active therapy, and this trend was maintained at least until the 12-month point. This clearly contrasted with the families whose coping abilities did not change throughout the 12-month period. Goldstein et al. (1978) did not report whether they had succeeded in achieving their intervention goal.

Let us now turn to the *patient-focused studies*. As regards prevention of relapse, Liberman et al.'s (1986a) social skill training and Buchkremer and Fiedler's cognitive therapy appeared to be most successful. Brenner et al. (1980, 1985) also report that during the 18-month follow-up period the rehospitalization rate for the experimental group was significantly lower than that for the control groups. In all three studies the specified intervention goals were at least partly achieved at the end of the treatment period. In addition, Liberman et al. as well as the Brenner group report that persisting training effects could still be observed at follow-up. The remaining patient-focused interventions were less successful in terms of relapse prevention. It is mostly unclear whether this was because the declared goals of intervention were not achieved. If for example, Bellack et al. (1984) found no differences in social skills between the experimental group and the control group at follow-up 6 months after treatment, this does not necessarily indicate a failure of the intervention in view of the high drop-out rates. Although Buchkremer and Fiedler (in press) observed a significant increase of social skills by the end of the training, it remains open whether this effect persisted over the follow-up period. Patients seemed to profit immediately from the holistic health program, but apparently practically never used the stress-reduction techniques they had learnt after discharge from impatient treatment. The second objective (positive influence on attitude to self and the illness) was obviously not achieved. Hartwich and Schumacher (1985) did not even bother to attempt to examine whether they had succeeded in increasing patients' acceptance of the consequences of their illness.

In summary we can say that there are still many unanswered questions as regards the relationship between outcome, in terms of relapse, and success or failure in achieving the intervention goals. Consequently, in most cases the studies do not enable any conclusions as to the relevance of the "mechanisms of action" on which they are based.

Conclusions To Be Drawn from the Intervention Studies

1. One result of the studies discussed in this review stands out: interventions proved to be successful if they aimed not explicitly at treating specific etiological factors in schizophrenia, but rather at manipulating and/or modifying *unspecific* factors considered to be stressors or moderators of social stress. It would thus seem legitimate to see these findings as arguments in favor of the vulnerability-stress model. However, one important qualification must be added: the results of interventions may tell us something about possible determinants of the *course* of the illness but nothing about which factors may have played a role in the development of the illness itself. This proviso seems necessary mainly for the following reasons:

- The psychosocial situation of schizophrenic individuals undergoes radical changes in the course of the illness, including the stigma of being a mental patient, increasing everyday life stress (Serban 1975), social isolation, and lack of social support (Lipton et al. 1981; Angermeyer and Lammers 1986). It is thus inadmissible to extrapolate their psychosocial status prior to the first psychotic manifestation.
- The same applies for the families of schizophrenic patients. The illness also induces significant changes here: emotional problems of individual family members (e.g., anxiety, guilt, shame, frustration, anger, feelings of inadequacy), behavioral changes in response to the patients's illness (e.g., overprotective tendencies, curtailing own activities in order to care for the patient), changes in intrafamilial relationships and family role structure (e.g., if the patient is living with his/her parents, growing intensity in the relationship between patient and mother while father and siblings take a marginal position; increasing maternal dominance), social isolation of the family (e.g., Angermeyer and Döhner 1980; Katschnig and Konieczna 1984).

If one examines the detailed objectives of family-focused interventions, one notices that they are to a considerable extent identical to the above aspects. Here are some examples from the Anderson et al. (1980, 1981, 1986a, b) intervention catalog: decreasing guilt, anxiety, and other negative emotional reactions to illness; increasing self-confidence and providing a sense of cognitive mastery; reinforcing interpersonal boundaries between family members and generational boundaries between parents and offspring; deisolation of the family and enhancement of social network. The intervention focused on the effect the illness had on the family. These results thus also do not allow conclusions to be drawn about the role of psychosocial factors when psychosis is first manifested. This is all the more true as the family problems described above are by no means typical of schizophrenia. Similar phenomena, with certain variations, can be observed in other chronic illnesses, regardless of any differences in etiology and no matter whether they are psychiatric, psychosomatic, or somatic in nature. Therefore it is only natural that similar goals have been formulated for interventions with families of patients who were suffering from cancer, rheumatism, diabetes, or other forms of chronic illness (Angermeyer and Döhner 1981; Angermeyer and Freyberger 1982). The decisive feature is most certainly chronicity. One argument for this assumption might be that the two family-focused intervention studies conducted with samples with a very high number of first admissions were less successful (disregarding the methodological objections outlined above).

2. The results of studies conducted to date do not suffice to validate any particular version of the vulnerability-stress model. As Dohrenwend and Dohrenwend (1981) were able to demonstrate, the literature contains widely varying concepts for the interplay between the single components of the vulnerability-stress model. Neither are the interventions discussed here based on a uniform concept. Whereas, for example, Leff et al. adopt an "additive burden model," Falloon et al. and Liberman et al. endorse an interactive "vulnerability" and "stress-coping competence model" (or in Dohrenwend and Dohrenwend's terminology, "vulnerability model"). There are especially four problems worth mentioning here:
– As described above, it must be doubted whether most interventions actually achieved their declared goals. Only if they can prove that they have done so can they be considered as test for the validity of the assumed pathogenic model.
– The concepts for the individual components of the vulnerability-stress model leave many questions unanswered. EE is just one example: Despite considerable research efforts, Kuipers' (1979) assertion that EE remains an esoteric measure still seems to hold true. This may in part explain why at present three different conceptual versions of the EE measure exist in the literature: (1) In the original conceptualization EE is considered a stressor particularly noxious to schizophrenic patients due to their high sensitivity to their social environment. The theory is that under overstimulating conditions, such as living with high-EE relatives, schizophrenic patients are likely to have heightened arousal levels over longer periods of time and that residual or latent thought disorders may become manifest as psychotic symptoms. In contrast to acute stress in the form of life events, EE is viewed as chronic stress (Brown et al. 1972). (2) Recently, Greenley (1986) proposed the reconceptualization of EE as an indicator of

family attempts to socially control the schizophrenic person's behavior in a particular way. Relatives' efforts at control are viewed as a coping response and not as a stable attribute of the family. This implies that EE is sensitive to changes in the patient's symptoms. Based on an analysis of data from the 1972 study by Brown et al., Greenley was able to provide support for the social control conceptualization. As hypothesized, the more anxious and fearful the family, the more it was likely to attempt to control the patient's behavior. Family recognition of the schizophrenic's problem as mental illness reduced the likelihood of a social control coping response as measured by EE. (3) Contrary to the common view of EE as a measure of chronic stress, some authors subsume EE under the rubric of social support. According to them, EE stands for a deficit in social support provided by significant others. In their survey of research instruments for investigating social support in schizophrenia, Beels et al. (1984), for example, designate EE as "probably the most quoted and best replicated measure of the quality of social supports in schizophrenia" (p. 406). Böker and Brenner (1983) also concur in suggesting a redefinition of EE as a negative component of social support. This redefinition of EE has the advantage that it seems better equipped to explain the puzzling finding that for patients with depressive neurosis (Vaughn and Leff 1976) and major depression (Hooley et al. 1986) and for obese women (Havstadt 1979), the crucial number of critical comments is only one-third or one-half of that for schizophrenic patients. Psychodynamic theory, for example, leads one to expect that depressives or persons with eating disorders are more sensitive to deficits in social support than schizophrenic patients.

– In spite of the various labels – "crisis-oriented family therapy," "psychoeducational family treatment," "behavioral family therapy," etc. – a comparison of individual elements of each family-focused intervention reveals more similarities than differences (Leff 1986). It is thus not particularly surprising that, for example, the studies by Leff et al. and Falloon et al., which – as we discovered – were based on different models and pursued different intervention goals, were equally successful in preventing relapses. Ironically, despite the explicit denial of having intended to reduce EE, the Falloon et al. project has provided the most convincing evidence to date for the thesis that psychosocial interventions are capable of exercising positive influence on the family's emotional atmosphere. In an investigation of family interaction 3 months after treatment had begun a significant reduction in the behavioral correlates of the EE attitudes was found (Miklowitz et al. 1984; Goldstein and Doane 1985; Goldstein and Strachan 1986). As Falloon and Pederson (1985) somewhat resignedly concluded, considering how tightly emotional attitude and problem-solving behavior are interwoven, it remains to be seen to what extent the benefits reported in family-focused studies are the result of reductions in the negative emotions directed towards the patient, or the result of increases in the constructive problem-solving behavior.

– Finally, influences given little or no attention so far may be at least partially responsible for the results of intervention studies (see below).

3. Fears that success in relapse prophylaxis might detract from the level of social adaptation or lead to an increase in negative symptoms, and vice versa, do

not seem to have gained substance. In any case, several authors report positive results in both areas (Falloon et al. 1985; Liberman et al. 1986 a, b; Stramke and Hodel-Oprecht 1983).

4. Interventions that focus on the patient can be just as successful as those that aim at manipulating or modifying the family environment. This conclusion is at least suggested by the results of the study by Hogarty et al. (1986) in which both family treatment and social skills training were conducted with patients under comparable conditions. Both modes of treatment had a similarly positive effect on relapse rate. When they were combined, an additive effect was observed.

5. A connection between degree of vulnerability and "toxicity" (Day 1986) of the family environment can also be empirically demonstrated. Falloon et al. (1985) report that patients in the group where family therapy – as we saw – was conducted with great success needed less neuroleptic medication than patients in the control group.

6. The issue seems to be psychosocial *"maintenance"* rather than brief intervention. Hogarty et al. (1986), for example, emphasized that the early prophylactic effects observed in family intervention studies were more likely related to the delay of schizophrenic relapse than to its prevention. One of their arguments is that as patients approached the end of the 2nd year of treatment, relapse continued to rise in all experimental groups. The frequently weaker results of patient-focused interventions than of family-focused interventions support this view. The former employed "real" follow-ups (with one exception), i.e., course of illness was observed over a specified period *after* completion of psychosocial treatment; in the latter, however, the intervention and follow-up periods were to a large extent identical. Liberman (1986) even believed that "it is likely that indefinite, if not lifelong, psychosocial support, guidance, and training may be optimal for most chronic patients" (p. 214).

7. Contrary to what one might expect according to the tenets of labeling theory, the explicit labeling of the illness as schizophrenic psychosis as well as the definition of behavioral deviances as schizophrenic symptoms (McGill et al. 1983; Berkowitz et al. 1984; Cozolino and Goldstein 1986) had no negative effect on the course of the illness. The opposite was the case, as demonstrated by the success of intervention programs which included a formal education component (Leff et al., Falloon et al., Hogarty et al.). In this context, Greenley's findings seem interesting: the family's recognition of the schizophrenic's problem as mental illness reduced the fearful and anxious family's likelihood to employ intense interpersonal social control as measured by EE.

Suggestions for Further Research

Future research in psychosocial interventions for schizophrenic patients should in my opinion direct more attention above all to the following three aspects:

1. Studies completed so far that aimed at modifying the patient's social milieu concentrated on the family. They did so for the good reason that the family, given the conditions of modern psychiatric care, is certainly the most important source of psychosocial support for patients. This insight is being increasingly accepted

in the profession which until recently was more or less sceptical toward and rejected patient family members. This was particularly due to the adoption of vulgarized concepts of family research which, explicitly or implicitly, sought the cause for the development of schizophrenic disturbances in the family (Angermeyer 1982). The discovery of the positive aspects of the family should not, however, distract one from two facts: Many, even the majority of schizophrenic patients do not live with their parents and do not have families of their own. Sooner or later their parents become old and frail and eventually die, and this resource is no longer available to them. Many parents are painfully aware of this distressing fact, which in my view is all too gladly forgotten by professional helpers in their enthusiasm for a new form of treatment for schizophrenia. The objective of future intervention must therefore be to influence the patient's social environment outside the family positively and to create a suitable way of life, with the emphasis on living conditions and job situation.

2. Recent research findings suggest that schizophrenic patients spontaneously develop self-help methods during the course of their illness. If their psychological balance threatens to decompensate, patients employ certain self-healing strategies (Böker and Brenner 1983, 1984; Böker et al. 1984; Brenner et al. 1985; Böker 1986) which act as a "buffer" against negative stressor effects, thus reducing the danger of a psychotic breakdown. According to Breier and Strauss (1983) three "mechanisms of self-control" are particularly common: self-instruction, reduced involvement in activity, and increased involvement in activity.

This presents a promising perspective for future interventions. The studies cited above by Buchkremer and Fiedler (in press) and Lukoff et al. (1986) represent first steps in this direction. However, before programs for systematic training of patients in the use of cognitive and behavioral control mechanisms can be developed, investigators will have to research more closely which strategies prove particularly effective with regard to relapse prophylaxis. This new therapeutic approach is especially worthy of note, as it could help patients toward more competence and autonomy in dealing with their disturbance.

3. Emotional coping with illness has received relatively little attention so far. The reason might be that it would prove particularly difficult to help patients effectively in coping and that one frequently runs the risk of being very easily confronted by the limits of therapy. The process of learning to accept the illness with all its negative effects on the individual as a person, current situation, and future perspectives in life is long and painful and is probably never quite mastered by some patients. It also seems that the psychosocial interventions discussed in this paper can do little to change this. For example, Leff et al. (1985) report that two patients in the experimental group committed suicide during the 2-year follow-up. Research will have to make added effort to find out how one can help patients not to lose their morale, to regain courage and develop a new perspective for their life. Whether this can succeed may also decide to what extent patients defend themselves against the psychosis or, instead, passively give in to their fate or even seek shelter from a reality experienced as depressing in the illness (Strauss et al. 1986).

In analogy to what was said above about the family, the psychosocial situation of patients can by no means be seen as specific to schizophrenia, but is in many aspects comparable with that of patients who suffer from other chronic illnesses. My plea is, therefore, for close cooperation with social scientists who are researching this field in other areas of medicine. Furthermore, results of sociological research on unemployment may be of use.

How important the patients themselves consider the problems discussed here is well illustrated by the answer of one patient to the question: What do you suffer from most of all? "It's not that sometimes I go crazy. It's more knowing that I am probably going to be living here in this hostel for ever, alone, without the chance of finding a partner for life, of having children, and having no hope of ever finding qualified work."

Acknowledgements. The author would like to thank Dietrich Klusmann and Johann-Jürgen Rohde for helpful comments.

References

Anderson CM, Hogarty GE, Reiss DJ (1980) Family treatment of adult schizophrenic patients: a psycho-educational approach. Schizophr Bull 6:490–505

Anderson CM, Hogarty GE, Reiss DJ (1981) The psychoeducational family treatment of schizophrenia. In: Goldstein MJ (ed) New developments in interventions with families of schizophrenics. Jossey-Bass, San Francisco, pp 79–84

Anderson CM, Hogarty GE, Reiss DJ (1986a) Schizophrenia and the family. Guilford Press, New York

Anderson CM, Griffin S, Rossi A, Pagonis I, Holder DP, Treiber R (1986b) A comparative study of the impact of education vs. process groups for families of patients with affective disorders. Fam Process 25:185–205

Angermeyer MC (1982) Der theorie-graue Star im Auge des Psychiaters. Zur Rezeption der Wissensbestände der Familienforschung in der Sozialpsychiatrie. MMG Medizin Mensch Gesellschaft 7:55–60

Angermeyer MC, Döhner O (1980) Die Familie in der Auseinandersetzung mit der schizophrenen Erkrankung des Sohnes. Gruppenpsychother Gruppendynamik 16:35–59

Angermeyer MC, Döhner O (eds) (1981) Chronisch kranke Kinder und Jugendliche in der Familie. Enke, Stuttgart

Angermeyer MC, Freyberger H (eds) (1982) Chronisch kranke Erwachsene in der Familie. Enke, Stuttgart

Angermeyer MC, Lammers R (1986) Das soziale Netzwerk schizophrener Kranker. Z Klin Psychol Psychopathol Psychother 34:100–118

Beels CC, Gutwirth L, Berkeley J, Struening E (1984) Measurements of social support in schizophrenia. Schizophr Bull 10:399–411

Bellack AS, Turner SM, Hersen M, Luber RF (1984) An examination of the efficacy of social skills training for chronic schizophrenic patients. Hosp Community Psychiatry 35:1023–1028

Berkowitz R, Eberlein-Fries R, Kuipers L, Leff J (1984) Educating relatives about schizophrenia. Schizophr Bull 10:418–429

Böker W (1986) Zur Selbsthilfe Schizophrener: Problemanalyse und eigene empirische Untersuchungen. In: Böker W, Brenner HD (eds) Bewältigung der Schizophrenie. Huber, Bern, pp 176–188

Böker W, Brenner HD (1983) Selbstheilungsversuche Schizophrener. Nervenarzt 54:578–589

Böker W, Brenner HD (1984) Über Selbstheilungsversuche Schizophrener. Schweiz Arch Neurol Neurochir Psychiatr 135:123–133

Böker W, Brenner HD, Gerstner G, Keller F, Müller J, Spichtig L (1984) Self-healing strategies among schizophrenics: attempts at compensation for basic disorders. Acta Psychiatr Scand 69:373–378

Breier A, Strauss JS (1983) Self-control in psychotic disorders. Arch Gen Psychiatry 40:1141–1145

Brenner HD (1986) Zur Bedeutung von Basisstörungen für Behandlung und Rehabilitation. In: Böker W, Brenner HD (eds) Bewältigung der Schizophrenie. Huber, Bern, pp 176–188

Brenner HD, Seeger G, Stramke WG (1980) Evaluation eines spezifischen Therapieprogramms zum Training kognitiver und kommunikativer Fähigkeiten in der Rehabilitation chronisch schizophrener Patienten in einem naturalistischen Feldexperiment. In: Hautzinger M, Schulz W (eds) Klinische Psychologie und Psychotherapie. GwG/DGVT, Köln, pp 32–47

Brenner HD, Böker W, Andres K, Stramke WG (1985) Efforts at compensation with regard to basic disorders among schizophrenics. In: Laaser U, Senault R, Viefhues H (eds) Primary health care in the making. Springer, Berlin Heidelberg New York Tokyo, pp 267–273

Brown GW, Mock EN, Carstairs GM, Wing JK (1962) Influence of family life on the course of schizophrenic illness. Br J Prev Soc Med 16:55–68

Brown GW, Birley JLT, Wing JK (1972) Influence of family life on the course of schizophrenic disorders: a replication. Br J Psychiatry 121:241–258

Buchkremer G, Fiedler P (in press) Kognitive vs handlungsorientierte Therapie: Vergleich zweier psychotherapeutischer Methoden zur Rezidivprophylaxe bei schizophrenen Patienten

Ciompi L (1986) Auf dem Weg zu einem kohärenten multidimensionalen Krankheits- und Therapieverständnis der Schizophrenie: Konvergierende neue Konzepte. In: Böker W, Brenner HD (eds) Bewältigung der Schizophrenie. Huber, Bern, pp 47–61

Cozolino LJ, Goldstein MJ (1986) Family education as a component of extended family-oriented treatment programs for schizophrenia. In: Goldstein MJ, Hand I, Hahlweg K (eds) Treatment of schizophrenia. Family assessment and intervention. Springer, Berlin Heidelberg New York Tokyo, pp 117–128

Day R (1986) Social stress and schizophrenia: from the concept of present life events to the notion of toxic environments. In: Burrows GD, Norman TR, Rubinstein G (eds) Handbook of studies on schizophrenia, part 1. Elsevier, Amsterdam, pp 71–82

Doane JA, Goldstein J, Miklowitz DJ, Falloon IRH (1986) The impact of individual and family treatment on the affective climate of families of schizophrenics. Br J Psychiatry 148:279–287

Dohrenwend BS, Dohrenwend BP (1981) Hypotheses about stress processes linking social class to various types of psychopathology. Am J Community Psychol 9:146–159

Dulz B, Hand I (1986) Short-term relapse in young schizophrenics: Can it be predicted and affected by family (CFI), patient, and treatment variables? An experimental study. In: Goldstein MJ, Hand I, Hahlweg K (eds) Treatment of schizophrenia. Family assessment and intervention. Springer, Berlin Heidelberg New York Tokyo, pp 59–75

Falloon IRH, Pederson J (1985) Family management in the prevention of morbidity of schizophrenia: the adjustment of the family unit. Br J Psychiatry 147:156–163

Falloon IRH, Boyd JL, McGill CW, Strang JS, Moss HB (1981) Family management training in the community care of schizophrenia. In: Goldstein MJ (ed) New developments in interventions with families of schizophrenics. Jossey-Bass, San Francisco, pp 61–77

Falloon IRH, Boyd JL, McGill CW, Razani J, Moss HB, Gilderman AM (1982) Family management in the prevention of exacerbations of schizophrenia. N Engl J Med 306:1437–1440

Falloon IRH, Boyd JL, McGill CW (1984) Family care for schizophrenia. Guilford Press, New York

Falloon IRH, Boyd JL, McGill CW, Williamson M, Razani J, Moss HB, Gilderman AM, Simpson GM (1985) Family management in the prevention of morbidity of schizophrenia. Arch Gen Psychiatry 42:887–896

Goldstein MJ, Doane JA (1985) Interventions with families and the course of schizophrenia. In: Alpert M (ed) Controversies in schizophrenia. Guilford Press, New York London, pp 381–397

Goldstein MJ, Kopeikin HS (1981) Short- and long-term effects of combining drug and family therapy. In: Goldstein MJ (ed) New developments in interventions with families of schizophrenics. Jossey-Bass, San Francisco, pp 5–26

Goldstein MJ, Strachan AM (1986) Impact of family intervention programs on family communication and the short-term course of schizophrenia. In: Goldstein MJ, Hand I, Hahlweg K (eds) Treatment of schizophrenia. Family assessment and intervention. Springer, Berlin Heidelberg New York Tokyo, pp 185–192

Goldstein MJ, Rodnick EH, Evans JR, May PRA, Steinberg MR (1978) Drug and family therapy in the aftercare of acute schizophrenics. Arch Gen Psychiatry 35:1169–1177

Gottesman I, Shields J (1982) Schizophrenia: the epigenetic puzzle. Cambridge University Press, London

Greenley JR (1986) Social control and expressed emotion. J Nerv Ment Dis 174:24–30

Hartwich P, Schumacher E (1985) Zum Stellenwert der Gruppenpsychotherapie in der Nachsorge Schizophrener. Nervenarzt 56:365–372

Havstad LF (1979) Weight loss and weight loss maintenance as aspects of family emotional processes. PhD thesis, University of Southern California, Los Angeles

Hogarty GE, Anderson C (1986) Eine kontrollierte Studie über Familientherapie, Training sozialer Fertigkeiten und unterstützende Chemotherapie in der Nachbehandlung Schizophrener: vorläufige Effekte auf Rezidive und Expressed Emotion nach einem Jahr. In: Böker W, Brenner HD (eds) Bewältigung der Schizophrenie. Huber, Bern, pp 72–86

Hogarty GE, Anderson CM, Reiss DJ, Kornblith SJ, Greenwald DB, Javna CD, Madonia MJ (1986) Family psychoeducation, social skills training, and maintenance chemotherapy in the aftercare treatment of schizophrenia. Arch Gen Psychiatry 43:633–642

Hooley JM, Orley J, Teasdale JD (1986) Levels of expressed emotion and relapse in depressed patients. Br J Psychiatry 148:642–647

Katschnig H, Konieczna T (1984) Angehörigenprobleme im Spiegel von Selbsterfahrungsgruppen. In: Angermeyer MC, Finzen A (eds) Die Angehörigengruppe. Enke, Stuttgart

Köttgen C, Sönnichsen I, Mollenhauer K, Jurth R (1984 a) The family relations of young schizophrenic patients: results of the Hamburg Camberwell Family Interview Study I. Int J Fam Psychiatry 5:61–70

Köttgen C, Sönnichsen I, Mollenhauer K, Jurth R (1984 b) Families' high-expressed-emotions and relapses in young schizophrenic patients: results of the Hamburg Camberwell Family Interview Study II. Int J Fam Psychiatry 5:71–82

Köttgen C, Sönnichsen I, Mollenhauer K, Jurth R (1984 c) Group therapy with the families of schizophrenic patients: results of the Hamburg Camberwell Family Interview Study III. Int J Fam Psychiatry 5:83–94

Kuipers L (1979) Expressed emotion: a review. Br J Soc Clin Psychol 18:237–243

Leff J (1986) Family therapy. In: Burrows GD, Norman TR, Rubinstein G (eds) Handbook of studies on schizophrenia, part 2. Elsevier, Amsterdam, pp 101–113

Leff J, Vaughn C (1981) The role of maintenance therapy and relatives' expressed emotion in relapse of schizophrenia: a two-year follow-up. Br J Psychiatry 139:102–104

Leff J, Kuipers L, Berkowitz R, Eberlein-Vries R, Sturgeon D (1982) A controlled trial of social intervention in the families of schizophrenic patients. Br J Psychiatry 141:121–134

Leff J, Kuipers L, Berkowitz R, Sturgeon D (1985) A controlled trial of social intervention in the families of schizophrenic patients: two year follow-up. Br J Psychiatry 146:594–600

Liberman RP (1986) Coping and competence as protective factors in the vulnerability-stress model of schizophrenia. In: Goldstein MJ, Hand I, Halweg K (eds) Treatment of schizophrenia. Family assessment and intervention. Springer, Berlin Heidelberg New York Tokyo, pp 201–215

Liberman RP, Evans CC (1985) Behavioral rehabilitation for chronic mental patients. J Clin Psychopharmacol 5:8S–14S

Liberman RP, Wallace CJ, Falloon IRH, Vaughn CE (1981) Interpersonal problem-solving therapy for schizophrenics and their families. Compr Psychiatry 22:627–630

Liberman RP, Mueser KT, Wallace CJ (1986 a) Social skills training for schizophrenic individuals at risk for relapse. Am J Psychiatry 143:523–526

Liberman RP, Jacobs HE, Boone SE, Foy DW, Donahoe CP, Falloon IRH, Blackwell G, Wallace CJ (1986 b) Fertigkeitstraining zur Anpassung Schizophrener an die Gemeinschaft. In: Böker W, Brenner HD (eds) Bewältigung der Schizophrenie. Huber, Bern, pp 96–112

Lipton FR, Cohen CI, Fischer E, Katz ST (1981) Schizophrenia: a network crisis. Schizophr Bull 7:144–151

Lukoff D, Wallace CJ, Liberman RP, Burke K (1986) A holistic program for chronic schizophrenic patients. Schizophr Bull 12:274–282

McGill CW, Falloon IRH, Boyd JL, Wood-Siverio C (1983) Family educational intervention in the treatment of schizophrenia. Hosp Community Psychiatry 34:934–938

Miklowitz DJ, Goldstein MJ, Falloon IRH, Doane JA (1984) Interactional correlates of Expressed Emotion in the families of schizophrenics. Br J Psychiatry 144:482–487

Nuechterlein KH, Dawson M (eds) (1984) Vulnerability and stress factors in the developmental course of schizophrenic disorders. Schizophr Bull 10:158–312

Serban G (1975) Stress in schizophrenics and normals. Br J Psychiatry 126:397–407

Stramke GW, Brenner HD (1983) Psychologische Trainingsprogramme zur Minderung defizitärer kognitiver Störungen in der Rehabilitation chronisch schizophrener Patienten. In: Brenner HD, Rey E-R, Stramke WG (eds) Empirische Schizophrenieforschung. Huber, Bern, pp 182–201

Stramke GW, Hodel-Oprecht B (1983) Untersuchungen zur Wirksamkeit psychologischer Therapieprogramme in der Rehabilitation chronisch schizophrener Patienten. In: Brenner HD, Rey E-R, Stramke WG (eds) Empirische Schizophrenieforschung. Huber, Bern, pp 216–234

Strauss JS, Harding CM, Hafez H, Lieberman P (1986) Die Rolle des Patienten bei der Genesung von einer Psychose. In: Böker W, Brenner HD (eds) Bewältigung der Schizophrenie. Huber, Bern, pp 168–175

Vaughn CE, Leff JP (1976) The influence of family and social factors on the course of psychiatric illness. Br J Psychiatry 129:125–137

Zubin J (1986) Models for the aetiology of schizophrenia. In: Burrows GD, Norman TR, Rubinstein F (eds) Handbook of studies on schizophrenia, part 1. Elsevier, Amsterdam, pp 97–104

Zubin J, Spring B (1977) Vulnerability – a new view of schizophrenia. J Abnorm Psychol 86:103–126

Zubin J, Magaziner J, Steinhauer S (1983) The metamorphosis of schizophrenia: from chronicity to vulnerability. Psychol Med 13:551–571

Clinicopsychological Factors in the Development and Prognosis of Schizophrenia

M. M. Kabanov, G. V. Burkovsky, and K. V. Korabelnikov

The study of the clinical and psychological factors in the development of and prognoses in schizophrenia is one of the priorities of contemporary psychiatry. This is due to a number of circumstances, among which perhaps the most important is that its therapeutic goals include not only the prevention and control of psychological manifestations but also the partial or complete restoration of the personal and social status of the patient, which is in fact the supreme goal of rehabilitation. Rehabilitation is a wider concept than treatment (Kabanov and Weise 1981; Kabanov 1985). There is no doubt that almost all mental disorders including schizophrenia are related in their development in three categories: clinicobiological factors, personality factors and social and psychological factors. As regards the latter two groups, a vast body of scientific evidence already exists that an important role in the development of schizophrenia can be attributed to the influence of the environment as well as to the premorbid influences (especially to the stress-related forms) of social functioning which can be corrected in the course of treatment only through special, goal-directed, micro-social interventions. Psychosocial factors to a large extent determine the success or not of the functioning of schizophrenic patients in society. Thus an analysis of the causes of rehospitalisations has demonstrated that, along with the biological severity of the disease, a significant role in the patients's instability in the community is played by loss or insufficiency of: (1) professional instrumental skills (2) social interaction skills in professional activity, family life and leisure; (3) behavioural adequacy; (4) ability to use social support after discharge from an inpatient facility (Hagen 1975; Paul and Lentz 1977; Wallace et al. 1980). To a great extent, the role of psychosocial factors in the course and outcome of schizophrenia has been dealt with in numerous prognostic studies summarised in various reviews (Shternberg 1978; Khramelashvili 1978; Strauss and Carpenter 1978; Beck 1978; Kringlen 1980; Jonsson and Nyman 1984).

In the rehabilitation department of the Bekhterev Institute in Leningrad a number of studies have dealt with the impact of psychosocial factors on the outcome of restorative therapy of schizophrenic patients. By restorative therapy we mean the initial stage in the rehabilitation process which usually is initiated in an inpatient environment. The objective of the study was not only to collect evidence to compare with the available data from the literature but also to apply such findings in addition to the available clinical information in the individual prediction of course outcome and degree of success in rehabilitation.

The Leningrad V. M. Bekhterev Psychoneurological Research Institute, 3 Bekhterev Street, 193019, Leningrad, USSR

The series of studies was carried out on a cohort of 768 schizophrenic patients with the support of the so-called rehabilitation automated information system (RAIS), which uses a structured case history composed of 995 items (Kabanov et al. 1984). In addition to clinical information this instrument contains detailed data on all spheres of personal and social functioning of the patient at various periods and points of his life and in various points of the evolution of his disorder. This allows the establishment of correlations of prognostic significance concerning the various factors involved, all carried out in a single design. Findings of the individual automated prediction, as based on these materials, demonstrated that the computerised prognosis agreed with the observed treatment outcome in 67%, was erroneous in 15% and indefinite in 18% of the cases.

The information employed is based on 40 informative indices which were used in correlation analysis. These include 15 clinical characteristics, for example age at onset, severity of symptomatology, rate of progression, length of psychotic states, etc. There were 25 characteristics related to personality or psychosocial sphere or functioning. Examples of the latter are the range of communication and the communication skills of the patient with special attention to communication with the opposite sex, aspects of the patient's work pattern, range of interests, habits concerning spending leisure time, etc. A special comparison of the prognostic informativeness of the clinical and psychosocial indices was made. Computerised prognosis, as based on psychosocial indications alone, agreed with reality in 58%, was erroneous in 15% and indefinite in 27% of the cases. The prognosis based on the clinical indications alone was true in 63%, erroneous in 15% and indefinite in 22% of the cases. Thus, the obtained findings suggest that psychosocial factors are no less informative prognostically than clinical ones. It may also be suggested that these factors determine, to a significant degree, the outcome of the restorational treatment. This stresses the necessity of a wider application of psychosocial methods to schizophrenic patients.

We should note that the effect of psychosocial factors on the treatment outcome is presented here as just an aggregate of the effects of separate personality characteristics and social functioning. To accomplish the research tasks of a purely pragmatic nature (prognosis) this may be sufficient; in more theoretically oriented works associated with attempts to identify pathogenetic mechanisms of the disease, it seems significant to consider not separate personality characteristics but the integral personality structure as a system of qualities that have definite, relatively stable correlations with each other.

To implement this methodological approach a study of 250 schizophrenic patients was carried out in collaboration with the Bekhterev Institute in Leningrad and the Karl Marx University in Leipzig in the German Democratic Republik. Its aims were to identify the role of premorbid personality structures in schizophrenic patients and their effects on the psychopathological manifestations of the disorder. It also considered a number of problems related to the question of how this personality structure had emerged. In the course of the study 15 six-point bipolar scales were used to evaluate the premorbid personality of the patients. In 38% of the cases this personality structure was characterised by a combination of an inclination to emotional delay and kindness without passivity. The presence of such a personality structure (conventionally designated as AIK – activity, inclination to emotional delay and kindness) was revealed to be interrelated with indices of the conditions of family upbringing, the character of premorbid social functioning and clinical manifestations registered in the formal case history.

A comparison of schizophrenics with or without the AIK premorbid personality structure has shown that in childhood, patients with AIK are more often found in conflictless families with a high cultural standard and a stable relationship of the mother to the child. It implies that the formation of such a personality structure takes place in definite family settings marked by a developed but often potentially contradictory system of cultural moral standards including both the demand for an active social position and increased limitations in the ways of reaching goals.

The presence of the AIK structure in the premorbid personality affects the psychosocial functioning of the future schizophrenic in a contradictory way. This is displayed by the fact that the same AIK structure is simultaneously found in both individuals with more and with less successful psychosocial functioning prior to disease manifestation. Indeed, patients with the AIK structure were significantly more satisfied than patients without it in regard to their social functioning and environment, namely the range of their personal contacts, financial and family situations, interrelations with their parents, colleagues, managers, and friends. Also, they were characterised by a higher premorbid level of social functioning. In particular, their range of personal contacts was wider, their grades in school and working productivity were higher, and they spent their leisure time more actively. At the same time, patients with AIK displayed indirect signs of an increased self-dissatisfaction and inner discomfort prior to disease onset. This was revealed in lowered self-evaluation, in a need for a different professional activity despite high achievement in the current one, in doubts concerning realisation of family plans and in a decreased level of contacts with the opposite sex.

Such an opposing nature of psychosocial functioning may be explained by a contradiction in the very structure of the premorbid personality demonstrated, on the one hand, in an increased emotional sensitivity and hence a greater need for emotional acting out and, on the other, in a reduced capability for alleviating negative emotions. This probably results in a chronic imbalance of emotional processes, overload of the brain symstems responsible for maintenance of emotional homeostasis and, therefore, accumulation and aggravation of mental tension and discomfort which provoke involvement of psychological defences aimed at their elimination and compensation. Lowered self-evaluation and increased self-dissatisfaction become stimuli for compensation of this negative emotional experience by a positive one. Thus, the individual reinforces activity aimed at making new progress in social functioning since it provides satisfaction. He also practises the socially approved style of sympathetic, kind behaviour which also gives satisfaction. However, such a modification of behaviour and activity creates a vicious circle of mental responses and provides constant repetition and reinforcement of the basic peculiarities in the personality structure and therefore of the mental tension and discomfort.

Also, a still greater role is played by another psychological defence mechanism of an intrapsychic nature which constitutes inner acting out of emotional redundancy through day dreaming and fantasy. This autistic mode of personality defence against frustration promotes temporary stabilisation of the mental state while resulting in abundant development of the fantasy apparatus, which predisposes the mental sphere to autism. It is possible that in the case of triggering the schizophrenic process and under its effect, the fantasy products may acquire a self-contained, autonomous character and present in the contex of hallucinations and delusions.

Our research has identified a number of peculiar features in patients with the AIK structure as compared with other schizophrenics. They more often than not present with severer symptomatology such as autism, withdrawal, increased expressivity, hypersexuality, delusions and hallucinations. This group of patients also usually has had longer hospitalisation and a greater decrease in the quality of their clinical remission.

The results of the present study may become a foundation of a hypothesis that formation of the AIK premorbid personality structure of a schizoid type is conditioned, excluding the effect of constitutional peculiarities, by definite conditions of family upbringing and his specific mode of interaction with the social environment in accordance with the positive feedback principle. Such an interaction of the developing personality with the environment may promote constant irritation and then development of the basic schizoid peculiarities in the individual's personality. During formation of this premorbid personality structure, reinforcement of the psychological defences takes place which may subsequently aggravate some psychological manifestations of the schizophrenic process and prevent their alleviation or elimination. Summarising our findings, we would like to stress that our results provide an additional empirical support of the biosocial model of schizophrenia upon which the concept of rehabilitation is based.

References

Beck IG (1978) Social influences on the prognosis of schizophrenia. Schizophr Bull 4(1):86–101

Hagen RL (1975) Behavioral therapies and the treatment of schizophrenics. Schizophr Bull 13(3):70–96

Jonsson H, Nyman AK (1984) Prediction of outcome in schizophrenia. Acta Psychiatr Scand 69(4):274–291

Kabanov MM (1985) Rehabilitation of the mentally ill (in Russian). Meditsina, Leningrad

Kabanov MM, Weise K (1981) Klinische und soziale Aspekte der Rehabilitation psychisch Kranker. Thieme, Leipzig

Kabanov MM, Burkovsky GV, Buks AY, Iovlev BV, Korabelnikov KV, Lavrushin AA (1984) Research into the rehabilitation process of the mentally ill with the aid of the rehabilitological automated information system (RAIS). SS Korsakov J Neuropathol Psychiatr (USSR) 5:735–739

Khramelashvili VV (1978) Some problems of schizophrenia prognosis in current literature (a review). SS Korsakov J Neuropathol Psychiatr (USSR) 5:755–768

Kringlen E (1980) Schizophrenia: research in the Nordic countries. Schizophr Bull 6(4):566–578

Paul GL, Lentz RJ (1977) Psychosocial treatment of chronic mental patients: milieu versus social-learning programs. Harvard Univ Press, Cambridge

Shternberg EY (1978) New studies of the course and outcome in schizophrenics abroad. SS Korsakov J Neuropathol Psychiat (USSR) 1:135–151

Strauss JS, Carpenter WT (1978) The prognosis of schizophrenia: rationale for multidimentional concept. Schizophr Bull 4(1):56–67

Wallace CJ, Nelson CJ, Liberman PP, Aitchson RA, Lukoff D, Elder JP, Ferris C (1980) A review and critique of social skills training with schizophrenic patients. Schizophr Bull 6(1):42–63

Vulnerability and Trigger Models/
Rehabilitation: Discussion

H. KATSCHNIG

The papers presented in this session are of different characters, including a review of the literature on the one hand and reports about original research carried out by very different methods (clinical, experimental, psychological, and epidemiological) on the other. I do not intend to discuss each of the papers in turn but have, instead, selected three topics on which to structure my discussion: the concept of vulnerability, the difficulties of defining and measuring triggers, and, finally, the specificity of research findings on vulnerability and triggers in relation to the phenomenology of schizophrenia.

The Concept of Vulnerability

Several times throughout this symposium allusion has been made to so-called vulnerability factors, and a comment on th proper use of the concept seems appropriate (Zubin and Spring 1977). Factors such as abnormalities in smooth-pursuit eye movements, attention, spontaneous fluctuations of skin conductance, IQ, p300, dopamine concentration in the left amygdala, specific personality features (AIK), social class and genetic factors have been mentioned as correlating with schizophrenia, i.e. as possible aetiological variables or as "markers", and they are certainly also possible candidates for vulnerability factors. However, in order to qualify as a vulnerability factor, certain requirements have to be fulfilled.

Etymologically, "vulnerability" implies that an individual is specifically susceptible to an external influence. It is not justifiable to call variables which have been found to be correlated simply with an increased risk of developing schizophrenia vulnerability factors. If no theoretical model comprising a mechanism of how an external factor affects a vulnerable individual can be formulated, such factors should be rather regarded as simple "risk factors", and the size of their contribution to the onset of schizophrenia should be expressed in calculating the "relative risk", which does not imply any theoretical assumption.

Nuechterlein's distinction between "stable vulnerability indicator", "mediating vulnerability factor" and "episode or symptom indicator" is quite helpful for clarifying the field. Clearly an "episode marker" as that presented in Leff's paper is, at best, a correlate of the psychopathological state. That such correlates may be some indication of an underlying "weakness" which manifests itself during an episode is a different question; since this underlying weakness is not measured by the indicator, we should not apply the term "vulnerability factor."

Psychiatrische Universitätsklinik, Währinger Gürtel 18–20, 1090 Vienna, Austria

One minimum requirement of vulnerability factor research is that only those variables which were measured before the outbreak of schizophrenia can be called potential vulnerability factors. The problem of measuring onset is already in itself a complex one (von Cranach et al. 1981). Measurements which have been carried out after disease onset may find just an episode indicator (state marker) or – if the measured phenomenon persists after remission – a consequence of the disease or its treatment. The increase of dopamine receptors in the brain of schizophrenics treated with neuroleptics is a typical example of these possibilities.

Finally, it has to be considered that vulnerability may change with age and stage of life, either because of slow psychological changes in personality or, e.g., because of a "burn out" of biological vulnerabilities in the dopaminergic neurone systems.

Unfortunately, in prospective studies of at-risk populations, not enough time has elapsed so far for the identification of vulnerability factors. It is true that in a proportion of children of schizophrenic mothers certain deficits, such as abnormalities in information processing and attentional functioning and also autonomic nervous system anomalies, have been reported, but it is not yet known whether these children will later develop schizophrenia. Information processing, attention and autonomous nervous system functioning could be called vulnerability factors, since they would constitute a specific susceptibility to environmental stimuli such as information overload.

It seems clear that the title of this last session ought not to have been "Vulnerability and Trigger Models" but "Vulnerability/Trigger Models" since vulnerabilities and triggers are necessary for each other: a vulnerability factor requires a trigger and a trigger needs a specific vulnerability on which to act. Such a model can only be tested empirically, if the trigger or stressor to which an individual is vulnerable is taken seriously. A loose attitude can be found among genetic researchers who, while applying very sophisticated methods to identify the contribution of hereditary factors to the relative risk of schizophrenia, generally refer only vaguely to social factors and triggers when concluding that there must be other influences if persons with identical genetic equipment, such as monozygotic twins, have less than 100% concordance rates.

If applied in the proper sense, the concept of vulnerability may prove to be fruitful for scientific progress in psychiatry. Although "boxologies" such as those presented by Nuechterlein may be criticised – since boxes connected with arrows do not explain anything – they have the merit that they draw attention to factors other than those which are a specific researcher's interest. Vulnerability models may thus serve to bring those who work in very different fields closer together and help understanding of other approaches.

Difficulties in Defining and Measuring Triggers

First, if a vulnerability/trigger model is to be tested empirically, the vulnerability and triggering factors should be clearly distinguished. It makes sense to assume that external influences which can act as triggering factors, such as life events, may leave a kind of vulnerability behind in an individual who may then be more likely to be vulnerable to subsequent stressors than before. Nevertheless, in carrying out empirical research, one should be as precise as possible in separating the different aspects. I do not see that Nuechterlein in his graphs really separates these issues, and there are also problems with Leff's and Dohrenwend's papers. Leff seems to regard "expressed emotion" and "life events" as belonging to the same dimension, while in a vulnerability/trigger model, high expressed emotion could be regarded as contributing to the vulnerability of an individual to develop schizophrenia if life events occur.

If life events are to be embedded in a vulnerability/trigger model and not just regarded as "risk factors" without being built into a theory, it is problematic to measure life events which have occurred as far back as 1 year before the onset of schizophrenia, as Dohrenwend has done in his study. The life events must be recent if their stress value is to be built into a vulnerability/trigger model. It would, therefore, be necessary to know whether, as has been found by Brown and Birley (1968), life stress increases just before the onset of a schizophrenic episode.

This brings us to a general problem of life stress studies. As Tsuang pointed out yesterday, it is extremely difficult to date onset precisely for many psychotic episodes, and clear rules have to be laid down. If onset was 1 year before the study interview, as in the case in Dohrenwend's study, a precise dating of the onset becomes even more difficult. However, such precision in dating the onset is essential for identifying life events which have occurred before the onset and thus have contributed to it, and for distinguishing them from those life events which may already be a consequence of the disease (Katschnig 1986).

Tsuang has indicated that the occurrence of life events may depend on the patient's social network and on his personality. This point is very important if the interplay between personality factors and the social network on the one hand – they may have the status of vulnerability or protective factors – and life stress is regarded. The number and type of life events occurring to a person may very well be dependent on the size of his social network, which in turn can depend on his personality. If specific personality features, which are connected with small and distorted social networks, are also concerned with a predisposition for developing schizohrenia, it may become very difficult to disentangle predisposing and precipitating factors. Also, other relationships between life events and these variables, which might obscure correlations, are possible. For instance, a life event occurring a few months back, such as a divorce, may reduce substantially the social support and social network of a patient and thus deprive him of possible protective and coping factors (Monroe and Steiner 1986).

Having mentioned the interdependence of stressful life events, social network and personality, which basically means that many life events are not "independent", i.e., they are not fateful blows out of the blue but are somehow self-inflicted, I would like to stress, nevertheless, that we have to take such events seriously. A vicious circle might be operating in which a person with specific personality traits may produce his own life events which in turn make the situation more difficult, creating further life events and so on. I do not see, therefore, the importance of separating dependent from independent life events at the onset of schizophrenia.

The Specificity Problem: Psychopathology, Vulnerability and Stressors

The issues of specificity brings us back to the very first papers of this conference, in which the phenomenology and definition of schizophrenia were discussed. It is trivial to say that it must at least be clear what we want to explain when we look for causes. However, the critical points on diagnosis raised in the first papers were not taken into consideration later; most of the other papers more or less spoke of "schizophrenia" assuming that we were all talking of the same dependent variable. In fact, in different studies presented here, very different diagnostic definitions of schizophrenia were used. What is even more striking, if we look at the problem in terms of a vulnerability/trigger model, is that the studies by Leff and Dohrenwend use diagnostic criteria which have either no or only marginal correlations with the deficit in information processing and attention that suits such a model.

It does make sense theoretically that changes in the social environment, and not necessarily severe stresses or losses, act as triggering factors in people who have a vulnerability in terms of coping with new information and new situations, such as are always involved in life events. In contrast, the schizophrenic patients studied by Leff were defined by the CATEGO system, which only uses first-rank symptoms (basically delusions and hallucinations) and does not rely on thought disorders or attentional deficit disorders at all. Similarly, Dohrenwend in using DSM-III definitions of schizophrenia (and other non-affective and non-organic psychoses) relies on a set of criteria in which thought disorders play only a minor role. This absence of a relationship to cognitive disturbances in these two very important definitions of schizophrenia looks rather strange, particularly within the framework of our discussions on vulnerability/trigger models. It would also be important in the study of high-risk populations to look at which kind of schizophrenia they develop and whether there is indeed a relationship with the cognitive disturbances identified in the children of schizophrenic mothers.

In separating positive-symptom from negative-symptom schizophrenics Nuechterlein gives an example of how specificity in symptomatology might be introduced into vulnerability models. He identifies partly different and partly similar risk factors which contribute to the occurrence of negative and positive symptoms, respectively. However, it is not clear from his graphs whether he regards these as two, different, non-overlapping syndromes. This distinction would not be in agreement with clinical experience since both types of symptoms may coexist in the same patient. It would be more meaningful to speak of two different processes instead of two distinct syndromes, whereby a combination of these processes would be possible.

This takes me to a suggestion recently put forward by Liddle (1987) at Charing Cross Hospital in London. In subjecting his data from chronic schizophrenics to a factor analysis, he identified three meaningful factors: a psychomotor poverty syndrome, a disorganisation syndrome and a reality distortion syndrome. He argues convincingly that so far cognitive disturbances have been arbitrarily attributed either to the negative-symptom or to the positive-symptom snydrome without any clear-cut theoretical background. From psychological tests and experiences with brain lesions, Liddle argues that while the reality distortion syndrome must be due to a temporo-limbic disturbance – several findings presented in this symposium support this view – the psychomotor poverty syndrome has its cortical representation in the dorsolateral prefrontal area, and the disorganisation syndrome could be due to orbital frontal cortex dysfunction.

Though very preliminarily, Liddle also reports that the psychomotor retardation syndrome seems to be connected with problems in psychosocial relationships, while the disorganisation syndrome is related more to problems of professional performance. This "triaxial" classification of schizophrenic symptomatology has yet to be tested for specific relationships to environmental influences. One may, however, speculate that it is especially the disorganisation syndrome which correlates with a poor capability to cope with life changes. It may also be that the psychomotor retardation syndrome specifically provokes high expressed emotion in relatives, which in turn may contribute to relapses with perhaps an activation of reality distortion symptoms.

This is clearly speculative, but I have chosen this example since it points in a direction which we must pursue: discovering whether a specific symptomatology is connected with certain vulnerability factors and also correlated in some way with psychosocial stressors. Two examples of such relationships can be mentioned. It is imaginable that patients with a specific disturbance in the dorsolateral prefrontal cortex are already premorbidly disturbed and are not able to build up social networks which would be of help in coping with later stress. Thought-disordered people may be especially vulnerable to minor life changes, in which adaptation and change per se are important and not just the undesirability of the life event as Dohrenwend has presumed when confining his analysis to severe disruptive losses.

Concluding Remarks

In conclusion, a few words about rehabilitation seem appropriate. If the vulnerability/trigger model of schizophrenia is correct, there are two possibilities for preventing relapse: reducing vulnerability or reducing external stress. Leff and his co-workers have clearly demonstrated that reducing the stress of an overinvolved environment either by removing the patient from it for some time or by changing the environment itself, decreases the risk of relapse. What is still unknown is whether it is patients with specific syndromes who profit most from such a reduction of environmental stress. In general, the idea of providing a structured environment seems most reasonable for patients suffering from a disorganisation syndrome. It should be clear that a large social network as such is not necessarily supportive and may create more stress. Social networks may play a double role, as a "safety net" and as a "spider web". It is probably the quality of the interaction which matters and not the number of relationships, at least for a subgroup of schizophrenic patients.

Even though we do not yet know what the causes of schizophrenia are, the few findings available to date about the prevention of relapse should encourage us to take action. We could act in a similar manner to John Snow in the middle of the last century, when he removed the handle from Broadwick Street pump in

London after discovering that people who had taken water from it had died from cholera. This was over 20 years before the infection theory of cholera was confirmed. Reportedly, the action was very effective.

References

Brown GW, Birley JLT (1968) Crises and life changes and the onset of schizophrenia. J Health Soc Behav 9:203–214

Katschnig H (ed) (1986) Life events and psychiatric disorders – controversial issues. Cambridge University Press, Cambridge

Liddle PF (1987) Schizophrenic syndromes, cognitive performance and neurological dysfunction. Psychol Med 17:49–57

Monroe SM, Steiner S (1986) Social support and psychopathology: interrelations with preexisting disorder, stress, and personality. J Abnorm Psychol 95:29–39

von Cranach M, Eberlein R, Holl B (1981) The concept of onset in psychiatry. In: Wing JK, Bebbington P, Robins LN (eds) What is a case – the problem of definition in psychiatric community surveys. Grant McIntyre, London

Zubin J, Spring B (1977) Vulnerability – a new view of schizophrenia. J Abnorm Psychol 86:103–126

Closing Comments

J. ZUBIN

Closing comments, by the very nature of their temporal placement, are intended not to summarize the rich harvest of the symposium but to pick off the most luscious fruit and display them for their brilliance and excellence.

I wish I had been worthy of such a task. Unfortunately it would have taken a renaissance man to accomplish it. Instead, I have undertaken a more modest if perhaps more imaginative task. I have asked my colleagues to climb down from the shoulders of the giants on which we have stood during the last 3 days. The trouble with sitting on their shoulders is that you can't see them or speak to them. We need to look them straight in the eye and inquire what they thought of our attempts to pursue the causes of schizophrenia into the lair of the still unknown. It is a risky business on this hallowed ground, but it may provide an opportunity to observe what progress we have made through the eyes of the founders of the schizophrenia syndrome. I would thus like to present an interview with each of our three giants.

Interviewer: Emil Kraepelin, you have sat through our sessions, burdened with the weight of our considerations. Was there anything that you could be happy about?

Emil: Well, I am very happy about the progress you report on the revival and standardization of diagnosis of schizohrenia. We now have at least a reliable system if not yet a valid one. I wonder, however, why you call the method neo-Kraepelinian. It seems to me that after some wandering and loosening of the diagnostic schema following the efforts of Eugen Bleuler to assimilate psychoanalysis into the diagnostic fold, you have returned to the original Kraepelin system.

Interviewer: Do you approve of the more rigorous limitations on the diagnosis?

Emil: Well, I do, but I am somewhat perplexed by the extreme rigor you have applied. I am afraid this rigor may lead to rigor mortis for schizophrenia, since even I found that some 13% of my patients recovered, something which your definitions do not allow for.

Interviewer: Why did you generally lean in the direction of a dire outcome even though your own data were somewhat benign in outcome?

VA Medical Center, Highland Drive, Pittsburgh, PA 15206, USA, and Department of Psychiatry University of Pittsburgh School of Medicine, Pittsburgh, Pennsylvania, USA

Emil: I always had the suspicion that those who improved were not really *"echte"* schizophrenics. Besides, as some of you have pointed out, I dealt probably with a biased sample of only very severe long-term cases for the most part, since the milder cases that my good friend Eugen's son, Manfred, dealt with either never came to me or did not leave a deep impression on me because of their disappearance from my clinic. Besides, I may have been unconsciously (to borrow a Freudian term) influenced by the powerful folk belief in the Degeneration Theory, which, though I disavowed it, may have led me to believe in the deteriorating quality in the families of schizophrenics. This persistent zeitgeist in the folk lore may be responsible for the fear which schizophrenia still arouses in family members of a patient.

Interviewer: What about the report on the state of the dopamine hypothesis and the discovery of the role of brain anatomy?

Emil: I had for a long time looked for the toxin of schizophrenia which I thought should be found in somewhat the same way that the spirochete of syphilis was found for general paresis. I had almost given up hope of finding it and was gladdened to hear of the dopamine hypothesis status reported here as well as the anatomical findings and the infectious viral hypothesis. It makes me feel that regarding schizophrenia as a disease may have some validity, and that my attempts to induce psychosis-like states by chemical means may have been on the right track.

Interviewer: In one of your papers you intimated that we could probably find, in groups of normal persons, individuals who would be at the extreme ends of the distribution on psychological tests and that these individuals might be at high risk of, or vulnerable to, schizophrenia. This idea has been followed up by the biometric approach to psychopathology and has led to the development of the "marker" movement for identifying vulnerability to schizophrenia. What led you to consider the importance of psychological tests as vulnerability markers?

Emil: Well, as I have indicated in my *Lebenserinnerungen* (my autobiography, which is soon to appear in English translation) I was a devoted disciple of Wilhelm Wundt, the founder of modern experimental psychology, and my original career ambition was to follow in his footsteps. One day Wundt noticed that I was wearing a new ring on my finger and inquired „Bist du verlobt?" I admitted that I was in love and was planning to get married. He looked at me with some astonishment and said "You know, Emil, I cannot guarantee you a chair as Professor of Philosophy, and I wonder whether you are not undertaking new responsibilities which you may find difficult to carry out." Well, after this warning I felt compelled to accept a post in the clinic when the next offer came. Thus not logic, but love, as it should, made the career decision for me. I, of course, carried into the clinic the experimental methods I learned from my master, Wundt, but I often muse as to what might have happened if I remained a psychologist? Perhaps we would have been further ahead with your markers and laboratory experiments, but what would have happened to diagnosis? Without improved diagnosis we could not have made much headway.

Interviewer: What do you think of the WHO cross-cultural studies?

Emil: I had tried to do cross-cultural comparisons myself, as you will remember during my visit to the East Indies. That is why I am very happy to see the tremendous effort in the cross-cultural direction. I still believe that schizophrenia defies cultural boundaries, but whether it has a constant incidence of 0.1% may be debatable.

Interviewer: Why does it take so long to make progress in the field of schizophrenia?

Emil: Well, it may be the case that we "knew" more in the early part of this century than we "know" now. In the USA I once heard someone say "It ain't ignorance that causes all the trouble. It's knowing things that ain't so!" Perhaps we had to unlearn the false knowledge before we could advance to the new, cut down the underbrush before the new plants could thrive.

Interviewer: Thank you Emil, for sharing your thought with us. Now we shall turn to your colleague Karl Jaspers. Karl, how did you come to write such a wonderful book on general psychopathology when you had so little personal experience with mental patients?

Karl: Well, one day, my Director, Franz Nissl, informed me that Springer-Verlag had asked him to write a new Textbook and asked me whether I would be willing to untertake it. I agreed, and began to delve into the case histories of patients in the clinic. These records were rich in the exact description of psychopathology and provided me with the individual case material on which the phenomenology of psychopathology was based.

Interviewer: How do you feel about the impact that the book has had?

Karl: I had never thought that the book would have such an impact in Europe, but apparently it did not have a great impact in the USA until very recently.

Interviewer: Yes, its translation into English came much later than its original appearance. However, it has been screened for its content in the making of the systematic interviews such as the PSE, the SADS, and the other instruments now in vogue.

Karl: I am surprised to hear you say that, because as I see these interviews, they can hardly reveal the rich phenomenology which patients experience.

Interviewer: You are quite right. Some of these interviews, and the diagnoses they yield, do not reflect the rich inner life of the patient; they are also influenced by factors other than those which would lead to truth and scientific value. Some of the questions and their assessment are dictated not by science and truth, but by political and market-place considerations such as the use of diagnoses for third-party insurance payments and other economic and social considerations. Even those who were the originators of these interviews and diagnostic schemas feel like the *Zauberlehrling* who cannot stop the flood of new techniques that are threatening to engulf diagnosis. We must return to reading your phenomenology and record what we observe in patients in addition to going through the motions of formal diagnoses needed for economic record keeping.

Karl: I have looked through axis II in DSM-III dealing with personality disorders. These classifications do not seem to relate to my own assessment of personality disorders.

Interviewer: No, they do not, and it is quite apparent that they fail to present a basic rationale for making the distinction needed to separate functional disorders like schizophrenia and depression from functional personality disorders. The former are essentially states, waxing and waning with the episode, while the latter are traits, more or less personality characteristics, which remain relatively permanent though they can undergo exacerbation or diminution in intensity. You are known for your clinical and phenomenological contributions. Do you find any use for the biometric approach to psychopathology?

Karl: Why yes, very often. I have indicated in my book that "The biometric methods give us more than figures and correlations. They foster clarity in all fields in which biometric variations can be established. Moreover, through the application of these methods we have concrete experiences which we would never have had without them ..."

Interviewer: Thank you, Karl, for your willingness to share your opinions. We shall now turn to Kurt Schneider. Kurt, how do you feel about the way your first-rank symptoms were dealt with by the symposium.

Kurt: I was surprised to note that they did not turn out to be as specific to schizophrenia as I had hoped, and that they seemed to be unrelated to heredity, but I am encouraged to see that the WHO study seems to suggest that the first-rank symptoms could be viewed as measures of severity.

I have heard several references to vulnerability theory. Can you explain these new trends in the field of schizophrenia?

Interviewer: The vulnerability theory goes back to Griesinger[1], who wrote:

If one considers the extraordinary frequency of all the noxious influences which are mentioned as causes for mental illnesses and, at the same time, considers the relatively infrequent emergence of this illness which follows those influences, one necessarily reaches the assumption that certain predisposing (preparatory) circumstances are necessary that cause the appearance of the illness and specifically this illness; that a certain susceptibility and disposition for illnesses cooperate with the triggering causes, even though they are sometimes not even very strong.

Some of Emil's early writings, as I indicated before, also referred to vulnerability, and even Freud made some reference to it, when he pointed out that repression is not causally sufficient for neurosis but that hereditary vulnerability is causally relevant [1].

In its modern garb the theory states that schizophrenia represents a state of vulnerability which may remain latent or express itself phenotypically in the form of an episode when sufficient stress is brought to bear on the vulnerable individ-

---

[1] After this statement was set in print I received a letter from Professor Dr. C. Scharfetter indicating that priority for the use of the "vulnerability" concept belongs to Karl Friedrich C. Constatt (1807–1850). For fuller discussion of the devolopment of the vulnerability concept see: Zubin J. Schizophrenia: chronicity vs. vulnerability in Handbook of Schizophrenia. Volume 3. Nosology Epidemiology and Genetics. Ming T. Tsuang, Editor. (General Series Editor Henry A. Nassarallah). London: Elsevier Science Publishers, Biomedical Division, in press

ual. The episode is finally dissipated and the individual returns more or less to his premorbid level. The trigger necessary to elicit the episode could be either a dramatic life event, like a death in the family, or the effect of a long-enduring toxic environment which finally causes the accumulation of sufficient stress to elicit an episode. However, not all vulnerable individuals inevitably develop episodes under stress. If the social network, ecological niche, or premorbid personality (with its coping skills) can absorb the stress produced, the episode can be aborted.

One may wish to know how the vulnerability model differs from the prevalent medical model. The essential difference between the medical model and the vulnerability model consists of the following:
— According to the medical model a person diagnosed as suffering with schizophrenia is essentially a sick person who for longer or shorter periods may appear to be well (in remission).
— According to the vulnerability model, the person is essentially well, and would remain so were it not for the exigencies of living that induce stressors which elicit the vulnerability, producing longer or shorter episodes of illness. These episodes are not permanent irreversible states, but eventually disappear, though they may leave scarring.

Kurt: How do you know who is vulnerable?

Interviewer: In order to determine who is vulnerable, a search for markers of vulnerability has been launched. The first attempt was to determine whether the available clinical research tools could serve as markers. They turned out to be unsuitable for either diagnosis or prognosis. The second attempt was to apply the finding of experimental psychology to the problems of psychopathology, a process which Emil initiated. The paradigm of information processing was recently chosen and attempts made to tap the integrity of information processing procedures in the brain of schizophrenics as compared to normals. The first step was to limit the techniques to those in which the response occurred not later than 1000 ms following stimulation. Among such techniques were cross-modality reaction time, ERP, pupillography, heart rate, and critical duration for visual and auditory stimulations. It was thought that a response occurring within the first 1000 ms would be relatively freer of artifacts and perhaps also less dependent on culture. A second generation of markers has recently arisen, consisting of CPT, span of apprehension, SPEM, crossover reaction time, etc.

It has become apparent that the claim that schizophrenia must have a clear sensorium is no longer tenable. Objective indicators of differences between patients and controls with regard to thresholds, reaction time, etc. lead us to conclude that the sensorium of the schizophrenic is not as clear of deviations as had been thought, and that these deviations could lay the foundation for markers.

Your work on psychopathic personality was a landmark in the classification of the nonpsychotic disorders. How do you feel about its current status?

Kurt: Since the publication of my work on psychopathic personality several new trends in personality disorders have emerged. Among these are the pseudo-neurotic schizophrenias, borderline cases, and schizotypic personalities. The attempt on the part of DSM-III to classify the personality disorders through axis II is a step in the right direction, since when an episode descends on an individual he is already in possession of a primary personality which may color the nature of the episode, and some of these premorbid personalities may in themselves already be deviant though not psychotic. But it is difficult to predict from the premorbid personality whether an episode will occur, since 30% of the primary personalities of premorbid schizophrenics are perfectly normal according to Manfred Bleuler's findings. A new view of personality disorders must develop, taking into consideration the old typologies dating back to Kretschmer and his "sensitive personality syndrome," Janet and his various typologies, and the more recent developments of Sjöbring, MMPI, Eysenck, and the still untried applications to psychopathology of normative personality systems such as those of Auck Tellegen.

Interviewer: Thank you, Kurt, for your willingness to share your thinking with us. We must now turn to some of the colleagues of our three giants who lived in other countries but who contributed to the search for the causes of schizophrenia. Notable among these was Sir Aubrey Lewis, who brought back the soul to schizophrenia research by fostering the role of psychosocial variables in the developments of the disorder. This was transmitted to the next generation through such outstanding researchers as John Wing, Michael Shepherd, and George Brown and to the third generation by such men as Julian Leff.

In the area of genetics we owe a great debt to a compatriot of our three giants. Franz Kallmann, who trained under Rüdin, fought the good fight in the USA for the recognition of the genetic component, supported there by Gottesman and in the UK by Slater and by Shields.

In the area of biochemistry and psychopharmacology, beginning with Thudicum and going on to Delay and Deniker and Carlsson, we are greatly indebted for the introduction of neuroleptics and the clarification of the role of neurotransmitters in brain function with special reference to schizophrenia.

Janet, in the French School, provided a deep understanding of the personality traits which are often deviant in people who do not develop episodes of schizophrenia.

Last but not least, we must pay homage to the Zurich School, Eugen Bleuler and Manfred Bleuler; the former for bringing psychology back to schizophrenia and the latter for his long-term follow-up of schizophrenia. The chronic deteriorating aspects of schizophrenia which had become the earmark of the disorder were contradicted by the benign outcome of Manfred's long-term follow-up. He has provided a proclamation of emancipation for schizophrenia from the yoke of inevitable chronicity, not unlike Abraham Lincoln's proclamation of emancipation for the American slaves. And his work has inspired Huber, Ciompi, and Brooks and Harding in the USA to replicate his findings and help convince us that deterioration is not an indigenous part of schizophrenia, except perhaps in a very small proportion of the cases.

In summary, our three giants and their contemporary colleagues would have been very happy with our proceedings. Even though the progress viewed retrospectively would have gladdened their hearts, our own hearts become heavy when we see prospectively how much further we still have to go before our problem can be solved. Some of us leave with a heavy heart and in great confusion, but it is confusion on a higher level of discourse than the simple confusion of the first half of this century. Let us hope that out of this confusion some new ideas will emerge and that we will not have to wait for the Twelfth Centennial of Heidelberg before schizophrenia is conquered.

Reference

1. Grünbaum A (1984) The foundation of psychoanalysis. University of California Press, Berkeley, p 13

Search for the Causes of Schizophrenia: Summary and Outlook *

H. HÄFNER

The vast body of data presented in this volume provides a comprehensive view of the results of recent investigative work on various biological and psychological factors possibly contributing to the risk of onset, course and outcome of schizophrenia. Our knowledge of the aetiology of the "disease" called schizophrenia, as pointed out by Joseph Zubin in his fictitious dialogue with Emil Kraepelin, Karl Jaspers and Kurt Schneider, has not yet made much progress from Kraepelin's days. In several areas, i.e. psychology, physiology, neurobiochemistry, descriptive genetics and molecular biology, recent scientific findings have led us far beyond the knowledge available to Kraepelin. We have achieved these findings by applying new methods and, to a lesser extent, new theoretical approaches. It is a nuisance and a challenge that none of them has brought us but a few steps closer to a better understanding of the aetiology of the schizophrenic psychosis and the related impairments and social dysfunctioning.

The vast number of isolated results, achieved by various research groups applying different approaches, conveys the rather confusing impression of there being a plethora of unrelated data that cannot be integrated into one model. Our aim, which was to bring together the largely separate ways of schizophrenia research and to encourage discussion over the boundaries of distinct methods dealing with selective aspects of the disease, seems to have proven a success. This was clearly reflected in the contributions of the invited discussants included in the volume, and the free discussion among them, which could not be included in this book. We hope that the symposium, which the Central Institute of Mental Health will from now on organise at regular intervals, has given an impetus that will last and prove fruitful.

Attempting to formulate at the end of this volume and outlook for the next phase of the search for the causes of schizophrenia on the basis of the results reported and approaches discussed, we must confine ourselves to a handful of promising ones in order to avoid simple repetition. It is perforce a subjective undertaking that will reflect our own judgements rather than a representative view of the colleagues participating in the symposium.

---

* I am indebted to Professor W. F. Gattaz for suggestions and a critical perusal of the chapter

The Contribution of Improved Diagnosis and Epidemiology to Schizophrenia Research

The heterogeneity of the psychiatric diagnosis has frequently been evoked to explain contradictory findings among studies and the different areas of schizophrenia research. The introduction of standardised diagnostic criteria in the 1970s reduced to a considerable extent the source of inconsistency by enabling a more homogenous selection of patients. This improved scientific communication among different research groups and thus provided the possibility of a more reliable comparison of results and the establishment of multi-centre and multi-cultural studies. It finally became possible in epidemiological research to obtain sufficiently precise data on the incidence of schizophrenia and its distribution over populations, time, and stable (age, sex, etc.) and variable (single/married; social status) sociodemographic characteristics. It has obviously also offered a chance of arriving at more reliable conclusions after several decades of socioepidemiological schizophrenia research providing in part inconsistent distribution and association patterns difficult to subject to a causal interpretation. New light seems to be shed even upon the old controversy of the explanation of the uneven distribution of the incidence over social classes, i.e. the competition between the breeder hypothesis and the intra- and intergeneration selection hypothesis (Dohrenwend and Dohrenwend 1969). The advantage of a precise diagnosis for biological-psychiatric research is not so clear. It also remains an open question whether the homogenous population of precisely diagnosed schizophrenia phenotypes can be attributed to homogenous or heterogenous genotypes or to phenocopies of different aetiology. It would be at least difficult to interpret abnormalities of transmitter processes or structural changes in the brain as possible causes of schizophrenia with any certainty, even if they were observed in subjects clearly diagnosed as schizophrenic. They might just as well – as is probably the case with disturbed dopamine metabolism – represent only accompanying processes of the psychosis in the form of a relatively unspecific pattern of responses of the brain to various noxious agents.

The transnational schizophrenia studies of the World Health Organization (Sartorius et al., this volume), conducted after the development and international standardisation of diagnostic instruments, have yielded remarkable results. The symptomatology of the schizophrenic psychosis and the impairments and social dysfunctions related to its course show a high stability over countries and cultures. One surprising finding was that the incidence rates, collected in the course of the WHO Determinants of Outcome Study in ten countries with the aim of obtaining full information on all cases of schizophrenia, proved to be equally uniform. They vary only slightly (about 0.10/1000 population, 15–54 years of age) when the CATEGO class S+ (made up almost completely by nuclear syndrome patients) is used as a case definition. Since even the few studies based on fairly complete data which were comparable by the definition of diagnosis and age structure and collected over long time periods did not yield any indication of changes in the morbid risk over time, schizophrenia, as a disease category, has to be considered anew (Häfner, this volume). It seems to be the only disease so far known that shows almost identical incidence rates and a relative stability over time in very different geographical regions, populations and cultures. We are thus faced with the question of whether schizophrenia is a unique disease, incomparable with any other (Zubin, this volume).

If this finding of a stable morbid risk could be replicated further, Kraepelin's hopes of making essential contributions to a causal explanation by transcultural psychiatric research would no longer seem very promising. Given the cultural invariability of the incidence, we could not hope to make any decisive progress towards explaining the aetiology by studying the uneven distribution of incidence over sociocultural context variables, such as occupational status or socioeconomic class. An explanation for the uneven distribution over social classes at first onset could rather be expected to arise from testing intra- and intergenerational selection hypotheses, for example, by assuming an interaction between social structures and processes and socially relevant behavioural dispositions or personality traits, which in turn are associated with the risk of schizophrenia (Ødegard 1975).

The speculative assumption that the even distribution of schizophrenia risk over cultures and populations might be explained in the same way as that of moderately severe and severe mental retardation (Häfner, this volume) opens up interesting prospects for future research. The diagnosis "schizophrenia" of narrower or broader definition might, like mental retardation, defined by varying IQ threshold values, represent cut-off points at the extreme ends of a scale; in turn the scale might be characterised by the not yet validated dimension "schizothymic behaviour or disorder", as once assumed by E. Kretschmer (1921). Provided the values along this schizothymia dimension showed an identical distribution in various populations, schizohrenia could be expected to show approximately equal rates, if more or less precisely measurable threshold values were used. All psychometric and experimental findings, e.g. deficits in attentional, perceptional and cognitive functioning, and personality dimensions, are indeed continuously distributed between schizophrenics and non-schizophrenics.

If one or several dimensions existed whose extreme values corresponded to what we define as schizophrenic psychosis, they would have to be found at one of the following three levels: (1) in the manifest symptoms of the psychosis and related disorders, (2) in stable personality traits (e.g. "schizophrenia spectrum disorder") or psychophysiological deficits which are present prior to the onset of the psychosis and in the symptom-free interval and may become gradually reinforced during the psychotic episode, and (3) in a specific vulnerability for the onset of schizophrenic episodes under stress, such as adverse stimuli (Nuechterlein, this volume). In this case not the psychopathology itself but the disposition to respond with schizophrenic episodes – similar to an insufficient production of insulin, which leads to a diabetes mellitus syndrome when the intake of carbohydrates exceeds a certain level – would be distributed dimensionally.

With regard to the even distribution of the risk of psychosis in several populations, it should be assumed, when proceeding from a vulnerability model, that the lifetime risk for the onset of a schizophrenic psychosis would largely be determined by the degree or the threshold value of the existing vulnerability. This would be the case if the stress factors operating as precipitants – like the intake of carbohydrates in diabetes – were largely ubiquitous or, like intensive feelings in close relationships, so closely related with the biological origins of man that they were present in all cultures more or less without difference.

Genetics

One of the consistent data in research on the causes of schizophrenia is that the disease has an increased familial aggregation and that this is largely due to genetic factors (Kendler 1986; Kringlen, this volume). In accordance with genetic and epidemiological data T. Crow (this volume) has shown by investigating pairs of affected siblings that the familial sequence of onset is determined by age and so most likely by transmission through genes and not by the communication of contagious agents. However, two major questions remain yet to be clarified: (a) what is the mode of the genetic transmission and (b) what is the genetically determined abnormality that causes the development of the disease?

Several sophisticated models for the mode of genetic transmission have been proposed (Baron, this volume). Their validation or the refutation of alternative models have yet to be undertaken. This can be done satisfactorily only if we succeed in identifying true genetic markers for the disposition to schizophrenia, which can also be shown to exist in the gene carriers among the relatives of schizophrenics.

It seems that twin studies, adoption studies and descriptive genetics in general have already made their most important contributions to the clarification of the mode of genetic transmission of the phenotype "schizophrenia" and the differing risk of transmission in kin (Strömgren, this volume). We are thus faced with a new phase of genetic schizophrenia research, i.e. the necessity to look for genetic markers that are either directly linked with a genotype associated with the risk for schizophrenia or determined by a gene that is located in the immediate proximity of a "schizophrenia gene". Whether smooth pursuit eye movement (Venables, this volume), or increased binding of the dopamine-antagonist speperone, recently reported by Bondy et al. 1985) or HLA antigens (Gattaz et al. 1981), a finding still awaiting replication, represent latent genetic markers of a schizophrenia genotype or of a locally linked gene is a very interesting question in need of replication or careful further research. Indeed, the tools available in molecular genetics have for the first time raised hopes of making progress towards the clarification of the role of genetic factors in the genesis of schizophrenia (Rosenberg et al. 1985). However, the localisation and identification of schizophrenia genes will not be as easy as the localisation of a single gene responsible for the genesis of Huntington's chorea or for Alzheimer's disease on chromosome 21 (Kang et al. 1987). Nevertheless, we hope that the scientific revolution ushered into medical research by molecular genetics will help to identify the genes responsible for the vulnerability to schizophrenia and, thus, decisively contribute to the search for the causes of the disease.

Nature and Nurture (Biological Approaches)

The hypothetical analogy between schizophrenia and mental retardation (Häfner, this volume) might imply that the disposition to schizophrenia, like mental retardation, is attributable to several genetic factors. Since the expression rate of schizophrenia is 0.26 (Zubin, this volume) and the concordance rates for monozygotic twins are well below 1.0, noninherited factors must also be active in schizophrenia, as in severe and moderately severe mental retardation (Crow, this volume; Reynolds, this volume; Kringlen, this volume; Strömgren, this volume). This is indicated by the fact that the schizophrenia syndrome as symptomatic schizophrenia may occur – mainly transitorily – in association with various types of brain dysfunctions, e.g. cases of intoxication, long-term amphetamine overdosage and brain traumas. As in mental retardation, the share of environmental factors in the disposition to schizophrenia is probably mediated neither at the psychological (e.g. by learning deficits) nor the biological (e.g. various types of brain dysfunctions and substance deficits) levels exclusively.

The proof of such environmental factors and the assessment of their contribution to the disposition to schizophrenia requires longitudinal studies on high-risk children, commenced at an early age and conducted over long time periods. Such studies are now in progress, but they have not yet reached the stage of evaluating the outcome effects on the risk of first onset (Leff, this volume). It is quite possible that not only the environmental factors are relatively multifarious; the genetic factors may, as already mentioned, also be attributable to several, perhaps even to a large number of genes, similar to the aetiology of mental retardation. In that case the manifest schizophrenia syndrome would represent "the final common pathway of a range of different genetic and noninheritant factors" (Lewis et al. 1987).

This assumption might be partially supported, for example, if it were possible to examine the complementary hyperactivity of the dopaminergic system in productive symptoms and its insufficiency in negative symptoms of schizophrenia with a new class of dopamine agonists and antagonists (Carlsson, this volume). If it were also possible to precipitate the derangements in the dopaminergic system characteristic of the schizophrenia syndrome not only by biochemical, but also by mental stimuli, essential progress would be made towards the assumption of a relatively uniform neurobiochemical pattern of response to a fairly large number of unspecific stimuli. Such studies on pathogenetic models of schizophrenic syndromes, which might help to explain other types of psychoses as well, are of little relevance to the attempts to elucidate the causation of the disease "schizophrenia", as long as the biochemical links with the underlying aetiological or genetically determined processes remain hidden. However, they constitute an important basis for the generation of an aetiological hypothesis and provide decisive clues for the development of an effective symptomatic therapy.

The attempt to bridge the gap between the pathogenesis and the aetiology, between our limited knowledge of the psychophysiological, neurohormonal and transmitter dysfunctions in the central nervous system on the one hand and the structural and metabolic changes observed in CT, PET scan, NMR scan and postmortem studies on the other hand, is still a daring undertaking. There are no solid stepping stones yet between the far distant limits of morphology and dysfunction. The structural and functional, e.g. PET scan, findings on brain metabolism and receptor binding for hemispheric localisation are still rather inconsistent. The only thing we can do at present is to summon up our courage for critical speculation. Reynolds (this volume), representing a rather conservative position, assumes that the atrophic changes in the temporal limbic region and particularly in the parahippocampal gyrus (predominantly on the left side) might lead to a relative dopamine hyperfunction of the nucleus amygdalae and thus precipitate the psychosis. Carlsson (this volume), assuming an intermediate speculative position, conjectures that the functional integration between the evolving neocortex and older subcortical structures, as vulnerable processes, might remain incomplete during the evolutionary process. In this process the neostriatum is supposed to play a key role. This in turn may account for the critical role of dopaminergic systems in the pathogenesis of the psychoses. The third speculative hypothesis (Gattaz et al., this volume) also refers to evolutionary processes: an acceleration of the neuronal elimination during the period of brain maturation may cause structural and functional abnormalities in schizophrenia. This could be due to innate or acquired biological abnormalities.

These speculative models are characterised by a certain remoteness from the actual biological and psychological processes of the psychosis that are known to us and which should go to explain it. The most simple way of bridging the gap between them and the schizophrenia syndrome is the dopamine hypothesis. However, it should be borne in mind that causality may basically run both ways. A disturbed maturation of specific brain structures may lead to psychological and neurobiochemical deficits, at least in childhood and probably also later in life. The underdevelopment of perception and other areas of mental functioning may lead to an underdevelopment of the neuronal network, later probably also to neuronal loss. Unfortunately, in the majority of the studies investigating these questions the methodological requirements at the clinical level have not kept pace with the growing sophistication of the biochemical and morphological research methods: sampling, measurement techniques and the examination of alternative explanations have been inadequate in many of these studies concerned with the clinical-psychological level.

One direction for further research is to distinguish between genetic and nongenetic schizophrenia (Lewis et al. 1987). This approach has already been applied in some studies, and preliminary evidence seems to suggest that it might be useful for the selection of more homogenous patient groups in regard to clinical and neurodiagnostic variables (Dworkin and Lenzenweger 1984; Reveley et al. 1984). If, however, it were expected that the disposition to schizophrenia is transmitted polygenetically and to some extent accounted for by heterogenous, noninherited factors, it would be at least difficult to identify homogenous genotypes within the spectrum of schizophrenia phenotypes. In particular the identification of genetically determined, isolated, biological abnormalities would be hindered by an aetiological heterogeneity. This could also account for the heterogeneity of findings among the different biological processes on the aetiology, mainly related to an isolated dysfunctioning in some neurotransmitter system or to an excess or deficiency of a determined substance (neurotransmitters, neuropeptides, etc.) in the central nervous system. Not only in the face of a possible aetiological hetero-geneity, but also in the face of the anatomical and functional interrelationships among the different neuronal systems in the brain, it is conceivable that many of the theories are not mutually exclusive, but represent different aspects of the same central dysfunction. The assumption of genetic and environmental heterogeneity, as already mentioned, does not rule out the hypothesis that the productive and possibly also the negative symptomatology of the psychosis are based on a rela-tively homogenous pattern of neurophysiological and neurobiochemical brain dysfunctions.

Approaches to the Generation of Testable Vulnerability Models

Zubin has described his vulnerability model in several publications. Later, he im-proved it to form a concept that can be operationalised (Zubin and Spring 1977). This is probably one of the reasons why only recently attempts have been made to test empirically the vulnerability models on the course of the psychosis (Nuech-terlein, this volume; Olbrich 1987). The disposition to schizophrenia, or better the threshold of vulnerability, probably changes with age and stage of life (Katschnig, this volume). The first onset of a schizophrenic psychosis usually takes place after puberty (in females, considerably later than in males; Häfner, this volume). In ad-dition, after a course of several decades both the risk of relapse and of developing psychotic symptoms become slightly reduced (Harding and Strauss 1985; Ciompi and Müller 1976; Janzarik 1968). Provided that vulnerability does not change during life course, it could be anticipated that the positive and the negative symp-tomatology become cumulatively reinforced in old age due to the addition of re-sidual states and new episodes triggered off by a life stress. But this is obviously not the case.

In the prospective studies conducted on representative groups of schizo-phrenics over long periods of time, trait markers and changes therein have not been investigated. This is a shortcoming inasmuch as, according to Zubin's vul-nerability model, stable abnormalities in information processing, attentional and autonomous nervous functioning probably constitute a specific susceptibility to environmental stimuli such as information overload and, thus, might support a plausible and testable vulnerability trigger model (Zubin, this volume; Katschnig, this volume). The difficulties of defining and measuring stimuli that might trigger off a schizophrenic episode are evident particularly in studies investigating the life-event paradigms among first-onset schizophrenics (Katschnig, this volume). Dohrenwend et al. (this volume), using a considerably improved methodology in their latest study, came to the conclusion that "recent environment induced stress from life events does not appear to be of primary importance as a risk factor for episodes of schizophrenia." Life events are only of secondary, inferred but not necessarily negligible importance, a conclusion well in agreement with the epi-demiological findings described at the outset.

Nevertheless, the Expressed Emotions (EE) concept introduced by G. Brown (1985) has enabled remarkable discoveries on the dependence of the risk of re-lapse in schizophrenics on external stressors, such as the quantity of critical remarks, hostility and emotional overinvolvement in close familial relationships. Studies conducted on this paradigm after the first onset of the disease and in which the measures of symptomatology and risk of relapse are used as outcome variables will, strictly speaking, not contribute to a causal explanation of the risk of developing schizophrenia (Leff et al., this volume). The design and findings of such studies, however, have assisted the authors consequently to improve upon and test the vulnerability trigger model, which is basically of heuristic value for the causal explanation of the morbid risk. After a successful replication of these results in several cultures, the model has received further support by the identification of protective effects: (1) neuroleptic permanent medication and (2) reduction of the time spent together with high-EE relatives.

The success of controlled experimental interventions – social treatment of high-EE families – has not only produced evidence for a causal link from the pathogenesis but also indicated an important direction for preventive measures. Finally, Leff et al. (this volume), by using a quasi-experimental design, have succeeded in identifying an indicator of the psychophysiological responsiveness to stressful life events and EE family contacts in schizophrenics: the frequency of spontaneous fluctuations of skin conductance seems to be associated with the symptom "acoustic hallucination" in the schizophrenic psychosis. These studies have remarkably contributed to the psychophysiological operationalisation of the vulnerability-trigger model. Their importance can be illustrated by drawing a parallel with the early risk predictors reported by Venables (this volume); hyperresponsive electrodermal activity and a low IQ seem to be the best predictors of schizophrenia in high-risk children at the age of 3. It should be noticed, however, that the enormous differences in the variables studied, their operationalisation and, in particular, the lack of clearly formulated models still considerably reduce the comparability of the results obtained in vulnerability research.

Course of Schizophrenia

Given the findings of the International Pilot Study on Schizophrenia and the WHO schizophrenia follow-up studies (Sartorius et al., this volume), we must assume that the course of schizophrenia, unlike the risk of first onset, is influenced by factors varying over different cultures. The factors responsible for differences in the quantity of the psychotic symptomatology, social impairment and completeness of remission at the 2- and 5-year follow-ups between developed and developing countries have not yet been elucidated satisfactorily (Sartorius et al., this volume). The differences persisted even after the representativeness of the cohorts in the schizophrenia follow-up study was carefully checked. None of the five hypotheses alone (differences in the number of stressful life events, in the emotional interaction of families, in the social processing of impairment, in survival rates and in the cultural perception of mental disease) put forward by the authors seems to explain the differences in course and outcome. We are thus looking forward to the final evaluation of the Determinants of Outcome study (Sartorius et al., this volume), which will provide information on the share of the variance accounted for by each of the factors, and the more so, as the elucidation of the causal relationships shows promise of new approaches to the prevention of unfavourable courses.

The use of standardised instruments for the measurement of symptomatology, impairment and social dysfunction, and the control of moderator variables, such as age, sex and environmental influences (Schubart et al., this volume) in carefully designed prospective longitudinal studies has considerably increased our knowledge of predictors of the course of schizophrenia. Plus symptomatology, minus symptomatology and social impairment or disability appear to be highly significant predictors of the course of the same measurement dimensions over 5 years. With regard to some other outcome variable, they seem to be predominantly of low predicitve power. It is remarkable that sociodemographic factors, apart from the relationship variables "warmth" and "key figure", show no predicitve power. Sex has a highly significant effect on the course only over 3 years, provided that age, marital status and frequency of utilization of health services are controlled for. At the 5-year follow-up the effect disappears. This illustrates the necessity to pay far more attention to the factor "time" in research on the course of schizophrenia. Particular other factors, such as being female, obviously have a marked effect on the course of symptoms and social disability in schizophrenia only for a limited period of time. This means that phase models or time series should be used in future research on factors influencing the course and outcome of schizophrenia.

The interpersonal and transcultural variability of the course of schizophrenia also supports process models proceeding from the assumption that personality and environmental factors influence the course of the disease (Strauss, this volume; Nuechterlein, this volume). Although it is an established finding that a high proportion of the offspring of schizophrenics and the high proportion who later fall ill with schizophrenia show more emotional instability, social withdrawal, isolation and/or an elevated level of aggressive and disruptive behaviour than the average, the relationship between these characteristics and the individual vulnerability for schizophrenia has not yet been elucidated. The same applies, to a greater extent, to the assumption of protective factors that, either in the form of an adequate coping repertoire or good social support, buffer stressful life events or help to prevent the onset of a psychosis at the prodromal stage. Detailed analyses (Strauss, this volume; Nuechterlein, this volume) have been conducted mainly on approaches involving an adequate coping with the onset of a psychosis and the illness itself or its direct corollaries. We are still at the stage of describing these phenomena. Already, they can be taken into account in therapeutic strategies, but it has not yet been possible to test them adequately on the basis of heuristic models. In this field, too, improved knowledge will be of considerable practical value (Strauss, this volume; Carpenter, this volume).

To explain the pathogenetic processes operating in the course of a schizophrenic psychosis, the findings of experimental-psychological research are also important (Hemsley, this volume; Cohen and Borst, this volume). The attempts to provide a limited causal explanation of the abnormalities by referring to disrupted information processing, recall deficits or just minus symptomatology are marred by several inconsistencies (Cohen and Borst, this volume). Cohen and Borst therefore propose the employment of more complex models, like motivation, regression, interference and attention deficit, which in their view were discarded without any good reason. The opportunity of imaging cerebral blood flow in the brain (PET) during test performance seems to be promising to them as the blood flow in the dorsolateral prefrontal area increases in normal controls when doing the Wisconsin Card Sorting Test, whereas in schizophrenics no such increase takes place and is associated with a low test performance. Controlled studies of schizophrenics in various states of mental activity by means of functional-analytical brain imaging techniques, especially if their resolution can be improved, will no doubt contribute to a better understanding of the functional abnormalities in the psychoses and of their relatedness to mental and cerebral functioning (Hirsh, this volume).

The aim of a symposium which focussed on the search for causal hypotheses explaining the morbid risk and the course of schizophrenia was to promote plausible speculations. Such contributions were made by A. Carlsson, G. P. Reynolds and W. F. Gattaz among others, reporting on morphogenetic or evolutionary theories. T. Crow undertook the attempt to explain the aetiology of schizophrenia by assuming one single, though not ordinary, disease cause. Since the onset of schizophrenia appears to be determined by age and not by common exposure to an environmental pathogen, he does not take the conservative step of looking for ordinary genes. He assumes a retrovirus or another type of mobile element integrated in the genome. If this assumption proves correct (and it is in agreement with the genetic transmission from parents to offspring), schizophrenia would again basically be a homogenous disease in the Kraepelinean sense, which has so far been impossible to show through any level of research. T. Crow's theory would solve a considerable number of research problems, but it is still in need of validation.

Closing Remarks

The present state of schizophrenia research, which is reflected in this symposium in an impressive way, is characterised by the accumulation of a wealth of data on the morbid risk, symptomatology, course and outcome of this disease process. The variety of data and the variety of approaches pursued in aetiological schizophrenia research are extraordinary. It is unlikely that all these approaches will be successful, especially those limited to one single method and ignoring other important aspects. Another important characteristic of the present situation is the lack of precise, empirically testable models and theories leading to a concise description of data and their interrelationships in a clear and operationalisable form. It is very likely that only such models that focus on more than one aspect, i.e. biological and psychological, and describe the interrelatedness of the processes at the most important levels of research will contribute to a better understanding of the causal relationships. The requirement for any comprehensive theory of the schizophrenic disease process is that it must allow a sensible organisation of data and relationships by taking into account the most important research areas.

We hope that the contributions to and the discussion at this symposium, "Search for the Causes of Schizophrenia", have given impetus to work for this aim.

References

Bondy B, Ackenheil M, Wildenauer D (1985) Biochemical alterations in lymphocytes of schizophrenic patients: a state or trait marker. In: Shagass C, Josiassen RC, Bridger WH, Weiss KJ, Stoff D, Simpson GM (eds) Biological psychiatriy. Elsevier, New York, pp 1068–1070

Brown GW: The discovery of "Expressed Emotion": Induction or deduction? In: Leff J and Vaughn C: Expressed emotion in families: Its significance for mental illness. Guilford Press: New York, 1985, pp 7–25

Ciompi L, Müller C (1976) Lebensweg und Alter der Schizophrenen. Monographien aus dem Gesamtgebiet der Psychiatrie 12. Springer, Berlin Heidelberg New York

Dohrenwend BP, Dohrenwend BS (1969) Social status and psychological disorder: a causal inquiry. Wiley, New York

Dworkin R, Lenzenweger M (984) Symptoms and the genetics of schizophrenia: implications for diagnosis. Am J Psychiatry 141:1541–1546

Gattaz WF, Beckmann H, Mendlewicz J (1981) HLA antigens and schizophrenia: a pool of two studies. Psychiatry Res 5:123–128

Harding CM, Strauss JS (1985) The course of schizophrenia: an evolving concept. In: Alpert M (ed) Controversies in schizophrenia – changes and controversies. Guilford, New York, pp 339–350

Janzarik W (1968) Schizophrene Verläufe. Springer, Berlin Heidelberg New York

Kang J, Lemaire H-G, Unterbeck A, Salbaum JM, Maasters CL, Grzeschik K-H, Multhaup G, Beyreuther K, Müller-Hill B (1987) The precursor of Alzheimer's disease amyloid A4 protein resembles a cell-surface receptor. Nature 325:733–736

Kendler KS (1986) The genetics of schizophrenia: a current perspective. Psychopharmacol Bull 22:918–922

Kretschmer E (1921) Körperbau und Charakter. Springer, Berlin

Lewis SW, Reveley AM, Reveley MA, Chitkara B, Murray RM (1987) The familial-sporadic distinction as a strategy in schizophrenia research. Br Psychiatry (to be published)

Ødegard Ø (1975) Social and ecological factors in the etiology, outcome, treatment and prevention of mental disorders. In: Kisker KP, Meyer JE, Müller C, Strömgren E (eds) Psychiatrie der Gegenwart, vol III, 2nd edn. Springer, Berlin Heidelberg New York, pp 151–198

Olbrich R (1987) Die Verletzbarkeit des Schizophrenen. Zubins Konzept der Vulnerabilität. Nervenarzt 58:65–71

Reveley AM, Reveley MA, Murray RM (1984) Cerebral ventricular enlargement in non-genetic schizophrenia: a controlled twin study. Br J Psychiatry 144:89–93

Rosenberg MB, Hansen C Jr, Breakefield XO (1985) Molecular genetic approaches to neurologic and psychiatric diseases. Prog Neurobiol 24:95–140

Zubin J, Spring B (1977) Vulnerability – a new view of schizophrenia. J Abnorm Psychol 86:103–126

Author Index

Razani J   346
Redd WH   191, 201
Redick RW   72
Redlich FC   48, 71
Redmond DE   240
Reich T   148, 150, 156, 159, 170
Reider RO   206, 213
Reimann H   48, 71
Reiss DJ   345, 347
Reveley AM   28, 52, 72, 140, 142, 155, 206, 213, 255, 259, 376
Reveley MA   142, 213, 259, 371, 376
Reynolds GP   197, 217, 236, 237, 238, 239, 240, 243, 248, 268, 269, 371, 375
Reynolds IJ   234
Reynolds JR   16
Rice J   169, 170
Richardson PH   181, 187
Richardson SA   70
Rieder RO   165, 170, 240
Riederer P   233, 240
Riley GJ   240
Risch N   159, 169, 170
Rist F   196, 201
Ritzler BA   86
Robertson GS   227
Robertson HA   227
Robins E   24, 25, 26, 28, 97, 144, 155, 156, 170, 249
Robins L   279, 295
Rochester SR   192
Rock DR   213, 315
Rodnick EH   298, 313, 315, 347
Rodriso A   215, 218
Roe BA   265
Roff JD   192
Rogat E   71
Rogers AW   248
Rogler LH   277, 288
Rohde A   218
Rohde PD   295, 330
Rolf J   87, 305
Roos BE   249
Ros E   233
Rosado V   200
Rosanoff AJ   125, 126, 127, 142
Rose M   247
Roseman RH   295
Rosen WG   193, 201
Rosenberg MB   369, 376
Rosenberg S   199

Rosenhan D   22, 28
Rosenthal D   27, 124, 126, 129, 132, 133, 134, 137, 139, 141, 142, 146, 155, 156, 213, 298, 306, 314, 316
Rosenzweig L   201
Ross HS   72
Ross JS   183, 188
Rossi A   345
Rossor M   240
Roth RH   130, 240
Roth WT   194
Rotrosen J   233
Rotter JB   281, 285, 318
Roux JT   249
Rüdin E   123, 364
Rush MG   266
Rutschmann J   212, 301, 313, 315
Rutter M   291

Saavedra JM   248
Saccuzzo DP   195
Salbaum JM   375
Salokangas RKR   99, 106
Salzmann LF   315
Sandeer W   11, 18
Santana F   329
Sanua V   47, 73
Sartorius N   5, 7, 43, 49, 50, 60, 67, 73, 107, 108, 113, 156, 271, 293, 296, 330, 367, 373
Saß H   13, 17, 20, 28
Sauer HC   71
Scally B   55, 73
Schaefer C   295
Schaffer JW   28, 156
Schalling D   212
Scharfetter C   150, 156
Scheibel AB   197, 256
Schindler CW   266
Schlom J   265
Schmid GW   266
Schmueli J   314
Schneider C   19, 21, 28
Schneider K   4, 5, 7, 13, 14, 18, 19, 21, 22, 23, 30, 39, 42, 51, 73, 147, 148, 149, 156, 362, 263, 364, 366
Schneider LH   239, 240
Schneider SJ   303
Schneider W   182, 194
Schonfeldt-Bausch R   240, 258
Schooler C   196, 201
Schooler NR   71, 199, 329

Schrank-Fernandez G   188
Schröder P   13
Schubart C   61, 62, 70, 73, 100, 106, 374
Schüle H   11, 18
Schulsinger F   27, 38, 141, 155, 156, 205, 206, 210, 212, 213, 302, 305, 309, 314, 315, 316
Schulsinger H   213, 303, 315
Schultzberg M   232
Schulz SC   272
Schumacher E   332, 334, 335, 336, 337, 340
Schüttler R   27, 72, 86, 106, 259
Schwarz R   73, 100, 106
Schwatz MD   219
Scotch NA   47, 72, 275, 295
Sedvall G   224
Seeman M   69, 73
Seeman P   236, 240
Seidman LJ   197, 206, 251, 252
Sekerle HJ   249
Selemon LKD   219
Selva A   329
Seminario I   215, 218
Serafetinides EA   191, 201
Serban G   340
Shader R   60, 73
Shagass C   195
Shakow D   190
Shanley BC   249
Shapiro R   60, 73, 296
Sharpe L   26
Shaye J   137, 142
Shephard G   271
Shepherd M   31, 34, 38, 41, 43, 74, 364
Sherer M   200
Shields J   71, 124, 125, 126, 127, 128, 129, 130, 136, 137, 143, 144, 147, 150, 152, 155, 159, 170, 275, 297, 298, 306, 331, 464
Shiffrin RM   182, 194
Shimura M   64, 73
Shrout PE   279, 294, 296
Shternberg EY   349, 352
Siever LJ   20, 27, 138, 142, 209, 213
Silverman J   85, 87, 192
Silverstein ML   215, 218
Silverton L   213
Simanyi M   233
Simmens S   313

Subject Index